McLaughlin and Ka...

Continuous Quality Improvement in Health Care

FOURTH EDITION

William A. Sollecito, DrPH
Clinical Professor, Public Health Leadership Program
Director, Online Global Health Certificate Program
UNC Gillings School of Global Public Health
University of North Carolina at Chapel Hill
Chapel Hill, North Carolina

Julie K. Johnson, MSPH, PhD
Associate Professor and Deputy Director
Centre for Clinical Governance Research
Faculty of Medicine
University of New South Wales
Sydney, Australia

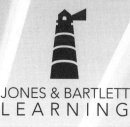

JONES & BARTLETT
LEARNING

World Headquarters
Jones & Bartlett Learning
5 Wall Street
Burlington, MA 01803
978-443-5000
info@jblearning.com
www.jblearning.com

Jones & Bartlett Learning books and products are available through most bookstores and online book-sellers. To contact Jones & Bartlett Learning directly, call 800-832-0034, fax 978-443-8000, or visit our website, www.jblearning.com.

Production Credits
Publisher: Michael Brown
Managing Editor: Maro Gartside
Director of Production: Amy Rose
Production Manager: Tracey McCrea
Production Editor: Tiffany Sliter
Marketing Manager: Grace Richards
Manufacturing and Inventory Control Supervisor: Amy Bacus
Cover and Title Page Design: Scott Moden
Composition: Cenveo Publisher Services
Cover and Title Page Image: © gualtiero boffi/ShutterStock, Inc.
Printing and Binding: Malloy, Inc.
Cover Printing: Malloy, Inc.

Library of Congress Cataloging-in-Publication Data

Sollecito, William A.
   Mclaughlin and Kaluzny's continuous quality improvement in health care
/ William A. Sollecito, Julie K. Johnson.—4th ed.
       p.; cm.
   Continuous quality improvement in health care
   Includes index.
   ISBN-13: 978-0-7637-8154-5 (pbk. : alk. paper)
   ISBN-10: 0-7637-8154-1 (pbk. : alk. paper)
   1. Medical care—United States—Quality control.   2. Total quality
management   United States.   I. Johnson, Julie K.   II. Title.   III. Title:
Continuous quality improvement in health care.
   [DNLM: 1. Delivery of Health Care—organization & administration.   2. Quality Assurance,
Health Care—methods. W 84.1]
   RA399.A3C66 2012
   362.1068'4—dc22   2011012724

6048
Printed in the United States of America
15 14 13 12   10 9 8 7 6 5 4 3 2

Dedication

To Michele, Maria and Rosalinda, for their never-ending patience, support, and love, through every new adventure.

WS

To my team at home—Paul, my husband and best friend; Harrison, our master-in-charge of juggling; Tore, our world traveler; and Elijah, who proves that it takes longer to edit a book than to have a baby.

JJ

Table of Contents

Acknowledgments

The production of this book and its companion casebook has been the backdrop to many life events that our team has experienced. These include the marriage of one of us, the birth of two children, and the graduation of another from UNC, the alma mater of both editors. All these joyous occasions we have celebrated and accepted along with the numerous personal and professional challenges that we faced as well. This has truly been a productive and life affirming time and we are greatly appreciative to everyone who inspired and supported us in our lives and our work.

We have benefited greatly from the feedback of students who have provided insight and understanding of the importance of making this book a practical teaching tool that addresses the continuing challenges of improving health quality and safety in the future. We are most appreciative to our friends and colleagues around the globe who authored chapters. The coordination and integration of the contributing authors was a tremendous undertaking and we were privileged to work with excellent colleagues, who are truly expert practitioners of continuous quality improvement in health care. The production of the book required a team effort at all levels and in multiple locations. We would first like to acknowledge the assistance and guidance of the editorial team at Jones & Bartlett Learning. In Chapel Hill, special appreciation goes to Dean Barbara Rimer, of the UNC Gillings School of Global Public Health, whose leadership inspires a learning environment that stimulates innovations and the motivation to pursue them. Deep appreciation is also given to Public Health Leadership Program Director, Anna Schenck, not only for making resources available to support this project, but also for her contribution as an author to both this book and its companion casebook. Also important was the contribution of PHLP staff members who gave their time and energy, including Chantal Donaghy, and especially Damian Gallina, who was an invaluable member of our team and who, as project coordinator, was the voice of experience and encouragement throughout the process. In Sydney, Australia we appreciate the support, encouragement, and contributions of Jeffrey Braithwaite, Director of the Australian Institute of Health Innovation. We benefited from the expertise of Joanne Travaglia and Hamish Robertson in developing the Instructor's Manual, and we thank them for those efforts, as well as for their contributions as chapter authors. Finally, we are most grateful for the mentorship and confidence of Drs. McLaughlin and Kaluzny, who entrusted us with what has clearly been one of the passions and great successes of their careers.

William A. Sollecito, Chapel Hill, NC
Julie K. Johnson, Sydney, Australia

Contributors

Paul Barach, MD, MPH
Department of Anesthesia and Center for Patient Safety
University of Utrecht, Netherlands
University of South Florida, Florida

Pierre M. Barker, MD, MB, ChB
Senior Vice President
Institute for Healthcare Improvement
Cambridge, MA
Clinical Professor of Pediatrics, School of Medicine
University of North Carolina at Chapel Hill
Chapel Hill, NC

Paul Batalden, MD
Professor of Pediatrics, Community and Family Medicine
The Dartmouth Institute for Health Policy and Clinical Practice
Dartmouth Medical School
Hanover, NH

Shulamit Landau Bernard, PhD, RN
Director, Clinical Research Program
Duke University School of Nursing
Durham, NC

Jeffrey Braithwaite, PhD
Foundation Director, Australian Institute of Health Innovation
Director, Centre for Clinical Governance Research
Professor, Faculty of Medicine
University of New South Wales
Sydney, Australia

Carol E. Breland, MPH, RRT, RCP-NPS
Project Manager, Chiltern International Ltd.
Slough, Berkshire, England, UK
Local Field Office: Chapel Hill, NC, USA

William R. Carpenter, PhD, MHA
Assistant Professor, Department of Health Policy and Management
UNC Gillings School of Global Public Health
University of North Carolina at Chapel Hill
Chapel Hill, NC

Susan I. DesHarnais, PhD, MPH
Professor, Program Director
Healthcare Quality and Safety
Jefferson School of Population Health
Thomas Jefferson University
Philadelphia, PA

Bruce Fried, PhD
Associate Professor & Director, Residential Masters Programs
Department of Health Policy & Management
UNC Gillings School of Global Public Health
University of North Carolina at Chapel Hill
Chapel Hill, NC

David Greenfield, PhD
Senior Research Fellow, Centre for Clinical Governance Research
Australian Institute for Health Innovation
Faculty of Medicine, University of New South Wales
Sydney, Australia

Susan Paul Johnson, PhD, MBA
Consultant
Decatur, Georgia

Cheryl B. Jones, PhD, RN, FAAN
Associate Professor in Health Care Systems, School of Nursing
Research Fellow, Cecil B. Sheps Center for Health Services Research
University of North Carolina at Chapel Hill
Chapel Hill, NC

Diane Kelly, DrPH, MBA, RN
Associate Professor (Clinical)
Director, Clinical Nurse Leader Program
University of Utah College of Nursing
Salt Lake City, Utah
Adjunct Assistant Professor, Public Health Leadership Program
UNC Gillings School of Global Public Health
University of North Carolina at Chapel Hill
Chapel Hill, NC

David C. Kibbe, MD, MBA
Director, Center for Health Information Technology
American Academy for Family Physicians
Washington, DC

Cheryll D. Lesneski, DrPh, MA
Clinical Assistant Professor
UNC Gillings School of Global Public Health
University of North Carolina at Chapel Hill
Chapel Hill, NC

Sara E. Massie, MPH
Program Director, Quality Improvement Research Partnership
UNC Health Care System
University of North Carolina at Chapel Hill
Chapel Hill, NC

Jill A. McArdle, RN, MSPH
Director, Federal Programs and Services
The Carolinas Center for Medical Excellence
Cary, NC

Curtis P. McLaughlin, DBA
Professor Emeritus of Business Administration
Kenan-Flagler Business School
Senior Research Fellow Emeritus
Cecil B. Sheps Center for Health Services Research
University of North Carolina at Chapel Hill
Chapel Hill, NC

Mike Newton-Ward, MSW, MPH
Social Marketing Consultant
North Carolina Division of Public Health
Raleigh, NC

Marjorie Pawsey, AM, MBBS, FAAQHC
Senior Visiting Fellow, Centre for Clinical Governance Research
Australian Institute of Health Innovation
Faculty of Medicine, University of New South Wales
Sydney, Australia

Rohit Ramaswamy, PhD, MPH
President
Service Design Solutions, Inc.
Des Moines, IA
Gillings Visiting Clinical Associate Professor
Public Health Leadership Program
UNC Gillings School of Global Public Health
University of North Carolina at Chapel Hill
Chapel Hill, NC

Greg Randolph, MD, MPH
Director
NC Center for Public Health Quality
Raleigh, NC
Adjunct Associate Professor, Public Health Leadership Program
UNC Gillings School of Global Public Health
Co-Director, NC Children's Center For Clinical Excellence
Associate Professor, Department of Pediatrics

University of North Carolina School of Medicine
Chapel Hill, NC

Hamish Robertson
Ageing Research Centre, Neuroscience Research Australia
University of New South Wales
Sydney, Australia

Lucy A. Savitz, PhD, MBA
Director of Research and Education
Institute for Health Care Delivery Research
Intermountain Healthcare
Associate Professor, Clinical Epidemiology
Director, CCTS Community Engagement Core
University of Utah
Salt Lake City, UT

Anna P. Schenck, PhD, MSPH
Associate Dean for Practice
Professor of the Practice
Director of the Public Health Leadership Program and the
    North Carolina Institute for Public Health
UNC Gillings School of Global Public Health
University of North Carolina at Chapel Hill
Chapel Hill, NC

Gwen Sherwood, PhD, RN, FAAN
Professor and Associate Dean for Academic Affairs
Co-Investigator, Quality and Safety Education for Nursing (QSEN)
School of Nursing
University of North Carolina at Chapel Hill
Chapel Hill, NC

Donna Slovensky, PhD
Professor, Department of Health Service Administration
School of Health Related Professions
University of Alabama at Birmingham
Birmingham, AL

Leif I. Solberg, MD
Director for Care Improvement Research
Health Partners Research Foundation
Minneapolis, MN

David P. Steffen, DrPH, MSN
Clinical Assistant Professor and
Leadership Master's Concentration Director
Public Health Leadership Program
UNC Gillings School of Global Public Health
University of North Carolina at Chapel Hill
Chapel Hill, NC

Joanne F. Travaglia, PhD
Acting Director, Health Management Program
Senior Lecturer, School of Public Health and Community Medicine
Senior Research Fellow, Australian Institute of Health Innovation
Faculty of Medicine
University of New South Wales
Sydney, Australia

Vaughn Mamlin Upshaw, EdD, DrPH
Lecturer in Public Administration and Government
School of Government
University of North Carolina at Chapel Hill
Chapel Hill, NC

Joseph G. Van Matre, PhD
Professor, School of Business
University of Alabama at Birmingham
Birmingham, AL

Robert Weiser
Chief Operations Officer
The Carolinas Center for Medical Excellence
Cary, NC

Preface

Through 15 years and three editions we have presented an interdisciplinary perspective on continuous quality improvement in health care, taking into account a number of disciplines including operations management, organizational behavior, and health services research. Special attention was given to the tools and approaches fundamental to quality improvement within a variety of health care settings. That approach has been well received and we hope that it has provided insight and useful practices for students, practicing clinicians, health service managers, and those involved with policy decisions.

The passage of health care reform legislation in the United States and the global reach of quality improvement bring a new set of challenges and opportunities. It seems now is the appropriate time to examine the topic with a fresh perspective. With this edition, we handed over the editorial reins to Bill Sollecito and Julie Johnson. Under their very able leadership, the contributing authors have again provided a thoughtful examination of the major contemporary issues affecting the implementation, management, and institutionalization of quality improvement's concepts and methods.

While maintaining the framework of previous editions, the fourth edition includes several new chapters and a number of significant revisions. With the present edition the cases are presented in a companion text, *Implementing Continuous Quality Improvement in Health Care: A Global Casebook* (McLaughlin, Johnson, and Sollecito, 2012) to better describe the varied situations where quality improvement has been implemented and to give the reader an opportunity to apply the principles and concepts in depth to a wider variety of operational settings.

This book, like the prior editions, is divided into four sections. The first section provides an overview of the underlying issues of quality improvement, its evolution, adaptation, and implementation within health care organizations. The second section—Basics of Quality and Safety— details and updates the concepts and tools fundamental to quality improvement initiatives, providing an understanding of variation and process improvement, managing teams, assessing outcomes, measuring consumer satisfaction, and a new approach using social marketing. It also addresses the growing role of patients in continuous quality improvement.

The third section—Implementation—focuses on the unique challenge of translating concepts and tools into operations. Here attention is given to designing the learning organization, the reality of medical error, and the role of information technology.

The final section—Applications—presents the workings of quality improvement in a variety of health care settings, including primary care, public health, nursing, quality improvement organizations, as well as emerging initiatives in resource poor countries. The book concludes with a forward look at the future of quality improvement in a changing health care system with global implications. Quality improvement as we know it faces new challenges with the focus on "value added," which includes consideration of the ratio of quality to cost. While there are few certainties in the road ahead, Sollecito and Johnson clearly identify the issues and provide insights into how to navigate the changing landscape where quality improvement must be managed within the context of available resources as well as the context of the local setting.

Quality improvement, with its underlying concepts and methods, has become an integral part of contemporary thinking in health care, perhaps verging on becoming a cliché. Its potential remains great and the engines for disseminating experiences and training professionals is ever expanding. Its effective use still remains the issue of the day and is the responsibility of individuals at all levels of the delivery system. More than ever quality improvement requires a working partnership between clinicians, managers, economists, and financial experts. We truly hope the fourth edition again contributes to this ongoing interdisciplinary dialogue and to society's ability to sustain and expand the concepts and methods of quality improvement in an ever changing, complex, and global health care world. It is a worthy cause and we wish you well.

Curtis P. McLaughlin
Arnold D. Kaluzny

Foreword

Francis Bacon observed, "Some books are to be tasted, others to be swallowed, and some few to be chewed and digested." Serious students of quality improvement owe it to themselves to make *Continuous Quality Improvement in Health Care* a main course in their intellectual diet. At its heart, quality improvement theory argues that all health delivery activities—structure, data systems, planning, accountability, etc.—should build up from value-adding work. Value-adding work occurs through defined (and, hopefully, designed) work processes. On that foundation, improvement is prediction about transformation. It starts with a vision of what could be. Iterative experimentation, informed by quantitative and qualitative measurement and integrated learning, builds a better reality over time. It is a race without a finish line. No process is ever perfect; so it is always possible to conceive and test changes that could make it better.

You hold in your hands an example of continuous improvement principles applied to the explication of the principles themselves. Now in its fourth edition, *Continuous Quality Improvement in Health Care* adds new insights and findings to a core resource. When it first appeared in 1994, under the editorship of Curtis McLaughlin and Arnold Kaluzny, this book was well before its time but it essentially got the entire structure right. It first appeared before a health care world where clinical quality improvement was, at best, skeptically questioned. Ideas that today are widely accepted could then still provoke impassioned debate. They laid out the core principles of process management and improvement and they correctly anticipated much of the fine detail—the elegant subtleties—that later years would validate. Now, almost two decades later, the fourth edition of *Continuous Quality Improvement in Health Care*, with new editors Bill Sollecito and Julie Johnson, once again brings together the core principles of quality improvement, but this time with new ideas, and new contributing authors to help create a new vision of health care delivery.

Russell Ackoff wrote about "power over" versus "power to." "Power over" is the exercise of authority, to punish or reward. "Power to" is the force of ideas to inspire, coordinate, and transform. As a workforce increases in education, the success of organizations shifts from "power over" to "power to," from management to leadership. While there is little question that quality improvement lies at the heart of a major shift in how people think about and execute health care delivery, it is a massive transformation that could well span a full generation. The ideas in this book could not be more timely. It presents a road map and a "how to" guide for the leadership of a health care transformation that is the core work of this generation of caring professionals.

Brent James
IHC Institute for Health Care Delivery Research

Introduction

The Global Evolution of Continuous Quality Improvement: From Japanese Manufacturing to Global Health Services

William A. Sollecito and Julie K. Johnson

"We are here to make another world."

—W. Edwards Deming

Continuous quality improvement (CQI) comes in a variety of shapes, colors, and sizes and has been referred to by many names. It is an example of the evolutionary process that started with industrial applications, primarily in Japan, and has now spread throughout the world, affecting many economic sectors, including health care. In this introductory chapter, we define CQI, trace its history and adaptation to health care, and consider its ongoing evolution. References to subsequent chapters and the companion casebook (McLaughlin et al., 2012) provide greater detail and illustrations of CQI approaches and successes as applied to health care.

It is clearly illustrated throughout this text that despite the evolution and significant progress in the adoption of CQI theory, methods, and applications, the need for greater efforts in quality improvement in health care continues unabated. For example, a major study from 2010 encompassing more than 2,300 admissions in 10 North Carolina hospitals demonstrated that much more needs be done in improving the quality and safety in U.S. hospitals, and it may have implications for health care globally. It found that "patient harms," including preventable medical errors and other patient safety measures, remained common with little evidence of improvement during the 6-year study period from 2002 to 2007 (Landrigan et al., 2010). The challenge of how to cross the quality chasm (Institute of Medicine [IOM], 2001) in health care clearly remains, and hopefully some of the material in this text and its companion case-book (McLaughlin et al., 2012) will help to shed light on the scope of the problem and potential solutions.

DEFINITION OF CONTINUOUS QUALITY IMPROVEMENT

What was originally called *total quality management* (TQM) in the manufacturing industry evolved into *continuous quality improvement* as it was applied to health care administrative and clinical processes. Over time the term continued to evolve, and now the same concepts and activities are referred to as *quality improvement* or *quality management*, or even sometimes simply as *improvement*, as in the Model for Improvement (Langley et al., 2009). In keeping with the previous editions and to focus on the unique challenges within health care, the term *CQI* will be used primarily throughout this text.

In health care, CQI is defined as a structured organizational process for involving personnel in planning and executing a continuous flow of improvements to provide quality health care that meets or exceeds expectations. CQI usually involves a common set of characteristics, which include the following:

- A link to key elements of the organization's strategic plan
- A quality council made up of the institution's top leadership
- Training programs for personnel
- Mechanisms for selecting improvement opportunities
- Formation of process improvement teams
- Staff support for process analysis and redesign

- Personnel policies that motivate and support staff participation in process improvement
- Application of the most current and rigorous techniques of the scientific method and statistical process control

Institutional Improvement

CQI, under its various labels, is both an approach, or perspective, and a set of activities applied at various times to one or more of the four broad types of performance improvement initiatives undertaken within a given institution:

1. Localized improvement efforts

2. Organizational learning

3. Process reengineering

4. Evidence-based medicine and management

Localized improvement occurs when an ad hoc team is developed to look at a specific process problem or opportunity. Organizational learning occurs when this process is documented and results in the development of policies and procedures, which are then implemented. Examples include the development of protocols, procedures, clinical pathways, and so on. Process reengineering occurs when a major investment blends internal and external resources to make changes, often including the development of information systems, which radically impact key organizational processes. Evidence-based medicine and management involve the selection of best clinical and management practices; these are determined by examination of the professional literature and consideration of internal experience. The lines of demarcation between these four initiatives are not clear because performance improvement can occur across a continuum of project size, impact, clinical content, external consultant involvement, and departure from existing norms.

Societal Learning

In recent years, the emphasis on quality has increased at the societal level. The U.S. Institute of Medicine (IOM) has issued a number of reports critical of the quality of care and the variability of both quality and cost across the country (2000, 2001). This concern has increased with mounting evidence of the societal cost of poor-quality care in both lives and dollars (Brennan et al., 2004). It builds on the pioneering work of Phillip Crosby (1979), who provided a focus on the role of cost in quality initiatives, which is quite relevant today. Crosby's writings emphasize developing an estimate of the *cost of nonconformance*, also called the *cost of quality*. Developing this estimate involves identifying and assigning values to all of the unnecessary costs associated with waste and wasted effort when work is not done correctly the first time. This includes the costs of identifying errors, correcting them, and making up for the customer dissatisfaction that results. Estimates of the cost of poor quality range from 20% to 40% of the total costs of the industry, a range widely accepted by hospital administrators and other health care experts.

This view leads naturally to a broadening of the definition of quality by introducing the concept of *adding value*, in addition to ensuring the highest quality of care, implying greater accountability and a cost benefit to enhance the decision-making and evaluation aspects of CQI initiatives. This concept has seen a resurgence in recent years as national health plans, for example in the United States and the United Kingdom, look to minimize cost and increase value while providing the highest quality of care. For example, several leading experts propose refocusing on quality and accountability simultaneously, noting that "improving the U.S. health care system requires simultaneous pursuit of three aims: improving the experience of care, improving the health of populations, and reducing per capita costs of health care" (Berwick et al., 2008, p. 759). These same sentiments are echoed by Robert Brook, of the RAND Corporation, who proposes that the future of CQI in health care requires a focus on the concept of *value*, with consideration of both cost and quality (Brook, 2010). These concepts are discussed in greater detail throughout this book, particularly in the final chapter (Chapter 20).

Concerns about linking quality and value are not limited to the United States; similar evidence and concerns have been reported from the United Kingdom, Canada, Australia, and New Zealand (Baker et al., 2004; Davis et al., 2002; Kable et al., 2002). This newer emphasis has played out in studies, commissions, and reports as well as the efforts of regulatory organizations to institutionalize quality through their standards and certification processes. As you will see throughout this book, concern for quality and cost is a matter of public policy.

Professional Responsibility

As further explored in Chapter 2, health care as a whole is often likened to a cottage industry with overtones of a medieval craft guild, with a bias toward treatment rather than prevention and a monopoly of access to and implementation of technical knowledge. This system reached its zenith in the mid-20th century and has been under pressure ever since (McLaughlin and Kaluzny, 2002; Rastegar, 2004; Schlesinger, 2002; Starr, 1982). It is reinforced by the concept of *professionalism*, by which service providers are assumed to have exclusive access to knowledge and competence and, therefore, take full responsibility for self-regulation and for quality. However, much of the public policy debate has centered on the weaknesses of the professional system in improving quality of care. Critics point to excessive professional autonomy; protectionist guild practices, such as secrecy, restricted entry, and scapegoating; lack of capital accumulation for modernization; and economic self-interest as major problems. As we will see, all of these issues impinge on the search for improved quality. However, we cannot ignore the role of professional development as a potential engine of quality improvement, despite the popular emphasis on institutional improvement and societal learning. This too will be addressed in subsequent chapters.

RATIONALE AND DISTINGUISHING CHARACTERISTICS

As health care organizations and professions develop their own performance improvement approaches, their management must lead them through a decision process in which activities are initiated, adapted, and then institutionalized. Organizations embark on CQI for a variety of reasons, including accreditation requirements, cost control, competition for customers, and pressure from employers and payers. Linder (1991), for example, suggests that there are three basic CQI strategies: true process improvement, competitive advantage, and conformance to requirements. Some institutions genuinely desire to maximize their quality of care as defined in both technical and customer preference terms. Others wish simply to increase their share of the local health care market. Still others wish to do whatever is necessary to maintain their accreditation status with bodies such as The Joint Commission (TJC), National Committee on Quality Assurance (NCQA), and others, after which they will return to business as usual. As you might imagine, this book is written for the first group—those who truly wish to improve their processes and excel in the competitive health care market by giving their customers the quality care that they deserve.

Although CQI comes in a variety of forms and is initiated for a variety of reasons, it does have distinguishing characteristics and functions. These characteristics and functions are often defined as the essence of good management. They include (1) understanding and adapting to the external environment; (2) empowering clinicians and managers to analyze and improve processes; (3) adopting a norm that customer preferences are important determinants of quality and that the term *customer* includes both patients and providers in the process; (4) developing a multidisciplinary approach that goes beyond conventional departmental and professional lines; (5) adopting a planned, articulated philosophy of ongoing change and adaptation; (6) setting up mechanisms to ensure implementation of best practices through planned organizational learning; and (7) providing the motivation for a rational, data-based, cooperative approach to process analysis and change.

What is perhaps most radical vis-à-vis past health care improvement efforts is a willingness to examine existing health care processes and rework these processes collaboratively using state-of-the-art scientific and administrative knowledge and relevant data-gathering and analysis methodologies. Many health care processes have developed and expanded in a complex, political, and authoritarian environment, acquiring the patina of science. The application of data-based management and scientific principles to the clinical and administrative processes that produce patient care is what CQI is all about. Even with all the public concern about medical error and patient safety, improvement cannot occur without both institutional will and professional leadership (Millenson, 2003).

CQI is simultaneously two things: a management philosophy and a management method. It is distinguished by the recognition that customer requirements are the key to customer quality and that ultimately customer requirements will change over time because of changes in education, economics, technology, and culture. Such changes, in turn, require continuous improvements in the administrative and clinical methods that affect the quality of patient care. This dynamic between changing expectations and continuous efforts to meet these expectations is captured in the Japanese word *kaizen*, translated as continuous improvement (Imai, 1986). Change is fundamental to the health care environment, and the organization's systems must have both the will and the way to master such change effectively.

Customer Focus

The use of the term *customer* presents a special challenge to many health professionals. For many, it is a term that runs contrary to the professional model of health services and the idea that "the doctor knows best." Some health professionals would prefer terms that connote the more dependent roles of *client* or *patient*. In CQI terms, *customer* is a generic term referring to the end user of a group's output or product. The customer can be external or internal to the system—a patient, a payer, a colleague, or someone from another department. User satisfaction then becomes one ultimate test of process and product quality. Consequently, new efforts and new resources must be devoted to ascertaining what the customer wants through the use of consumer surveys, focus groups, interviews, and various other ways of gathering information on customer preferences, expectations, and perceived experiences. Chapter 6 provides a more detailed discussion of how to measure customer satisfaction, and Chapter 7 discusses the role of the patient in quality and safety.

System Focus

CQI is further distinguished by its emphasis on avoiding personal blame. The focus is on managerial and professional processes associated with a specific outcome—that is, the entire production system. The initial assumption is that the process needs to be changed and that the persons already involved in that process are needed to help identify how to approach a given problem or opportunity.

Therefore, CQI moves beyond the ideas of participative management and decentralized organizations. It is, however, participative in that it encourages the involvement of all personnel associated with a particular work process to provide relevant information and become part of the solution. CQI is also decentralized in that it places responsibility for ownership of each process in the hands of its implementers, those most directly involved with it. Yet this level of participation and decentralization does not absolve management of its fundamental responsibility; in fact, it places additional burdens on management. Where the problem is with the system (the usual case), management is responsible for change. CQI calls for significant amounts of managerial thought, oversight, flexibility, and responsibility.

CQI inherently increases the dignity of the employees involved because it not only recognizes the important role belonging to each member of the process improvement team, but it also involves them as partners and even leaders in the redesign of the process. In some cases, professionals can also serve as consultants to other teams as well as to management. Not surprisingly, organizations using CQI often experience improvements in morale. When the level of quality is being measured, workers can rightly take pride in the quality of the work they are producing.

Measurement and Decision Making

Another distinguishing feature of CQI is the rigorous belief in fact-based learning and decision making, captured by the saying, "In God we trust. All others send data." Facts do include perceptions, and decisions cannot all be delayed to await the results of scientifically correct, double-blind studies. However, everyone involved in CQI activities is expected to study the multiple causes of events and to explore a wide array of system-wide solutions. The primary purpose of data and measurement in CQI is learning—how to make system improvements and what the impact of each change that we have already made has had on the overall system. Measurement is not intended to be used for selection, reward, or punishment (Berwick, 1996). It is surprising and rewarding to see a team move away from the table-pounding "I'm right and you're stupid" position (with which so many meetings in health care start) by gathering data, both qualitative and traditional quantitative data, to see what is actually happening and why. Multiple causation is assumed, and the search for answers starts with trying to identify the full set of factors contributing to less-than-optimal system performance.

Subsequent chapters refer to some of the inherent barriers that accompany CQI implementation. These include the tension between the professionals' need for autonomy and control and the objectives of organizational learning and conformance to best practices. Organizations can also oversimplify their environment, as sometimes happens with clinical pathways. Seriously ill patients or patients with multiple chronic conditions do not fit the simple diagnoses often assumed when developing such pathways; a traditional disease management approach may not suffice, and a broader chronic care model that incorporates a personalized approach may be necessary (Seidman and Wallace, 2004). There may also be a related tendency to try to overcontrol processes. Health care is not like manufacturing, and it is necessary to understand that patients (anatomy, physiology, psyche, and family setting), providers, and diagnostic categories are highly variable and that variance reduction can only go so far. One has to develop systems that properly handle the inherent variability (called common cause variability) after unnecessary variability (called special cause variability) has been removed (McLaughlin, 1996).

ELEMENTS OF CQI

Together with these distinguishing characteristics, CQI is usually composed of a number of elements, including:

- Philosophical elements, which for the most part mirror the distinguishing characteristics cited previously
- Structural elements, which are usually associated with both industrial and professional quality improvement programs
- Health care–specific elements, which add the specialized knowledge of health care to the generic CQI approach

Philosophical Elements

The philosophical elements are those aspects of CQI that, at a minimum, must be present in order to constitute a CQI effort. They include:

1. Strategic focus—Emphasis on having a mission, values, and objectives that performance improvement processes are designed, prioritized, and implemented to support

2. Customer focus—Emphasis on both customer (patient, provider, payer) satisfaction and health outcomes as performance measures

3. Systems view—Emphasis on analysis of the whole system providing a service or influencing an outcome

4. Data-driven (evidence-based) analysis—Emphasis on gathering and using objective data on system operation and system performance

5. Implementer involvement—Emphasis on involving the owners of all components of the system in seeking a common understanding of its delivery process

6. Multiple causation—Emphasis on identifying the multiple root causes of a set of system phenomena

7. Solution identification—Emphasis on seeking a set of solutions that enhance overall system performance through simultaneous improvements in a number of normally independent functions

8. Process optimization—Emphasis on optimizing a delivery process to meet customer needs regardless of existing precedents and on implementing the system changes regardless of existing territories and fiefdoms. To quote Dr. Deming: "Management's job is to optimize the system."

9. Continuing improvement—Emphasis on continuing the systems analysis even when a satisfactory solution to the presenting problem is obtained

10. Organizational learning—Emphasis on organizational learning so that the capacity of the organization to generate process improvement and foster personal growth is enhanced (see Chapter 10)

Structural Elements

Beyond the philosophical elements just cited, a number of useful structural elements can be used to structure, organize, and support the continuous improvement process. Almost all CQI initiatives make intensive use of these structural elements, which reflect the operational aspects of CQI and include:

1. Process improvement teams—Emphasis on forming and empowering teams of employees to deal with existing problems and opportunities (see Chapter 4)

2. Seven CQI tools—Use of one or more of the seven CQI tools so frequently cited in the industrial and the health quality literature: flowcharts, cause-and-effect diagrams, histograms, Pareto charts, run charts, control charts, and regression analyses (see Chapter 3 for these and other tools)

3. Parallel organization—Development of a separate management structure to set priorities for and monitor CQI strategy and implementation, usually referred to as a quality council

4. Organizational leadership—Leadership, at the top levels and throughout the organization, to make the process effective and foster its integration into the institutional fabric of the organization (see Chapter 2)

5. Statistical analysis—Use of statistics, including statistical process control, to identify and reduce unnecessary variation in processes and practices (see Chapter 3)

6. Customer satisfaction measures—Introduction of market research instruments to monitor customer satisfaction at various levels (see Chapter 6)

7. Benchmarking—Use of benchmarking to identify best practices in related and unrelated settings to emulate as processes or use as performance targets (see Chapter 5)

8. Redesign of processes from scratch—Making sure that the end product conforms to customer requirements by using techniques of quality function deployment and/or process reengineering (see Chapter 3)

Health Care–Specific Elements

The use of CQI in health care is often described as a major management innovation, but it also resonates with past and ongoing efforts within the health services research community. The health care quality movement has its own history, with its own leadership and values that must be understood and respected. Thus in health care there are a number of additional approaches and techniques that health managers and professionals have successfully added to the philosophical and structural elements associated with CQI, including:

1. Epidemiological and clinical studies, coupled with insurance payment and medical records data, often referred to as the basis of evidence-based medicine

2. Involvement of the medical staff governance process, including quality assurance, tissue committees, pharmacy and therapeutics committees, and peer review

3. Use of risk-adjusted outcome measures

4. Use of cost-effectiveness analysis

5. Use of quality assurance data and techniques and risk management data

EVOLUTION OF THE QUALITY MOVEMENT

"If you would understand anything, observe its beginning and its development."

—Aristotle

To fully understand the foundation of the CQI approaches that have developed over the years and the reasons for their successful implementation, it is important to understand the underlying philosophies of the founders of this "movement" and the way in which these methodologies that have been adapted to health care evolved from industry.

The application of quality improvement techniques has reached unprecedented levels throughout the world and especially in health care. What started as a "business solution" to address major weaknesses, including a reputation for poor quality, which Japan faced in its manufacturing after World War II, has spread beyond manufacturing to encompass both products and services. This proliferation includes multiple industries across the world and, most notably, all sectors of health care. W. Edwards Deming described what happened in Japan as a "miracle that started off with a concussion in 1950." This miracle was the beginning of an evolutionary process whereby the Japanese military was transformed after the war and given a new goal: the reconstruction of Japan. As a result, "Japanese quality and dependability turned upward in 1950 and by 1954 had captured markets the world over" (Deming, 1986, p. 486). Built upon the expertise of Japanese leaders from industry, science, and the military, and with the guidance of Deming, using his own ideas and those of his colleague, Walter Shewhart, this miracle would transform industry not only in Japan, but also in many other countries around the world.

Although Deming and Shewhart both had been advocating a statistical approach to quality for some time, the Japanese were the first to implement these ideas widely. In Japan, the use of these techniques quickly spread to both product and service organizations. Outside Japan, despite slow adoption at first, this movement spread to the United States and Europe in the 1960s and 1970s. But its large-scale adoption did not occur until the 1980s, in manufacturing, most notably due to competition from the Japanese automobile industry. In fact, the U.S. industry was perceived to be in a state of crisis when these methods began to receive wider acceptance. As Deming surmised, this crisis was due to poor quality that could be traced primarily to the incorrect belief that quality and productivity were incompatible. Deming demonstrated the fallacy of this notion in his landmark book, *Out of the Crisis*, first published in 1982 (Deming, 1986), thus forming the basis of what is now known as continuous quality improvement.

From this foundation, CQI has evolved exponentially—over time, across the world, and from industrial manufacturing to the provision of services. The beginning of the quality revolution occurred in America in 1980, when Deming was featured on an NBC television documentary, "If Japan Can, Why Can't We?" and a later PBS program, "Quality or Else," both of which had a major impact on bringing quality issues into the U.S. public's awareness (AmStat News, 1993).

Over many years, Deming made enormous contributions to the development of TQM/CQI, but he is perhaps best known for the 14-point program of recommendations that he devised for management to improve quality (see **Table 1–1**). His focus was always on processes (rather than organizational structures), on the ever-continuous cycle of improvement, and on the rigorous statistical analysis of objective data. Deming believed that management has the final responsibility for quality because employees work in the system; management deals with the system itself. He also felt that most quality problems are management controlled rather than worker controlled. These beliefs were the basis for his requirement that TQM/CQI be based on a top-down, organization-wide commitment.

The quality evolution later crossed fields as diverse as computer science, education, and health care; and within health care, it has evolved to encompass multiple levels and segments of health care delivery. As discussed earlier, this evolution has taken many forms and names over the years, encompassing and subsuming quality control, quality assurance, quality management, and quality improvement. Like the field itself, its name has evolved from total quality management to continuous quality improvement, or simply quality improvement.

TABLE 1-1 Deming's 14-Point Program
___

1. Create and publish to all employees a statement of the aims and purposes of the company or other organization. The management must demonstrate constantly their commitment to this statement.

2. Learn the new philosophy, top management and everybody.

3. Understand the purpose of inspection, for improvement of processes and reduction of cost.

4. End the practice of awarding business on the basis of price tag alone.

5. Improve constantly and forever the system of production and service.

6. Institute training.

7. Teach and institute leadership.

8. Drive out fear. Create trust. Create a climate for innovation.

9. Optimize toward the aims and purposes of the company the efforts of teams, groups, staff areas.

10. Eliminate exhortations for the work force.

11a. Eliminate numerical quotas for production. Instead, learn and institute methods for improvement.

11b. Eliminate management by objective.

12. Remove barriers that rob people of pride of workmanship.

13. Encourage education and self-improvement for everyone.

14. Take action to accomplish the transformation.

Source: Reprinted from *The New Economics for Industry, Government, Education* by W. Edwards Deming, with permission of MIT and W. Edwards Deming. Published by MIT, Center for Advanced Engineering Study, Cambridge, MA 02139. Copyright © 1993 by W. Edwards Deming.

From TQM to CQI

The evolution from TQM to CQI was more than a simple change in terminology; it represents a fundamental change in how organizations have come to recognize the importance of ensuring that changes are improvements and that the improvement processes are ongoing, requiring learning and involvement in the process at all levels, from the individual to the organization level. CQI has been directly linked to management and leadership competencies and philosophies that embrace change and innovation as the keys to a vision of value-driven growth. The fundamentals of TQM are based on the scientific management movement developed in the early 20th century. Emphasis was given to "management based on facts," but with management assumed to be the master of the facts. It was believed to be the responsibility of management to specify one correct method of work for all workers and to see that personnel executed that method to ensure quality. Gradually, that perspective has been influenced by the human relations perspective and by the recognition of the importance and ability of the people in the organization. **Figure 1–1** illustrates the wide range of leaders who were involved in the quality evolution, with an emphasis on health care. Some of the most notable contemporaries of Deming and Shewhart who were major contributors to the history of TQM and later CQI include Armand Feigenbaum, Joseph Juran, and Philip Crosby. Their contributions have been widely documented in the literature, as well as through organizations that continue to promote their ideas, such as the Juran Institute (see http://www.juran.com/). They are included, along with many others, in Web sites that profile these gurus of quality improvement and their individual ideas and techniques that form the basis of modern CQI (see http://www.qualitygurus.com/gurus/).

Ongoing Evolution in Japan

While the quality concepts originally applied in Japan were evolving across other countries, they continued to develop and evolve within Japan as well, with numerous original contributions to CQI thinking, tools, and techniques, especially since the 1960s. The most famous of the Japanese experts are Genichi Taguchi and Kaoru Ishikawa.

Taguchi was a Japanese quality expert who emphasized using statistical techniques developed for the design of experiments to quickly identify problematic variations in a service or product; he also advocated a focus on what he called a "robust" (forgiving) design. He emphasized evaluating quality from both an end-user and a process approach. Ishikawa is well known for developing one of the classic CQI tools, the fishbone (or Ishikawa) cause-and-effect diagram (see Chapter 3). Along with other Japanese quality engineers, Ishikawa also refined the application of the foundations of CQI and added the concepts described in **Table 1–2**.

Cross-Disciplinary Thinking

More than a historical business trend or a movement, the growth of quality improvement represents an evolution of both the philosophies and processes that have been studied and improved over the years, through application, review, feedback, and then broader application. There has

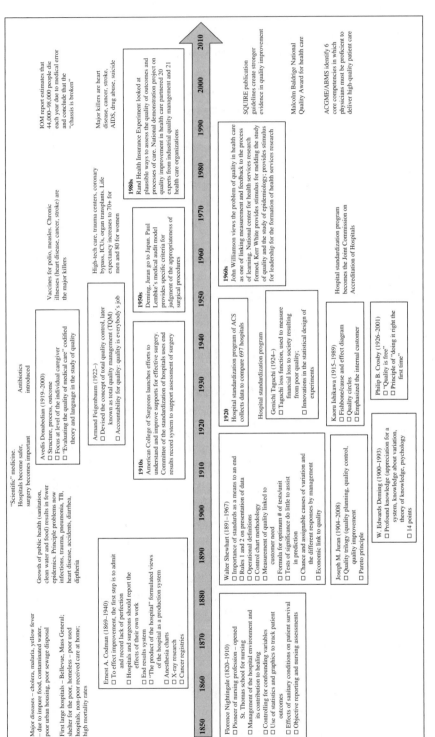

FIGURE 1-1 Some of the Evolutionary Context of Quality in Health Care

TABLE 1-2 Recent Contributions of Japanese Quality Engineers

1. Total participation is required of all members of an organization (quality must be company-wide).
2. The next step of a process is its "customer," just as the preceding step is its "supplier."
3. Communicating with both customer and supplier is necessary (promoting feedback and creating channels of communication throughout the system).
4. Emphasis is placed on participative teams, starting with "quality circles."
5. Emphasis is placed on education and training.
6. Instituted the Deming Prize to recognize quality improvement.
7. Statistics are used rigorously.
8. Instituted "just in time" processes.

Source: Adapted from McLaughlin and Kaluzny, 2006.

been a fair amount of scrutiny, and these approaches have not only stood the test of time but have evolved to address criticisms and have been adapted to meet specialized needs that are unique in some segments, especially in health care. This phenomenon has occurred naturally as a result of cross-disciplinary strategic thinking processes, where learning occurs by focusing not on what makes industries and disciplines different from each other, but rather on what they share in common (Brown, 1999). A good example of this commonality is a focus on adding value to products and services for customers, be they automobile buyers, airline passengers, or hospital patients. This notion can be directly extended to quality improvement (see **Figure 1-2**) by noting that industries—for example, automobile manufacturing vs. health care—may differ in terms of specific mission,

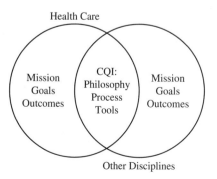

FIGURE 1-2 Cross-Disciplinary Strategic Thinking

goals, and outcomes but may share strategies to add value, including the philosophy, process, and tools of CQI. As a result, the common strategic elements of CQI have been adopted from diverse industrial applications and then customized to meet the special needs of health care.

Comparing Industrial and Health Care Quality

Cross-disciplinary learning between industry and health care was spurred during the 1990s and contributed to this evolutionary process. A comparison of quality from an industrial perspective vs. quality from a health care perspective reveals that the two are surprisingly similar and that both have strengths and weaknesses (Donabedian, 1993). The industrial model is limited in that it (1) ignores the complexities, including the dynamic character and professional and cultural norms, of the patient–practitioner relationship; (2) downplays the knowledge, skills, motivation, and legal/ethical obligations of the practitioner; (3) treats quality as free, ignoring quality–cost trade-offs; (4) gives more attention to supportive activities and less to clinical ones; and (5) provides less emphasis on influencing professional performance via "education, retraining, supervision, encouragement, and censure" (Donabedian, 1993, pp. 1–4). On the other hand, Donabedian suggested that the professional health care model can learn the following from the industrial model:

1. New appreciation of the fundamental soundness of health care quality traditions

2. The need for even greater attention to consumer requirements, values, and expectations

3. The need for greater attention to the design of systems and processes as a means of quality assurance

4. The need to extend the self-monitoring, self-governing tradition of physicians to others in the organization

5. The need for a greater role by management in assuring the quality of clinical care

6. The need to develop appropriate applications of statistical control methods to health care monitoring

7. The need for greater education and training in quality monitoring and assurance for all concerned (1993, pp. 1–4)

In reality, there is a continuum of TQM/CQI activities, with manufacturing at one end of the continuum and professional services at the other (Hart, 1993). The TQM/CQI approach should be modified in accordance with its position along this continuum. Manufacturing processes have linear flows, repetitive cycle steps, standardized inputs, high analyzability, and low worker discretion. Professional services, on the other hand, involve multiple nonstandardized and variable inputs, nonrepetitive operations, unpredictable demand peaks, and high worker discretion. Many organizations, including health care organizations, have processes at different points along that continuum that should be analyzed accordingly. The hospital, for example, has laboratory and support operations that are like a factory and has preventive, diagnostic, and treatment activities that are professional services. The objective of factory-like operations is to drive out variability to conform to requirements and to produce near-zero defects. At the other end, the objectives of disease prevention, diagnosis, and treatment are to do whatever it takes to produce improved health and satisfaction and maintain the loyalty of customers—including both patients (external customers) and employees (internal customers).

An important contrast between traditional industry and health care is evidence of the pace of quality improvement initiatives in health care relative to the traditional industries that spawned CQI methods globally. As described by a former director of the McKinsey Global Institute, William Lewis, "For most industry the benefits from the various quality movements have been quite large but . . . they are also largely in the past" with only incremental progress now being made, and he contrasts that development with health care, which is the "big exception" (Leonhardt, 2009, p. 11). So while health care has learned from manufacturing and commercial industry, its evolution in CQI has led to acceleration in comparison to the slowdown, and even reversal, seen in manufacturing and commercial industry; for example, consider the quality issues faced by Toyota in 2010 (Crawley, 2010), a manufacturing pioneer from which these approaches have evolved.

This evolution, or cross-disciplinary translation, continues within a variety of health care settings, as will be illustrated throughout this text, with some tools and techniques, such as the Plan, Do, Study, Act (PDSA) cycle originally developed by Shewhart (1931) for industry being especially amenable to widespread use and finding new applications to meet an ever-widening range of clinical and programmatic problems (see **Figure 1–3**). One very interesting example of the cross-disciplinary/industry phenomenon, which has been given much attention both in scientific journals and in

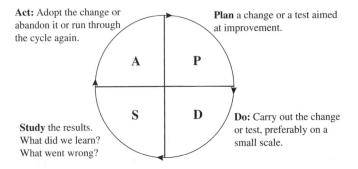

FIGURE 1–3 Shewhart (PDSA) Cycle

Source: Reprinted from *The New Economics for Industry, Government, Education* by W. Edwards Deming, with permission of MIT and W. Edwards Deming. Published by MIT, Center for Advanced Engineering Study, Cambridge, MA 02139. Copyright © 1993 by W. Edwards Deming.

popular media circles in 2009–2010, including both print and television, is the adoption of surgical checklists to prevent errors. This is based on a very simple but powerful device—the checklist—which has been used in many industries and has been both a project management and a safety tool, but it is probably most well known for its effectiveness in the airline industry. A strong case has been made in scientific publications and in the popular media for greater adoption of checklists in surgery (Haynes et al., 2009) and other medical specialties (Gawande, 2009; Pronovost et al., 2006). Although its adoption in a wide range of settings has been seen recently, the effectiveness of this tool, used by itself, has been questioned by some (Bosk et al., 2009). At the same time, practice-based research continues to explore its uses and to expand its applicability (de Vries et al., 2010). Checklists will be further discussed later in this text, both as an example of a quality improvement tool (in Chapter 3) and as an example of the broader issue of diffusion of CQI in health care (in Chapter 2); checklists are also the subject of an example in Chapter 8 and Case 9 in the companion casebook (McLaughlin et al., 2012).

New approaches, refinements of older concepts, and different combinations of ideas are occurring almost daily in this ongoing evolutionary process. As more and more organizations adopt CQI, we are seeing increasing innovation and experimentation with CQI thinking and its applications. This is especially true of the health care area, where virtually every organization has had to work hard to develop its own adaptation of CQI to the clinical process.

The Evolution Across Sectors of Health Care

The evolution in health care—which started in the most well-defined sector, hospitals—now includes all segments of the health care system and has become woven into the education of future practitioners, including not only administrators and physicians but also nurses, public health practitioners, and a wide array of other health professionals. It has spanned health care systems in many industrialized nations and now has become a way of meeting emerging crises, with widespread global health applications in resource-poor nations—for example, to help address the worldwide AIDS epidemic (see Chapter 19).

As illustrated in Figure 1–1, the health care evolution of CQI may be traced back to the work of Florence Nightingale, who pioneered the use of statistical methods to analyze variation and propose areas for improvement. As one of many quality improvement initiatives, Florence Nightingale used descriptive statistics to demonstrate the link between unsanitary conditions and needless deaths during the Crimean War (Cohen, 1984). The evolutionary context of quality in health care, described in Figure 1–1, has occurred at many different levels, spanning history and geography, and has included a broadening of applications and a sharpening of tools and techniques. Both within and outside health care, probably the most dramatic part of this evolution has been the wide dispersion of knowledge about how to use these techniques, first starting with a small group of expert consultants and later expanding to a broad range of practitioners with a common goal to make improvements in a diverse set of products and services. Coupled with that "practice" goal have been educational efforts to develop and disseminate quality improvement competencies by teaching these methods to an ever-widening range of health care professionals. For example, these efforts have included recent initiatives in nursing, the primary profession of Florence Nightingale (see Chapter 17).

In parallel with this broadening health care evolution over time and space, the same improvement processes were being applied to CQI tools and techniques, leading to improvements and greater precision relative to the measurement of outcomes and processes. The improvement processes also spawned international private and public sector organizations that can be thought of as "health care quality czars," which have applied and expanded these approaches. These organizations include the Institute for Healthcare Improvement (IHI) and both national and international regulatory agencies, such as the

CMS in the United States, which, with the establishment of Quality Improvement Organizations (QIOs), uses data from the Medicare and Medicaid system to monitor quality of care and, more importantly, to define improvement strategies (see Chapter 15). Similarly, local, national, and international accreditation agencies, such as TJC in the United States and its global counterparts (e.g., Joint Commission International [JCI]), have mandated the need for quality improvement in large health care systems (see Chapter 18). Ultimately, this has led to the emergence of quality leaders, with recognized achievements via a health care organization's eligibility to receive awards such as the Malcolm Baldrige National Quality Award (Hertz et al., 1994; McLaughlin and Kaluzny, 2006) (see http://www.nist.gov/baldrige/) and other awards, such as the annual NCQA Health Quality Awards (see http://www.ncqa.org/tabid/1117/Default.aspx).

Around the mid-1980s, CQI was applied in several health care settings. Most notable was the early work done by three physicians following the principles outlined by Deming: Paul Batalden at Hospital Corporation of America (HCA), Donald Berwick at Harvard Community Health Center and IHI, and Brent James at Intermountain Health Care. Examples of their work and ideas will be illustrated throughout this chapter and this book (see, for example, Chapter 13).

Armed with the ideas of these creative quality leaders who elaborated on techniques, such as the PDSA cycle, that were drawn originally from the pioneers of quality improvement, an acceleration marked by more widespread applications has occurred throughout all sectors of health care in the 21st century. That acceleration was spurred greatly by "a wake-up call" describing the crisis that health care quality was facing entering the new millennium.

THE BIG BANG—THE QUALITY CHASM

Quality under the rubric of patient safety suddenly came to dominate the scene following the two significant IOM reports *To Err Is Human* (2000) and *Crossing the Quality Chasm* (2001). Virtually all those concerns about cost and benefits and professional autonomy seemed swamped by the documentation of unacceptably high rates of medical errors. The recognition that needless human suffering, loss of life, and wasted resources were related to unnecessary variability in treatment and the lack of implementation of known best practices galvanized professional groups, regulators, and payers into action. Suddenly, quality improvement was acknowledged to be a professional responsibility, a quality-of-care issue rather than a managerial tactic. Current investment and involvement levels are high as evidence has mounted that the variability in clinical processes and the lack of conformance to evidence-based best practices has cost the public dearly. Many of the actors identified previously are demanding accountability for patient safety and for achieving acceptable levels of clinical performance and outcomes achievement. Adverse events are now undergoing extreme scrutiny, and a broad range of quality indicators are being reported, followed, and compared by payers and regulators (see Chapter 11). One important change that called even greater attention to the seriousness of medical errors was that effective October 1, 2008, the CMS adopted a non-reimbursement policy for certain "never events," which are defined as non-reimbursable serious hospital-acquired conditions. The goal is to motivate hospitals to accelerate improvement of patient safety. The rationale is that hospitals cannot bill CMS for adverse events and complications that are considered never events because they are preventable. A list of never events can be found at the AHRQ Web site (see http://psnet.ahrq.gov/primer.aspx?primerID=3), and a summary of how this step came about is offered by Michaels et al. (2007).

Local and regional variability in health care has long been known to exist, but the translation of that variability into missed opportunities for improved outcomes has been slow in coming. With that veil of secrecy about medical errors lifted, the demands for action and professional responsiveness have become extensive. This sea-change goes well beyond concerns about malpractice insurance to issues of clinical governance, professional training, certification, and continuity of care.

For a while, financial questions seemed to have dissipated as the social costs took precedence. However, these cost issues have certainly been revisited and have grown in importance as national health care reform initiatives undergo full implementation in the United States and other locations around the world, such as Australia and the United Kingdom, which is in the process of reviewing and reorganizing its National Health Service, largely to save money. Concerns about cost of care continue and need to be considered relative to CQI initiatives and the overall nature of the relationship of cost to quality.

FROM INDUSTRIALIZATION
TO PERSONALIZATION

Quality has been and continues to be a central issue in health care organizations and among health care providers. The classic works of Avedis Donabedian, Robert Brook, and Leonard Rosenfeld, to name a few, have made major contributions to the definition, measurement, and understanding of health care quality. However, the corporatization of health care in the United States (Starr, 1982) and health care change have redefined and will continue to redefine how we manage quality. Given the increasing proportion of the gross national product allocated to health services and the redefinition of health care as an "economic good," health care organizations are influenced to a growing extent by organizations in the industrial sector. As part of this process, health care organizations have become "corporations," with expansion goals to create larger hospital systems. The long-held perception of health care as a cottage industry persisted into the 1960s and 1970s. In this view, health care was seen as a craft or art delivered by individual professionals who had learned by apprenticeship and who worked independently in a decentralized system. These practitioners tailored their craft to each individual situation using processes that were neither recorded nor explicitly engineered, and they were personally accountable for the performance and financial outcomes of the care they provided.

The 1980s and 1990s witnessed a distinct change, which is often described as the "industrialization of health care" (Kongstvedt, 1997). This change affected almost all aspects of health care delivery, influencing how risks are allocated, how care is organized, and how professionals are motivated and incentivized. **Figure 1–4** outlines this industrialization process utilizing the dynamic stability model of Boynton et al. (1993). One route, marked A, follows the traditional route of industrialization as illustrated by the bundling of cataract operations into a few high-volume, specialized centers. However, most health care activities have followed the B route, bypassing mass production due to the high variability in patient needs and using techniques of CQI and process reengineering.

The Victor and Boynton (1998) model for the organization suggests an appropriate path for organizational development and improvement. As presented in **Figure 1–5**, health care processes and product lines have begun to move from the craft stage to positions in all of the other three stages of that model. Each of the four stages requires its own approach to quality.

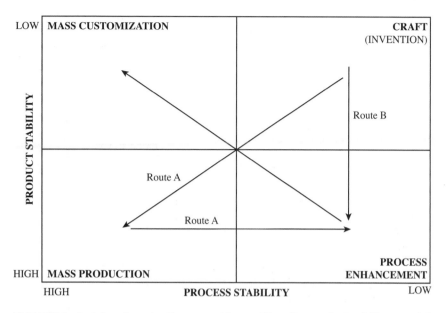

FIGURE 1–4 Adapting the Boynton-Victor-Pine Dynamic Stability Model to Health Care

Source: *OR/MS Today*, Vol. 25, No. 1. Reprinted with permission.

1. Craft requires that the individual improve with experience and use the tacit knowledge produced to develop a better individual reputation and group reputation. Craft activities can be leveraged to a limited extent by a community of cooperating and teaching craftspersons.

2. Mass production requires the discipline that produces conformance quality in high volume at low cost. Critics sometimes refer to this approach using terms such as *industrialization* or the *deskilling* of the profession and occasionally mention Henry Ford's assembly lines as a negative model.

3. Process enhancement requires that processes be analyzed and modified to develop a best-practice approach using worker feedback and process-owning teams within the organization.

4. Mass customization requires that the organization takes that best practice, modularizes and supports it independently, and then uses those modules to build efficient, low-cost processes that are responsive to individual customer wants and needs.

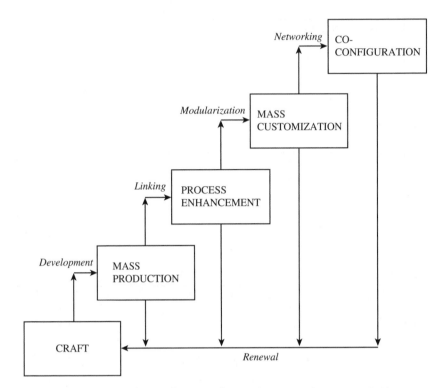

FIGURE 1–5 The Right Path Transformations Are Sequenced Along the Way

Source: Reprinted with permission from Victor, B., and Boynton, A. C. 1998. *Invented Here: Maximizing Your Organization's Internal Growth and Profitability*. Boston: Harvard Business School Press.

Because health care is a complex, multiproduct environment, various types of care can be found at each of the four stages, depending on the state of the technology and the strategy of the delivery unit. The correct place to be along that pathway depends on the current state of the technology. The revolution in health care organization is driven not only by economics, but also by the type of knowledge work that is being done. As described in Victor and Boynton:

> Managers take the wrong path when they fail to account for the fact that (1) learning is always taking place, and (2) what learning is taking place depends on the kind of work one is doing. The learning system we describe along the right path requires that managers leverage the learning from previous forms of work. . . . If managers attempt to transform without understanding the learning taking place . . . , then

> transformation efforts will be at best slightly off the mark and at worst futile. In addition, if managers misunderstand what type of work (craft, mass production, process enhancement, or mass customization) is taking place in a given process or activity when transformation starts, then they may use the wrong transformation steps (development, linking, modularization, or renewal). (1998, p. 129)

These authors, however, were referring to a single commercial firm with a relatively limited line of goods and services. In health care, a single organization such as a hospital might contain examples of multiple stages due to the variety of its products. There is a recognition that complexity is ever increasing; for example, one hears complaints that some traditional definitions apply to patients with only one diagnosis, whereas most very sick patients, especially the elderly, have multiple diagnoses. Therefore, the prevailing quality and performance enhancement systems have to be prepared with much greater levels of variability—in patient problem constellations, anatomy, physiology, and preferences, as well as in provider potentials and preferences (McLaughlin, 1996). Furthermore, increased availability of genetic information will further fractionate many disease categories, making the definitions of disease even more complex. Among other ideas, this has led to the concept of personalization of medicine and an associated concept, individualization of care, that will be discussed in greater detail in the next section.

Figure 1–6 suggests how this has and will occur in health care. As scientific information about a health care process accumulates, it shifts from the craft stage to the process enhancement stage. After the process is codified and developed further, it may shift into the mass production mode if the approach is sufficiently cut and dried, the volume is high, and the patients will accept this impersonal mode of delivery. If there is still too much art or lack of science to justify codification, the enhanced process can be returned to the craft mode or moved into the mass customization and co-configuration pathway.

The craft mode contains multiple delivery alternatives. If, for example, one were to decide to commission an artist to make a custom work of art, one has two ways to specify how it is to be controlled. The first is to say, "You are the artist. Do your thing and I will pay whatever it costs." This is fee-for-service indemnity. The other is to say, "You can decide what to do, but here is all that I can afford to pay." This is capitation. In both cases, the grand design and the execution are still in the hands of the artist.

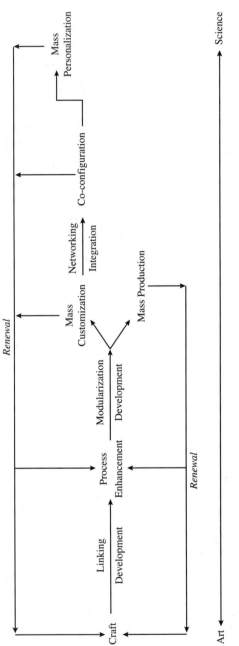

FIGURE 1-6 Revised Boynton and Victor Model for Health Care

Source: Adapted from McLaughlin and Kaluzny, 2006.

However, that does not preclude the artist from learning by doing or from vendors of materials and equipment or by observing and collaborating with colleagues. However, one does not commit to a one best way to do things, because one is not able to either articulate or agree on what is the best way.

The mass customization pathway has long been thought of as the best way to produce satisfied health care customers at low or reasonable relative costs. The organization develops a series of modular approaches to prevention and treatment, highly articulated and well supported by information technology, so that they can be deployed efficiently in a variety of places and configurations to respond to customer needs. Clinical pathways represent one example of modularization. They represent best practice as known to the organization, and they are applied by a configuror (the health care professional) to meet the needs of the individual patient. This requires an integrated information system that will give the configuror, usually a generalist, access to specialized information and to full information about the patient's background, medical history, and status; the system will also allow the configuror to synchronize the implementation of the modules of service being delivered. In a sense, mass customization represents a process that simulates craft but is highly science based, coordinated, integrated with other process flows, and efficient. How does this differ from the well-run modern hospital or clinic? As described by Victor and Boynton:

> The tightly linked process steps developed under process enhancement are now exploded, not into isolated parts, but into a dynamic web of interconnected modular units. Rather than the sequential assembly lines, . . . work is now organized as a complex, reconfigurable product and service system.
>
> Modularization breaks up the work into units that are interchangeable on demand from the customer. And everything has to happen fast. . . . Modularization transforms work by creating a dynamic, robust network of units.
>
> Within some of these units, . . . there may still be active craft, mass production, or process enhancement work taking place, but all the possible interfaces among modules must be carefully designed so that they can rapidly, efficiently, and seamlessly regroup to meet customer needs. (1998, pp. 12–13)

Where does science come in? Victor and Boynton refer to architectural knowledge, a much deeper process understanding than that needed for earlier stages of their model. Also at a practical level, it takes hard science to legitimize the conformance by providers required to make such a system work.

The remaining stage of this model has been called "co-configuration"—a system in which the customer is linked into the network, and customer intelligence is accessed as readily as the providers'. In a futuristic sense, one should also be able to include the patient in the decision-making network to a high degree. The future has arrived in the form of what many authors call "mass personalization." It represents an even more intense involvement of customers in product and service delivery choices; in health care, patient-specific needs and wants are being more directly addressed.

Mass Personalization

Personalization is an evolutionary concept that is not only having an impact on how industries deliver products and services but also on how organizations are structured, such as in learning organizations (see Chapter 10). It is an example of a business application that continues to evolve within the business world and is now beginning to evolve at its own pace within health care. In business, this evolution is especially apparent in service industries, where the morphing of mass customization into mass personalization has been fueled by the rapid growth of technology, especially the Internet, search engines, and personal media, to bring each customer's wants and needs in direct contact with service providers.

This phase of evolution has happened quite rapidly, and its speed of growth is directly correlated with technological advances. "Two decades after its conception there is growing evidence that mass customization strategy is transforming into a mass personalization strategy" (Kumar, 2007, p. 533). It was not until 1987 that the term *mass customization* was first introduced. However, from 1987 to 2008, more than 1,100 articles on mass customization appeared in scholarly journals, with exponential growth in the 1990s (Kumar, 2007).

Personalization of products began in the 1950s, with affordability being the key component that led to its popularity and growth. As computer technologies have become more personalized, the concepts of mass customization and co-configuration have evolved into personalization, at an accelerated pace. As Kumar explains, "Mass personalization strategy evolved from mass customization strategy as a result of strides in information and operational technologies" (2007, p. 536). Both strategies are in current use; while similar, they do have differences. As described by Tseng and Piller, who have written extensively on this trend:

> Personalization must not be mixed up with customization. While customization relates to changing, assembling, or modifying product or service components according to customers' needs and desires, personalization involves intense communication and interaction between two parties, namely customer and supplier. Personalization in general is about selecting or filtering information objects for an individual by using information about that individual (the customer profile) and then negotiating the selection with the individual. . . . From a technical point of view, automatic personalization or recommendation means matching meta-information of products or information objects against meta-information of customers (stored in the customer profile). (2003, p. 7)

This leads to strategies that are directed at what Kumar calls "a market of one" (Kumar, 2007, p. 533).

Health Care Applications of Personalization

That mass personalization is directly applicable to CQI is quite obvious due to their common focus on adding value and customer satisfaction and their common reliance on data and technology. What is a bit surprising is that personalization can be applied directly to CQI in health care and how rapidly this stage of evolution from business to health care is occurring. This concept is closely related to what Berwick calls "patient centeredness," a consumerist view of quality of care, which he describes as involving "disruptive shifts in control and power out of the hands of those who give care and into the hands of those who receive it" (2009, p. 555).

At first glance, the importance and reliance on evidence-based practice as part of CQI in health care might seem contradictory to personalization; however, as noted by Sackett and many others, the steps in applying evidence-based practice include evaluating the best data available but also using individual clinical judgment and patient input, including patient preferences, in making final treatment decisions (Sackett, 1996). The current definition of health care personalization encompasses the concepts of individualized care and shared decision making, in addition to personalized medicine (Barratt, 2008; Pfaff et al., 2010; Robinson et al., 2008). In all forms, these concepts lead to greater focus on patient characteristics, needs, and preferences in decision making about their care, and they are all closely associated with the customer focus concepts that are central to CQI. With greater availability of information, via the Internet and other more traditional sources, patients and their families are playing a greater role in health care decision making and quality of care. Sources of data and information abound in numerous easily accessible formats. For example, for many years the Agency for Healthcare Research and Quality (AHRQ) has provided information to encourage patient participation in their medical care and the quality of the medical care they receive; one example is the report "20 Tips to Help Prevent Medical Errors," which is available online (http://www.ahrq.gov/consumer/20tips.htm). Similar resources have long been provided by other organizations to support patients with specialty needs; for example, the National Cancer Institute's Cancer Information Service was established in 1975 to help cancer patients find information and treatment resources (http://www.cancer.gov/aboutnci/cis). What has contributed notably to the use of such information is that patients now have greater knowledge and access to technology, such as search engines to find medical information. This has led to input by patients and their families in their own health care decisions and in the quality of their care, which is discussed in greater detail Chapter 7.

But the growth in health care personalization goes beyond patients having access to medical information; it relates directly to medical strategies and emerging science for providing higher quality, safer, more personalized treatments. As described by Drs. Collins (Director of the U.S. National Institutes of Health) and Hamburg (Director of the U.S. Food and Drug Administration), we are now clearly on a path to personalized medicine (Hamburg and Collins, 2010). These distinguished health care leaders describe their vision of personalized medicine primarily in terms of genomic medicine; it is a means of "focusing on the best ways to develop new therapies and optimize prescribing by steering patients to the right drug at the right dose at the right time" (p. 301). They go on to describe a partnership among industry, academia, doctors, patients, and the public that will lead to a "national highway for personalized medicine." One of the earliest signs of success relates to identifying the optimal dosage and combination of treatments for cancer patients (Spector and Blackwell, 2009).

As in the business community, the personalization concept in health care has evolved to include broader components of health care, in part because of advances in research and technology. In medical care, this includes not only recent breakthroughs in genomics but also tools provided by computer technology, including greater use of electronic medical records. Individualized treatment strategies are further extensions of these concepts, going beyond genomics to include patients' preferences and experiences in shared decision making with their providers, allowing greater patient participation in choice of drugs and dosages and administration; even more broadly, individualization leads to patients being more proactive in regard to prevention, screening, and early treatment, through greater use of information technology, electronic medical records, and decision-making tools, such as patient decision support technologies (Pfaff et al., 2010).

Seidman and Wallace (2004) describe health care personalization more broadly as an extension of Wagner's chronic care model (1996), which focuses on the individual rather than the condition. This approach is especially useful when individuals have multiple chronic conditions leading to what these authors describe as "an evolution to mass personalized chronic condition care," encompassing both evidence-based medicine and self-management support, which relies on a collaborative approach between individuals and their physicians (Seidman and Wallace, 2004).

The evolutionary path of CQI within health care is an important catalyst to personalization that is reflective of broader societal trends spanning a wide range of businesses. These trends are reflected in the concept of customer relationship management (CRM). As described by Kumar (2007), "CRM is the philosophy, policy, and coordinating strategy connecting different players within an organization so as to coordinate their efforts in creating an overall valuable series of experiences, products, and services for the customer." Kumar notes that CRM also requires that the customer be integrated into all aspects of product and process design and that "customer driven innovation has become a key source of strategic advantage." This relates not only to health care personalization but also to the traditional focus on customers in CQI and on methods of gathering customer feedback, as described in Chapter 6.

With new opportunities come new challenges. The greater amount of information available and the increased role of "untrained" patients and their families in care decisions present the challenge of knowing how to evaluate the quality and appropriateness of treatment options. This has led to some level of conflict as the two extremes of standardization vs. personalization strain the boundaries and definitions of evidence-based medicine, with both extremes striving to achieve the highest quality of care. There is an ongoing broad discussion throughout health care, locally and globally, about how to balance these concepts (Pfaff et al., 2010; Robinson et al., 2008). What is clear is that these patient-centered concepts are here to stay and will lead to the next stages of the evolution in health care and, as with the previous stages, will continue to grow exponentially.

Likewise, as described in Chapter 7, and referring back to Berwick's notion of "patient centeredness" (2009), patients are playing—and should play—a greater role in health care quality improvement. These patient-centered trends have had an impact on quality improvement education for health care professionals. For example, they are being incorporated into nursing education, as described in Chapter 17. Day and Smith describe this need:

> Unfortunately there is wide variation in the quality of information provided by websites and no search engine screens for quality or accuracy. An important part of basic nursing education is helping students develop skills that enable them to evaluate web-based information, especially if that information is going to be passed on to a patient or family member or used as the basis for patient and family teaching. (2007, pp. 139–140)

Thus, as with other evolutionary stages in CQI, new challenges to quality management present themselves and will hopefully lead to new opportunities in an unending cycle of improvement.

BROAD-BASED APPROACHES/SUCCESSES

As CQI philosophies and processes have evolved within health care, a series of broad-based approaches have evolved and proven to be successful across a range of health care settings. These can be thought of as umbrella approaches under which specific change methods can be applied. The two most notable are the historically proven PDSA cycle and the quality improvement collaborative. These two broad approaches have proven to be particularly successful in health care as frameworks within which a variety of improvement methods have been applied to measure and further initiate improvement strategies.

The PDSA Cycle

Walter Shewhart, at Bell Laboratories, was the first to introduce the Plan, Do, Study, Act (PDSA) cycle, which was presented earlier in Figure 1–3. Although the PDSA cycle is often attributed to Deming, he attributes it to Shewhart (Deming, 1986). It should also be noted that over time, the abbreviation PDSA was changed by some to PDCA, the "S" for study being changed to "C" for check, as in *checking* what impact an improvement has made on the process being changed. Today the terms are used interchangeably, as we will do throughout this book. Either way, Shewhart's concept has become a very powerful and frequently used quality improvement methodology that has withstood the test of time.

The two very successful and well-known applications of the PDSA cycle that have evolved in health care are HCA's FOCUS–PDCA model (Batalden and Stoltz, 1993) and the Model for Improvement (Langley et al., 2009). In addition to these two major PDSA applications, numerous other CQI initiatives have centered around this basic improvement cycle.

The broad applicability of the PDSA cycle in health care can be traced directly to its roots as it was applied by Deming. One of Deming's major premises (1993) was that management needs to undergo a transformation. In order to respond successfully to challenges to organizations and their environments, the way to accomplish that transformation, which must be deliberately learned and incorporated into management, is by pursuing what he called "profound knowledge." The key elements of his system of profound knowledge are (1) appreciation for a system, (2) knowledge about variation, (3) theory of knowledge, and (4) psychology.

The Deming process is especially useful in health care because professionals already have knowledge of the subject matter as well as a set of values and disciplines that fit the Deming philosophy. Training in Deming methods adds knowledge of how to build a new theory using insights about systems, variation, and psychology, and it focuses on the answers given to the set of basic questions that center around knowing what is to be accomplished. Furthermore, it applies a cyclical process of testing and learning from data whether the change being made is an improvement and what improvements are needed in the future (Batalden and Stoltz, 1993). A Deming approach, as adopted by the HCA, is illustrated in **Figure 1–7**. It was referred to by the HCA as FOCUS–PDCA and provided the firm's health care workers with a common language and an orderly sequence for implementing the cycle of

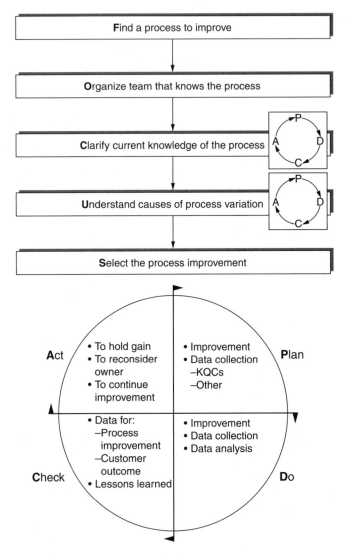

FIGURE 1–7 The FOCUS–PDCA Cycle

continuous improvement. It focuses on the answers given to the following basic questions (Batalden and Stoltz, 1993):

1. What are we trying to accomplish?

2. How will we know when that change is an improvement?

3. What changes can we predict will make an improvement?

4. How shall we pilot test the predicted improvements?

5. What do we expect to learn from the test run?

6. As the data come in, what have we learned?

7. If we get positive results, how do we hold on to the gains?

8. If we get negative results, what needs to be done next?

9. When we review the experience, what can we learn about doing a better job in the future?

In parallel with the FOCUS–PDCA model was the introduction in 1992 of the Model for Improvement by Langley et al. (2009). It includes a PDSA cycle as its core approach, returning to the traditional "S," emphasizing the importance of *studying* what has been accomplished before making further changes (**Figure 1–8**). Careful study and reflection are

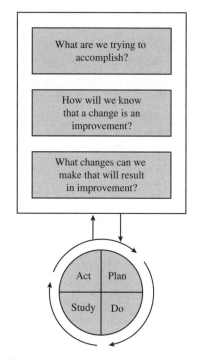

FIGURE 1–8 Model for Improvement

Source: The "Model for Improvement"—a systematic approach to rapid improvement of health processes (Langley et al., 2009).

points of emphasis made by Berwick (1996), who describes this model as "inductive learning—the growth of knowledge through making changes and then reflecting on the consequences of those changes." Central to this model are three key questions:

1. What are we trying to accomplish?

2. How will we know that a change is an improvement?

3. What change can we make that will result in an improvement?

The wide use of these approaches is due directly to the elegance and simplicity of the PDSA cycle. Likewise, the range of applications ties directly to the generalizability of the PDSA cycle. Recent applications have included public health (see Chapter 16), health care in resource-poor countries (see Chapter 19) and traditional medical care in industrialized settings, which are described throughout this book.

Quality Improvement Collaboratives

Quality improvement collaboratives (QICs) are another example of a broad-based approach that exemplifies the evolution of CQI methods across geographic boundaries and areas of health care, with applications that range from primary care to public health. Although some authors feel that clear evidence of their effectiveness, in terms of improved outcomes, is lacking, their widespread adoption is well documented (Schouten et al., 2008). Simply defined, QICs consist of "multidisciplinary teams from various health care departments or organizations that join forces for several months to work in a structured way to improve their provision of care" (Schouten et al., 2008, p. 1491). They have been described as temporary learning organizations (Ovretveit et al., 2002) and have also been described in the context of diffusion of innovation; more specifically, in their comprehensive review of the literature on diffusion of innovation in health service organizations (2005), Greenhalgh et al. describe the goal of QICs as "spread of ideas." These authors formally describe QICs as multi-organizational structured improvement collaboratives and provide a succinct description of how they work:

> Participants in a quality collaborative work together over a number of months, sharing ideas and knowledge, setting specific goals, measuring progress, sharing techniques for organizational change and

implementing rapid-cycle, iterative tests of change. Learning sessions are the major events of a Collaborative; these are 2-day events where members of the multi-disciplinary project teams from each health care organization gather to share experiences and learn from clinical and change experts and their colleagues. The time between learning sessions is called an action period in which participants work within their own organizations towards major, "breakthrough" improvement, focusing on their internal organizational agenda and priorities for changes and improvements whilst remaining in continuous contact with other Collaborative participants. (p. 163)

Introduced initially in the United States in the mid-1980s, QICs are now used in many countries with varying health care financing systems, including Canada, Australia, and European countries, where several national health authorities support nationwide quality programs based on this strategy. A similar approach has been used in the United Kingdom through its National Health Service Modernization Agency; it is called the Beacon Model and focuses on transfer of best practices, derived from Beacon organizations "that have achieved a high standard of service delivery and are regarded as centers of best practice" (Greenhalgh et al., 2005, p. 168).

QICs were initially developed and are still used in primary care. They have now evolved to a broader number of settings, and their widespread adoption in the United States has led to the formation of a national organization, the Network for Regional Healthcare Improvement; this is discussed in greater detail in Chapter 14 in relation to primary care.

One of the first uses of QICs was the Northern New England Cardiovascular Disease Study Group in 1986. Their continuing effective use within cardiovascular care is described in a systematic review of the management of heart failure, published in 2006, 20 years after its first introduction. This review concludes that the collaborative methodology "has significant potential to improve the outcomes of patients, particularly those with [heart failure] and chronic cardiovascular disease" (Newton et al., 2006, p. 161). The success and widespread adoption of QICs are directly related to the exchange and application of best practices by experts and peers to carry out improvement initiatives.

One notable contributor to the growth in use of QICs is the widespread application known as the Breakthrough Series, developed by the Institute for Healthcare Improvement in 1995 (Schouten et al., 2008).

Once again, QICs serve as an umbrella under which a broad array of specific methods can be used to carry out changes; these can also include the use of PDSA approaches, which have been a key feature of the collaborative methodology (Newton et al., 2006).

Referring to the work of Ovretveit et al. (2002), the reasons for the success of QICs can be grouped into four general categories: topics chosen for improvement, participant and team characteristics, skills of facilitator and expert advisers, and ensuring ways to maximize spread of ideas. Greenhalgh et al. explain that these success factors result from:

1. Clearly focused important topics that address clear gaps between current and best practice.

2. Highly motivated participants who clearly understand individual and corporate goals in a supportive organizational culture.

3. Effective teams and team leadership whose goals are in alignment with those of the organization.

4. Facilitation by credible experts, who provide adequate support outside as well as through the learning events.

5. Maximizing the spread of ideas through networking between teams and other mechanisms. (2005, p. 167)

Based on their systematic review of the literature, these authors conclude that QICs have been demonstrated to be successful and popular ways of implementing improvements in health service delivery; however, they also point out that two major criticisms are that they are expensive and that gains from them have been difficult to measure.

CONCLUSIONS

The examples of how CQI has evolved in an exponential manner, especially since the advent of the new millennium, are many and varied. Whether this trend is due to greater customer awareness and demands, technology improvements, greater competition, or a combination of these factors, what is clear is that the trend is continuing on a global scale. While some traditional industries that had incorporated CQI are now "making only incremental progress" (Leonhardt, 2009) and some sectors of industry that were once leaders, such as the automotive industry in Japan, have experienced back stepping (Crawley, 2010), CQI in health care is leaping forward, using examples and lessons from outside as well as inside health care. National developments (e.g., health care reform in the United States) and international developments (e.g., applications of CQI in resource-poor nations) have been both the result of and the source of global learning. This cycle of learning has led to innovations and paradigm shifts, such as mass personalization, that will ensure further evolution in the future.

The examples in this text of how CQI has spread and evolved are by no means exhaustive; improvements will continue to evolve at a pace that is difficult to capture in any snapshot in time. But the patterns of change that are described in the chapters of this text provide a strong basis for future models of health care and the challenges that come with these future models, as they address the questions of quality and cost and the issues of "value-added" care, leading to further learning and innovation to meet customer needs, improved health care, and outcomes on a global basis.

Cross-References to the Companion Casebook*

(McLaughlin, C. P., Johnson, J. K., and Sollecito, W. A. [Eds.]. 2012. *Implementing Continuous Quality Improvement in Health Care: A Global Casebook*. Sudbury, MA: Jones & Bartlett Learning.)

Case Study Number	Case Study Title	Case Study Authors
1	West Florida Regional Medical Center	*Curtis P. McLaughlin*
5	The Intermountain Way to Positively Impact Costs and Quality	*Lucy A. Savitz*
9	Forthright Medical Center: Social Marketing and the Surgical Checklist	*Carol E. Breland*
14	Continuing Improvement for the National Health Service Quality and Outcomes Framework	*Curtis P. McLaughlin*
17	Elk Hills Community Medical Center: Revisiting the Baldrige Award	*Curtis P. McLaughlin*

*Although there are other case studies that apply to this overview chapter, these are the cases with the most direct relevance to concepts presented in Chapter 1.

REFERENCES

AmStat News. 1993. *W. Edwards Deming to address members in San Francisco* (pp. 1–3). Washington, DC: American Statistical Association.

Baker, G. R., Norton P. G., Flintoft, V., et al. 2004. The Canadian adverse events study: The incidence of adverse events among hospital patients in Canada. *CMAJ*, 170: 1678–1686.

Barratt, A. 2008. Evidence-based medicine and shared decision making: The challenge of getting both the evidence and preferences into health care. *Patient Educ Counsel*, 73: 407–412.

Batalden, P., and Stoltz, P. 1993. Performance improvement in health care organizations. A framework for the continual improvement of health care: Building and applying professional and improvement knowledge to test changes in daily work. *Jt Comm J Qual Improvement*, 19: 424–452.

Berwick, D. M. 1996. A primer on leading the improvement of systems. *BMJ* 312: 619–622.

Berwick, D. M. 2009. What "patient-centered" should mean: Confessions of an extremist. *Health Aff*, 28(4): w555–w565.

Berwick, D. M., Nolan, T. W., and Whittington, J. 2008. The triple aim: Care, health, and cost. *Health Affairs*, 27(3): 759–769.

Bosk, C. L., Dixon-Woods, M., Goeschel, C. A., et al. 2009. The art of medicine: Reality check for checklists. *Lancet*, 374: 444–445.

Boynton, A. C., Victor, B., and Pine, B. J. 1993. New competitive strategies: Challenges to organizations and information technology. *IBM Systems J*, 32(1): 40–64.

Brennan, T. A., Leape, L. L., Laird, N. M., et al. 2004. Incidence of adverse events and negligence in hospitalized patients: Results of the Harvard medical practice study I. *Qual Safety Health Care*, 13(2): 145–151.

Brook, R. H. 2010. The end of the quality improvement movement: Long live improving value. *JAMA*, 304(16): 1831–1832.

Brown, M. 1999. *Strategic thinking*. Presentation at UNC School of Public Health.

Cohen, I. B. 1984. Florence Nightingale. *Sci Am*, 250: 128–137.

Crawley, J. 2010. Toyota's top U.S. exec warned about quality in 2006. Washington, DC: Reuters (March 2). Retrieved February 19, 2011, from http://www.reuters.com/article/idUSTRE6210JB20100302

Crosby, P. B. 1979. *Quality Is Free: The Art of Making Quality Certain*. New York: Mentor.

Davis, P., Lay-Yee, R., Briant, R., et al. 2002. Adverse events in New Zealand public hospitals I: Occurrence and impact. *New Zealand J Med*, 115(1167): U268.

Day, L., and Smith, E. 2007. Integrating quality and safety content into clinical teaching in the acute care setting. *Nurs Outlook*, 55: 138–143.

Deming, W. E. 1986. *Out of the Crisis*. Cambridge: Massachusetts Institute of Technology Center for Advanced Engineering Study.

Deming, W. E. 1993. *The New Economics for Industry, Government, Education.* Cambridge: Massachusetts Institute of Technology Center for Advanced Engineering Study.

de Vries, E. N., Prins, H. A., Crolla, R. M., et al. 2010. Effect of a comprehensive surgical safety system on patient outcomes. *N Engl J Med,* 363: 1928–1937.

Donabedian, A. 1993. *Models of quality assurance.* Leonard S. Rosenfeld Memorial Lecture, School of Public Health, University of North Carolina at Chapel Hill, February 26.

Gawande, A. 2009. *The Checklist Manifesto.* New York: Metropolitan Books.

Greenhalgh, T. Robert, G., Macfarlane, F., et al. 2005. *Diffusion of Innovations in Health Service Organizations.* Oxford, UK: Blackwell Publishing Inc.

Hamburg, M. A., and Collins, F. S. 2010. The path to personalized medicine. *N Eng J Med,* 363: 301–304.

Hart, C. 1993. Handout, Northern Telecom—University Quality Forum, Research Triangle Park, NC, June.

Haynes, A. B., Weiser, T. G., Berry, W. R., et al. 2009. A surgical safety checklist to reduce morbidity and mortality in a global population. *N Eng J Med,* 360: 491–499.

Hertz, H. S., Reimann, C. W., Bostwick, M. C. 1994. The Malcolm Baldrige National Quality Award concept: Could it help stimulate or accelerate health care quality improvement? *Quality Manage Health Care,* 2(4): 63–72.

Imai, M. 1986. Kaizen: *The Key to Japan's Competitive Success.* New York: Random House.

Institute of Medicine, National Academy of Sciences. 2000. *To Err Is Human: Building a Safer Health System.* Washington, DC: National Academies Press.

Kable, A. K., Gibbard, R., and Spigelman, A. 2002. Adverse events in surgical patients in Australia. *Int J Qual Health Care,* 14: 269–276.

Kongstvedt, P. R. 1997. *Essentials of Managed Health Care* (2nd ed.). Gaithersburg, MD: Aspen Publishers.

Kumar, A. 2007. From mass customization to mass personalization. *Int J Flexible Manufact Syst,* 19: 533–547.

Landrigan, C. P., Parry, G. J., Bones, C. B., et al. 2010. Temporal trends in rates of patient harm resulting from medical care. *N Engl J Med,* 363(22): 2124–2134.

Langley, G. L., Nolan, K. M., Nolan, T. W., et al. 2009. *The Improvement Guide: A Practical Approach to Enhancing Organizational Performance* (2nd ed.). San Francisco: Jossey-Bass Publishers.

Leonhardt, D. 2009. Making health care better. *New York Times,* November 8, 2009. Retrieved February 19, 2011, from http://www.nytimes.com/2009/11/08/magazine/08Healthcare-t.html

Linder, J. 1991. Outcomes measurement: Compliance tool or strategic initiative. *Health Care Manage Rev,* 16(4): 21–33.

McLaughlin, C. P. 1996. Why variation reduction is not everything: A new paradigm for service operations. *Int J Ser Ind Manage*, 7(3): 17–30.

McLaughlin, C. P., Johnson, J. K., and Sollecito, W. A. (Eds.). 2012. *Implementing Continuous Quality Improvement in Health Care: A Global Casebook*. Sudbury, MA: Jones & Bartlett Learning.

McLaughlin, C. P. and A. D. Kaluzny. 2002. Missing the middleman: Disintermediation challenges to the doctor-patient relationship, MGMA Connexion 2 (4):48–52.

McLaughlin, C. P., and Kaluzny, A. D. (Eds.). 2006. *Continuous Quality Improvement in Health Care* (3rd ed.). Sudbury, MA: Jones and Bartlett Publishers.

Michaels, R. K., Makary, M. A., Dahab, Y., et al. 2007. Achieving the National Quality Forum's "never events": Prevention of wrong site, wrong procedure, and wrong patient operations. *Ann Surg*, 245: 526–532.

Millenson, M. L. 2003. The silence on clinical quality failure. *Health Affairs*, 22(2): 103–112.

Newton, P. J., Davidson, P. M., Halcomb, E. J., et al. 2006. An introduction to the collaborative methodology and its potential use for the management of heart failure. *J Cardiovasc Nurs*, 21(3): 161–168.

Ovretveit, J., Bate, P., Cleary, P., et al. 2002. Quality collaboratives: Lessons from research. *Qual Saf Health Care*, 11: 345–351.

Pfaff, H., Driller, E., Ernstmann, U., et al. 2010. Standardization and individualization in care for the elderly: Proactive behavior through individualized standardization.*Open Longevity Sci*, 4: 51–57.

Pronovost, P. J., Needham, D., Berenholtz, S., et al. 2006. An intervention to reduce catheter-related bloodstream infections in the ICU. *N Engl J Med*, 355: 2725–2732.

Rastegar, D. A. 2004. Health care becomes an industry. *Ann Family Med*, 22: 79–83.

Robinson, J. H., Callister, L. C., Berry, J. A., et al. 2008. Patient-centered care and adherence: Definitions and applications to improve outcomes. *J Am Acad Nurse Pract*, 20: 600–607.

Sackett, D. 1996. Evidence-based medicine: What it is and what it isn't. *Br Med J*, 312: 71–72.

Schlesinger, M. 2002. A loss of faith: The source of reduced political legitimacy for the American medical profession. *Milbank Q*, 80(2): 185–235.

Schouten, L., Hulscher, M., Everdingen, J., et al. 2008. Evidence for the impact of quality improvement collaborative: systematic review. *Br Med J*, 336: 1491–1494.

Seidman, J., and Wallace, P. 2004. Improving population care and disease management using Ix principles. Retrieved March 19, 2011, from *http://www.ehealthinitiative.org/sites/default/files/file/IxPopulationCare.pdf*

Shewhart, W. A. 1931. *Economic Control of Quality of Manufactured Product*. Princeton, NJ: Van Nostrand Reinhold.

Spector, N., and Blackwell, K. 2009. Understanding the mechanisms behind trastuzumab therapy for human epidermal growth factor receptor 2–positive breast cancer. *J Clin Oncol,* 27(34): 5838–5847.

Starr, P. 1982. *The Social Transformation of American Medicine.* New York: Basic Books.

Tseng, M. T., and Piller, F. T. (Eds.). 2003. *The Customer Centric Enterprise: Advances in Mass Customization and Personalization.* Berlin: Springer-Verlag.

Victor, B., and Boynton, A. C. 1998. *Invented Here: Maximizing Your Organization's Internal Growth and Profitability.* Boston: Harvard Business School Press.

Wagner, E. 1996. Improving outcomes in chronic illness. *Managed Care Q,* 4(2): 12–25.

Factors Influencing the Application and Diffusion of CQI in Health Care

William A. Sollecito and Julie K. Johnson

"Change is the only constant."

—Heraclitus (Greek philosopher)

INTRODUCTION

Continuous quality improvement (CQI) has gained acceptance within all sectors of health care and across geographic and economic boundaries. It has evolved as a global strategy for improving health care in a variety of settings, spanning a broad number of issues and improving services to a variety of customers ranging from individual patients to communities. The range of applications covers not only direct patient care in primary care or hospital settings, but also disease prevention and population initiatives—such as HIV, childhood obesity, and influenza vaccination programs—under the domain of public health agencies at the local, national, and international levels. As described in Chapter 1, these applications are characterized by continuous, ongoing learning and sharing among disciplines about ways to use CQI philosophies, processes, and tools in a variety of settings. New applications continue to emerge, but at the same time, there are new challenges to the broad application of CQI. In this chapter, we examine the factors and processes that facilitate or impede the implementation of CQI as a dynamic programmatic innovation within a health care setting.

The Dynamic Character of CQI: The Case of the Safe Surgery Checklist

As a natural consequence of the scientific method, CQI methodology and applications continue to evolve and also continue to be challenged and debated before they are fully accepted as evidence-based practice. A recent example is a reemphasis on the use of a simple tool—the checklist—to improve patient safety. Checklists are a good example of the use of CQI philosophies and processes. They demonstrate leadership and interdisciplinary teamwork, using a form of the Plan, Do, Study, Act (PDSA) improvement cycle to test, learn, and improve by enlisting a broad range of expertise to improve safety on a global scale. The World Health Organization (WHO) initiative to promote use of the Surgical Safety Checklist is an excellent example of both the evolutionary process of spreading CQI in health care and, at the same time, the challenges to full diffusion and institutionalization of CQI (Gawande, 2009). This idea follows the same cross-disciplinary evolutionary path that has spurred so many recent CQI applications and has been well documented by Gawande.

The process for developing and proving the value of the surgical checklist was long and arduous. Checklists first contributed to improvements in safety and quality in other fields, most notably aviation, where they have made a dramatic impact on the testing and development of new aircraft as well as the safety of the thousands of people who travel by air on a daily basis (Gawande, 2009). The successful use of checklists in the aviation industry led to the initial efforts by Pronovost et al. (2006) to test the use of checklists to reduce central line infections and other adverse events in intensive care units (ICUs). This effort, which started in 2001, was successful and led to experimentation within medical care to extend the use of checklists to attack other inpatient medical safety issues, again following the same evolutionary model that has led to the expansion of CQI in other health care areas.

Following on the successful applications of Pronovost et al. to reduce central line infections, a global initiative was launched under the auspices of the WHO to develop and apply checklists to improve surgical safety. Enlisting safety and surgery experts from multiple countries and applying techniques learned from various medical applications, a quasi-experimental study was undertaken that encompassed a large number of medical facilities practicing surgery under a wide range of conditions. As a result, Haynes et al. (2009) demonstrated a statistically significant ($p < .001$) overall reduction in complication rates from 11.0% at baseline to 7.0% and a statistically significant ($p = .003$) reduction in death rates from 1.5% to 0.8% with the introduction of the surgical safety checklist in eight hospitals in eight cities, worldwide.

Similar results were demonstrated in a study in six hospitals in the Netherlands (the SURPASS collaborative group) including almost 4,000 surgical patients observed before and after implementation of a surgical checklist, extending the checklist process to activities both within and outside the operating room. Findings included a statistically significant ($p < .001$) decrease in the proportion of patients with one or more complications, from 15.4% to 10.6% (de Vries et al., 2010). The findings from both of these studies replicate earlier findings demonstrating reduction in catheter-related bloodstream infections associated with the use of checklists in ICUs (Pronovost et al., 2006).

Despite the successful adaptation of checklists from industry to health care, significant questions about the application of checklists and the adaptation and diffusion of quality improvement methods remain:

- Why aren't more health care providers using CQI tools and processes?
- Why is the gap between knowledge and practice so large?
- Why don't clinical systems incorporate the findings of clinical science or copy the "best known" practices reliably, quickly, and even gratefully into their daily work simply as a matter of course?

The answers to these questions, which have been raised by CQI leaders such as Dr. Brent James (Leonhardt, 2009) and Dr. Donald Berwick (2003), are multifaceted. For example, critics of checklists assert that the overemphasis on simple tools like the checklist is not without risks and instead advocate pursuing more complex system solutions for ensuring patient safety and the highest quality of care (Bosk et al., 2009).

The checklist example is only one very limited application but a good current illustration of some of the key issues surrounding the diffusion of CQI in health care. It is the tip of the iceberg for a set of much broader issues. These broader issues include, but are not limited to, process vs.

outcome, and cost vs. benefit vs. value. Also important in this debate are scientific issues regarding the minimum standards to define evidence for change, such as the use of double-blind randomized trials vs. quasi-experimentation. These issues are the direct result of the traditions of the scientific process guiding all we do in health care; this rich tradition requires rigor but also imposes buffers to quick decisions, including complex assumptions, different interpretations of causality, and, more simply, differences of opinion about findings. Also related is the question of how to influence practitioners to adopt new ideas and the broader topic of diffusion of innovation in health care.

The remainder of this chapter will address several questions:

- What is the current state of quality in health care, and what are the problems regarding implementation of CQI in health care?
- Given the widespread application of CQI in recent years, what are the factors that contribute to the implementation of CQI across industries and settings?
- Specifically for our application in health care, what are the factors that have influenced the rate of diffusion and spread of CQI in health care?

To answer these questions, we will consider the current state of health care, and we will consider the parallels between CQI and more general factors associated with the diffusion of innovation in health care, including factors associated with the business case for the use of CQI in health care.

THE CURRENT STATE OF CQI IN HEALTH CARE

Despite progress since the publication of the Institute of Medicine's landmark reports *To Err Is Human* (2000) and *Crossing the Quality Chasm* (2001), and the interprofessional as well as global dispersion of CQI techniques in various segments of health care, major gaps still exist in the quality of care and the functioning of the health care system. For example, qualitative assessments have characterized, or "graded," the progress of the patient safety movement to close the gap as a B– in 2009, compared to the C+ awarded 5 years earlier (Wachter, 2010). This qualitative assessment has been supported by numerous studies that present quantitative data confirming this lack of progress. For example, a 2010 study documented that little change occurred in "patient harms" during a 6-year review (from 2002 to 2007) of more than 2,300 admissions in 10 hospitals in North Carolina, a state chosen for study because it had shown a high level of engagement in patient safety efforts (Landrigan et al., 2010).

Although there is evidence that these are global trends, a group of learned and experienced experts assess the situation in the United States as follows:

> U.S. health care is broken. Although other industries have transformed themselves using tools such as standardization of value-generating processes, performance measurement, and transparent reporting of quality, the application of these tools to health care is controversial, evoking fears of "cookbook medicine," loss of professional autonomy, a misinformed focus on the wrong care, or a loss of individual attention and the personal touch in care delivery. . . . Our current health care system is essentially a cottage industry of nonintegrated, dedicated artisans who eschew standardization. . . . Growing evidence highlights the dangers of continuing to operate in a cottage-industry mode. Fragmentation of care has led to suboptimal performance. (Swensen et al., 2010, p. e12(1))

These statements were made at a time when the United States was launching the most major health reform in its history, amid great opposition. The challenge of the coming years is how to fix this broken system.

Rather than assume that we have any easy answers—which we do not—some time will be devoted in this chapter to further describe the scope of the problem, with a particular focus on CQI philosophies and processes and why they have not been more widely adopted. Hopefully this will give us some direction toward a set of ideas to expand the implementation of CQI across a broader range of providers.

Dr. Brent James is Executive Director of the Institute for Health Care Delivery Research and Vice President of Medical Research and Continuing Medical Education at Intermountain Health Care. He has demonstrated leadership in improving health care in many ways, not the least of which is his leadership by example at Intermountain Health Care (see Case 5 of the companion casebook [McLaughlin et al., 2012]). In an interview with the *New York Times*, Dr. James gives several examples of how Intermountain Health Care has led the way to value-based care through the use of CQI processes. He identifies the lack of widespread change as being directly related to the complexity of the health care system; a clear symptom of the depth of problems that persist is that the American health care system is vastly more expensive but not vastly better than the health systems of other countries (Leonhardt, 2009). Dr. Donald Berwick founded the Institute for Healthcare Improvement (IHI) more than 20 years ago and in 2010 was appointed by President Obama as Administrator of the Centers for Medicare and Medicaid Services (CMS). In 2003, he noted that "Americans spend almost 40% more per capita for health care than any other country, yet rank 27th in infant mortality, 27th in life expectancy, and are less satisfied with their care than the English, Canadians, or Germans" (Berwick, 2003, p. 1969). He is one of many to point out the gravity of this situation due to the fact that little change has occurred between 2003 and 2010. Two of the important issues at the heart of this problem, complexity and cost, were also key factors in the debate about health reform in the United States in 2009; as will be shown later in this chapter, they are also contributors to the explanation of why CQI has not been more widely adopted.

The complexity of the health care system is both a challenge and a source of ideas for how to make improvements (Plsek and Greenhalgh, 2001). Health care can be described as a complex adaptive system, a concept that has implications for how to improve the system. For example, the importance of leadership is critical, as are incentives for improvement. As a complex adaptive system, health care can only be designed to a certain extent and cannot be designed around minimizing costs; rather, the focus must be on maximizing value (Rouse, 2008). (See Chapter 20 for further discussion of the value proposition.)

CQI AND THE SCIENCE OF INNOVATION

While health care is unique in many ways, one commonality that it has with other complex endeavors is the difficulty surrounding diffusion of innovation, starting with simple resistance to change but including many other complex factors. Understanding these issues helps to provide pathways toward greater diffusion of CQI in health care.

The research and principles that are specific to diffusion of innovation of health services are summarized in a systematic review of the literature presented by Greenhalgh et al. (2005). From this review, it is noted that there is a wide range of literature using a variety of concepts and approaches that describe how to move along the spectrum from the initiation of a concept for change to the spread, diffusion, and institutionalization of innovation.

Diffusion theory is useful in understanding the factors that thwart or support the adoption of CQI in health care. Because of the complexity of health care and the added complexity of CQI, as alluded to earlier in this chapter, there are no simple answers about how to move CQI innovations into the mainstream of health care more quickly and efficiently. Complexity must be considered in understanding innovation. Although there are competing theories about how and why, innovation clearly does happen in "complex zones." There is some evidence that while innovation may not be susceptible to being managed, it is possible to design and control organizational conditions that "enhance the possibility of innovation occurring and spreading" (Greenhalgh et al., 2005, p. 80). Addressing this complexity requires, first and foremost, leadership, but also the creation of a receptive and even enthusiastic culture; one excellent example of how this has been accomplished in CQI in health care is the formation of quality improvement collaboratives, such as the SURPASS collaborative group, mentioned earlier in regard to the successful application of surgical checklists to improve patient safety (de Vries et al., 2010). These ideas and examples will be discussed further in this context later in this section.

The speed and overall adoption of any change, including CQI, can be influenced by the characteristics of the change and how it is perceived by those responsible for implementation. These characteristics include relative advantage, compatibility, simplicity, trialability, and observability (Rogers, 1995). All of these characteristics relate to changes and improvements in health care, and two, in particular, are directly relevant to the checklist example: compatibility, which relates to how closely the change ideas align with the existing culture and environment, and trialability, which addresses how the changes can be adapted and tested in the new environments in which they are being spread.

A further extension of these change concepts yields the following seven rules for dissemination of innovation in health care (Berwick, 2003):

1. Find sound innovations.

2. Find and support innovators.

3. Invest in early adopters.

4. Make early adopter activity observable.

5. Trust and enable reinvention.

6. Create slack for change.

7. Lead by example.

All of these rules are applicable to innovations around CQI; leadership, trust, and reinvention are fundamental. Reinvention has to do with the cross-disciplinary learning concept that has permeated CQI and, as described in Chapter 1, is responsible for its evolution across industries and across the globe. CQI cannot be a top-down mandate. It must be part of the vision of an organization and accepted by all who must implement CQI, thus requiring trust at all levels, which comes from leadership, teamwork, and Deming's concept of "constancy of purpose." Top leadership must be involved, supporting and communicating the vision for innovation and change; however, participation, buy-in, and support from opinion leaders at all levels within an organization are critical for successful implementation and the process to reinvention.

One size will not fit all. As described by Berwick, "To work, changes must be not only adopted locally, but also locally adapted" (2003, p. 1974). Berwick asserts that for this to happen, there must be reinvention. In his words, "Reinvention is a form of learning, and, in its own way, it is an act of both creativity and courage. Leaders who want to foster innovation . . . should showcase and celebrate individuals who take ideas from elsewhere and adapt them to make them their own" (Berwick, 2003, p. 1974).

Once again, the checklist example cited at the beginning of this chapter is a clear illustration of this process of reinvention and leadership. It was adapted from the airline and other industries, first to intensive care and later to surgery, with trusted leaders in their fields using scientific media and disseminating their ideas and successes. The fact that these evidence-based tools are not fully accepted and used returns us to the point that health care is complex and requires diligence to spread the improvement process. The systematic review of diffusion of innovation in health services identifies complexity as one of the key elements that is inversely associated with successful diffusion. Quite often, due to the complex nature of health care systems, equally complex quality improvement strategies are required, thus lessening their quick and easy adoption.

This helps to explain why simpler quality improvement processes, such as the use of PDSA cycles, have enjoyed broad success. However, resistance to the use of simple checklists defies this explanation.

A prospective study of the attributes of 42 clinical practice recommendations in gynecology (Foy et al., 2002) may help to explain this resistance to some degree. After review of almost 5,000 patient records, findings indicate two outcomes of relevance to the checklist example. First, recommendations that were compatible with clinician values and did not require changes to fixed routines (to some, the surgical checklist may be contrary to both of these notions) were associated with greater compliance. Second, initial noncompliance could be reversed after audit and feedback stages were carried out (indicating that perhaps more time will yield greater compliance). Although these findings may bode well for the long-term acceptance of the surgical checklist and the ICU checklist developed in 2006 by Pronovost et al., there is insufficient evidence at the time of this writing to make firm conclusions.

The techniques and philosophies described throughout this book provide some other examples of progress that has been made in specific segments of health care and also describe models that can be considered to increase diffusion of CQI ideas. For example, social marketing has been documented as being an effective tool for understanding ways to improve the impact of innovations in health care in general (Greenhalgh et al., 2005). In Chapter 8 of this text and in Case 9 of the companion casebook (McLaughlin et al., 2012), a novel social marketing approach is proposed as a technique for increasing compliance with checklists and other CQI innovations.

THE BUSINESS CASE FOR CQI

Health care delivery systems are large, decentralized, and complex, yet at their core they involve a fundamental personal relationship between providers and patients. Moreover, if this were not a sufficient challenge, rapid and uncertain changes in the structure and processes of providing and paying for care make measuring the effect of any single management intervention over time very difficult, if not impossible. Although evidence has been accumulated from both controlled trials (Goldberg et al., 1998; Mehta et al., 2000; Solberg, 1993) and survey data (Shortell et al., 1998) on the implementation process and perceived impact, much of the evidence remains anecdotal (Arndt and Bigelow, 1995; Bigelow and Arndt, 1995). Leatherman et al. (2003), for example, argue that the "business case" for quality improvement is yet to be proven, even while evidence mounts for the overall societal and economic benefits:

> A *business case* for a health care improvement intervention exists if the entity that invests in the intervention realizes a financial return on its investment in a reasonable time frame, using a reasonable rate of discounting. This may be realized as "bankable dollars" (profit), a reduction in losses for a given program or population, or avoided costs. In addition, a *business case* may exist if the investing entity believes that a positive indirect impact on organization function and sustainability will accrue within a reasonable time frame. (p. 18)

These arguments continue; the economic case includes the returns to all the actors, not just the individual investing business unit. The social case, as they define it, is one of measuring benefits, but not requiring positive returns on the investment. That has been overriding the consideration in the battle to control medical variation and medical errors (McGlynn et al., 2003). The business case for quality improvement suffers from the same negative factors as the business case for other preventive health care measures—namely, all or part of the benefits accruing to other business units or patients, and delayed impacts that get discounted heavily in the reckoning (Leatherman et al., 2003). The regulatory arguments for quality improvement efforts have generally been justified on the basis of social and economic benefits such as lives saved and overall cost reductions, but these arguments are not necessarily profitable to the investor. These authors also present a whole array of public policy measures that would overcome the barriers to a positive business case and encourage wider and more assertive implementation of quality improvement methods. Clearly economics alone does not provide an argument strongly for or against the use of CQI, but it does add to the complexity that pervades the wider and more rapid implementation of CQI in health care.

In summary, this brief overview indicates that a strong business case for CQI in health care cannot be made. Looking back over the past 40 years, Robert Brook, UCLA Professor of Medicine and Health Services and Director of the Health Sciences Program for the RAND Corporation, observes, "Although there are some examples in the literature to support the concept that better quality of care is less expensive, few studies have produced information that could be generalized across time and institutional settings" (2010, p. 1831). Building on the traditional business concepts that have been discussed and in consideration of the limited evidence to support the business case for CQI, a transformation that may support greater diffusion of CQI and the continuing need to bridge the quality chasm is to consider a more value-based approach to CQI in health care. This approach argues for simultaneous goals of higher quality and lower cost, which will only be achieved when there is a reorientation among CQI proponents that includes a thorough understanding of how to achieve a positive return on investment (Brook, 2010). This view will be discussed in greater detail in the final chapter of this text (Chapter 20), which will focus on future quality trends in health care.

FACTORS ASSOCIATED WITH SUCCESSFUL CQI APPLICATIONS

Despite the need for greater diffusion of CQI in health care, much progress has been made, suggesting a broad array of factors that can be associated with successful CQI implementation. The key to greater diffusion is understanding and emphasizing those factors that do work while exploring new concepts, such as the value focus described previously. This analysis starts with motivational factors but also includes regulatory (e.g., accreditation) factors and finally organizational factors such as leadership, organizational culture, and teamwork.

Motivational Factors

A number of motivational factors contribute to the sustained interest and enthusiasm for CQI for health care. These factors have an impact on the motivation of the management of the organization and its employees. The first argument for CQI is its direct impact on quality, usually a net gain to the customer and to the employees of the organization, the external and internal customers. The second argument relates to the set of benefits associated with a plan that empowers employees in health care through participation in decision making. These factors represent benefits for employees and management that can be classified as follows.

Intrinsic Motivation

The vast majority of health care workers support the concept of quality care and would like to see improvements and participate in a meaningful quality improvement process. Allowing personnel to work on their own processes, permitting them to "do the right thing," and then rewarding them for that behavior is almost sure to increase intrinsic motivation in employees, if done properly. It is a classic case of job enrichment for health care workers.

Capturing the Intellectual Capital of the Workforce

Industrial managers are increasingly recognizing that frontline workers know their work processes better than the management does. Therefore, management encourages workers to apply that knowledge and insight to the firm's processes. This is especially true in health care, where the professionals employed by or practicing in the institution control the technological core of the organization. Management that does not capitalize on this available pool of professional and specialized knowledge within the organization is naive at best.

Reducing Managerial Overhead

Some companies have been able to remove layers of management as work groups have taken responsibility for their own processes. Health care organizations are actually already limited in the number of staff positions, mostly because the professionals rather than the corporate staff have clinical process knowledge. Indeed, one might view the new investments in CQI as a catching-up process for the lack of process-oriented staff that are involved in process enhancement in most other industries. This is but another example of how the incentives in health care are misaligned. Since physicians are not employees in most community hospitals, they are not at risk when processes are suboptimal, unless the situation is so bad that it prompts a lawsuit.

Lateral Linkages

Health care organizations are characterized by their many medical specialties, each organized into its own professional fiefdom. Specialization is just one response to an information overload in the organization (Galbraith, 1973). By specializing, each unit tends to learn more and more about less and less. One way to offset the effects of this specialization is to provide lateral linkages—coordinators, integrating mechanisms—to get the information moving across the organization as well as up and down the chain of command (Galbraith, 1973; Lawrence and Lorsch, 1967). So far, that has proved very difficult in health care institutions. CQI, however, through its use of interdisciplinary teams and its focus on a broader definition of process and system as it affects customers rather than professional groups, presents one way to establish linkages. The technology of CQI focuses as much on coordination of the change process as on its motivation. In modern medicine, as practiced in the 21st century, this coordination and motivation of CQI is bolstered by the need for greater coordination in medical care in general and is therefore quite natural. There is a greater emphasis on interdisciplinary care, which leads to fostering interdependence and, in turn, better teamwork, including greater employee engagement and improvements in the patient experience and the financial performance of practices (Swensen et al., 2010).

Regulatory Agencies and Accreditation

Regulatory mechanisms such as accreditation are key factors that have led to greater diffusion of CQI and will continue to do so in the future as a direct result of mandated measurement and improvement of the quality of care. Chapter 18 will provide a broad overview of accreditation and its impact across the globe, but for the purposes of this discussion, a focus on the United States is illustrative.

In the United States, the efforts of The Joint Commission (TJC) and CMS have led to the implementation of a series of initiatives that require hospitals to report on quality measures; after a period of strong resistance, routine reporting of key metrics is now commonplace and required for accreditation by TJC. Likewise, CMS generates extensive CQI activities and associated reporting of findings via the efforts of Quality Improvement Organizations (QIOs). As described in Chapter 15 of this text and in Case 3 of the companion casebook (McLaughlin et al., 2012), QIOs represent a clear example of diffusion of CQI in health care and continue to play an important role in ensuring the highest quality of care to the 46 million beneficiaries covered by Medicare in the United States. QIOs are a clear example of diffusion, as they grew from what were in 1972 termed Professional Standards Review Organizations (PSROs).

In fact, QIOs may also provide a good model for how to ensure quality in a national health plan such as that which is being initiated in the United States. Also, as described in Chapter 16 of this text and in Case 15 of the companion casebook (McLaughlin et al., 2012), accreditation initiatives at the national and state levels have served as an impetus for CQI in public health agencies in the United States.

The processes for each of these regulatory mechanisms provide evidence for factors to be considered, as well as lessons learned, in regard to further diffusion of CQI in health care. For example, the impact of the measurement requirements has been notable. In a review published by members of TJC, this impact was described as being due to the use of robust, evidence-based measures, which link process performance and patient outcomes (Chassin et al., 2010). Despite extensive documentation of successes in the article, these authors also note the need and define a direction for further improvement, centered around process measurement. They point out that the focus of this measurement process is entirely on hospital care, leaving much to be done in regard to ambulatory care. They also note that the measures in place are process measures, not outcome measures. In the spirit of continuous improvement, they offer guidance in improving the measures that are currently in place.

Once again, this program, while not without problems, is a good model for further diffusion of CQI; early resistance to measurement no longer exists, and now the issue is more about finding the most effective measures, with little resistance from hospitals and physicians expected. In the language of diffusion of innovation, TJC has passed the early adoption stage and is now well into the instiutionalization stage, at least in the hospital sector, and relative to a subset of process measures. However, despite their optimism about the progress that has been made and the value of their proposed measurement framework, Chassin et al. close their discussion of these new accountability measures by realistically pointing out that perpetual vigilance is required to review and improve the measurement process via feedback from internal and external customers. So a partial answer to our question of how to "fix the broken system" is provided by accreditation, and much has been accomplished, with some guidance from TJC on what to do next.

However, these comments are specific to measurement of processes in hospitals, and a more general answer is still needed to truly address the broader health care system and its subcomponents.

Transformational Leadership, Teamwork, and a Culture of Excellence

Throughout the history of the application of CQI, one of the most important factors associated with successful applications of CQI has been the interaction of leadership, organizational culture, and teamwork. Transformational leadership, distinguished by its reliance on vision, is a starting point and a consistent factor in motivating change and improvement. To ensure CQI, the most important role of a leader is transformation (Deming, 1993), which starts with a motivating vision that must be developed, communicated, and embraced by all in the organization, which in turn leads to high levels of commitment to the vision of change and improvement (Melum and Sinioris, 1993; Tichy and Devanna, 1986). Leaders ensure commitment to the vision by shaping a culture that not only accepts but embraces change (Balestracci, 2009; Schein, 1991). **Figure 2–1** describes the way in which this is accomplished in an organization that is dedicated to CQI and thereby defines a set of factors that are critical to the greater diffusion of CQI in health care.

The development of a vision and the commitment to that vision lead to what Deming called constancy of purpose for all in the organization, referring to a clear sense of where the organization is going or what a system is intended to accomplish (Deming, 1986). The type of culture that is needed to succeed in an organization whose goal is to continuously improve can be called a "culture of excellence." This concept is similar to a "safety culture," defined as a culture in which "a commitment to

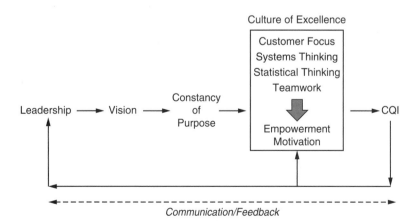

FIGURE 2–1 Factors Influencing Successful CQI Implementation

safety permeates all levels of the organization from frontline personnel to executive management" (AHRQ, 2011). Similarly, a culture of excellence is one that ensures excellence and high quality at every customer interface and in which a commitment to the highest quality—and CQI, in particular—is shared by all in the organization. Underlying the creation of a culture of excellence is a need for a systems view. A systems view of health care emphasizes the importance of adding value and the importance of leadership rather than management, influence rather than power, and the alignment of incentives focused on quality rather than quantity of services (Rouse, 2008). A culture of excellence embraces this view, is performance oriented, and at a minimum adopts a CQI philosophy (as defined in Chapter 1). It exemplifies the following elements outlined in Figure 2–1:

- *Customer focus*: Emphasizing the importance of both internal and external customers (see Chapter 1)
- *Systems thinking*: Maintaining a goal of optimizing the system as a whole and thereby creating synergy (Deming, 1986; Kelly, 2007)
- *Statistical thinking*: Understanding causes of variation and the importance of learning from measurement; having the ability to use data to make decisions (see Chapter 3 and Balestracci, 2009)
- *Teamwork*: Teams of peers working together to ensure empowerment, thereby creating the highest levels of motivation to ensure alignment of the organization, the team, and the individual around the CQI vision (see Chapter 4 and Grove, 1995)
- *Communication and feedback*: Maintaining open channels of communication and feedback to make adjustments as needed, including modifying the vision to achieve higher levels of quality in a manner consistent with a learning organization (see Chapters 6 and 10 and Senge, 1990), including feedback that is fact based and given with true concern for individuals' organizational success (Balestracci, 2009)

Leadership and Diffusion

In discussing factors that support the implementation of CQI, the theory of diffusion of innovation clearly supports the important role of leadership in CQI. Innovativeness, as described in the literature of organizational psychology, is seen as critically dependent on good leadership; one of the key factors to the implementation and routinization of innovation once adopted is the consultation and active involvement of leaders. Furthermore, organizational leadership is critical to the development of a culture that fosters innovation (Greenhalgh et al., 2005). CQI is a form of change and innovation that also requires cultural change driven by leadership. As Greenhalgh et al. explain, "Leaders within organizations are critical firstly in creating a cultural context that fosters innovation and secondly, establishing organizational strategy, structure, and systems that facilitate innovation" (2005, p. 69). This perspective ties directly back to Deming's point about leadership; leaders must know and understand the processes they are responsible for and lead by example, acting as part of the improvement effort and on the "corrections" required (Deming, 1986). This point was emphasized by Gawande in describing how the initial adoption of surgical checklists was accomplished:

> Using the checklist involved a major cultural change, as well—a shift in authority, responsibility, and expectations about care—and the hospitals needed to recognize that. We gambled that their staff would be far more likely to adopt the checklist if they saw their leadership accepting it from the outset. (2009, p. 146)

Leaders at All Levels

Various types of leaders can contribute to (or detract from) the innovation process. Traditional organizational and team leaders are most often associated with CQI initiatives; however, in regard to innovations, the terminology of "leader" can be expanded to include opinion leaders, champions, and boundary spanners.

Opinion leaders represent a broad range of leaders "within the ranks" as well as those at the top level. In clinical settings, opinion leaders have influence on the beliefs and actions of their colleagues, either positive or negative in regard to embracing innovation. Opinion leaders may be experts who are respected for their formal academic authority in regard to a particular innovation; their support represents a form of evidence-based knowledge. Opinion leaders may also be peers who are respected for their know-how and understanding of the realities of clinical practice (Greenhalgh et al., 2005).

Unlike opinion leaders, who may support or oppose an innovation, champions persistently support new ideas. They may come from the top management of an organization, including technical or business experts. Champions include team and project leaders and others who have perseverance to fight both resistance and/or indifference to promote the acceptance of a new idea or to achieve project goals (Greenhalgh et al., 2005).

Boundary spanners represent a combination of these various types of leaders and are distinguished by the fact that they have influence across organizational and other boundaries (Greenhalgh et al., 2005; Kaluzny et al., 1974). Boundary spanners play an important role in multi-organizational innovations and quality improvement initiatives, such as quality improvement collaboratives. Each of these types of leaders is found in the adoption of quality improvement initiatives in health care, and often these various types of leaders are found in combination.

Teamwork

CQI in health care is a team game. These teams are composed of peers who are highly trained technical experts supporting each other and empowered to take a leadership role as required to meet the needs of customers. Teamwork is one of the most important components of all successful CQI initiatives; team building centers on the ability to create teams of empowered and motivated people who are leaders themselves and who will take the lead as needed to foster change, innovation, and improvement (Byham and Cox, 1998; Grove, 1995; Kotter, 1996). The glue that holds a culture of excellence together and that ensures there will be quality at every interface is the link between leadership and teamwork—with leadership exhibited as called for at all levels within a team. As Deming states, "There is no substitute for teamwork and good leaders of teams to bring consistency of effort along with knowledge" (1986, p. 19).

Inherent in teamwork is a high level of empowerment of team members, which in turn leads to high levels of motivation. Empowerment implies that levels of authority match levels of responsibility and training. For example, suggestions and interventions can be made to allow improvements and prevent problems or errors; this initiative goes beyond simply allowing team members to speak up, but means providing comfort in speaking up when something seems wrong (Byham and Cox, 1998; Deming, 1986; Grove, 1995). This is illustrated in the surgical checklist example, which emphasizes that all members of the surgical team are responsible for the outcome, not just the surgeon, and all members have a role in preventing errors, which implies the empowerment to question traditional authority and take actions (Gawande, 2009).

Improved motivation is the direct result of empowerment, and both will interact to lead to higher quality; but to work, these elements require another aspect of cultural change and associated leadership responsibility—building a culture of trust. This is emphasized in Deming's 14 points, namely point number 8: Drive out fear. Create trust. Create a climate for innovation (see Chapter 1). Deming explains, "No one can put in his best performance unless he feels secure. . . . Secure means without fear, not afraid to express ideas, not afraid to ask questions" (1986, p. 59). This ties directly back to the surgical checklist example as well as the airline safety tradition, where use of a checklist implies responsibility to communicate and question each other as part of the checklist process, regardless of the team member's rank. A leader's goal must be to create a culture where people are empowered to do their jobs to the best of their abilities, with trust and a clear understanding of the vision that creates the constancy of purpose needed to achieve the highest quality.

Training is critical to the success of leaders and the ability to achieve constancy of purpose, not only training of employees in the skills required to do their jobs, but also training the future leaders of the organization. Training of future leaders is one of the most important responsibilities of a leader (Tichy, 1997). Several later chapters in this text discuss what is needed to train and educate health care professionals who are prepared to lead the improvement of health care. For example, in Chapter 17 the emphasis on quality improvement in the curriculum for the education of nurses is described; one critical goal described is to ensure that nurses, because of their close interaction with patients, can take a greater leadership role in ensuring the quality of care provided to patients and take more direct responsibility for identifying and leading, not merely participating in, quality improvement initiatives. Gawande (2009) addresses this issue in describing the process for testing and implementing the surgical safety checklist. Despite the obvious key role of the surgeon, it was decided that the "circulating nurse" on the surgery team would be the one to start the checklist process at the beginning of a surgery. This was done for several reasons, but one of the most important was "to spread responsibility and the power to question" (p. 137).

Examples of Leadership and Teamwork in CQI

The linkage between leadership and teamwork to ensure success in quality improvement in health care has been demonstrated in many instances, including the very successful implementation of quality improvement collaboratives (QICs), introduced in Chapter 1. QICs represent a form of virtual organizations (Byrne, 1993) whose effectiveness have been demonstrated in industry for many years. Part of the success of QICs can be tied to this effective team structure. For example, in describing the successful application of a QIC using the IHI Breakthrough series (Kilo, 1998) in 40 U.S. hospitals to reduce adverse drug events, Leape et al. (2000) identify strong leadership and teamwork among their most important success factors: "Success in making significant changes was associated with strong leadership, effective processes, and appropriate choice of intervention. Successful teams were able to define, clearly state, and relentlessly pursue their aims, and then chose practical interventions and moved early into changing a process" (Greenhalgh et al., 2005, p. 165).

In summary, leadership, effective teamwork, and the empowerment of teams have been critical factors in the evolution of CQI in health care and are directly related to the pace and broad adoption of CQI in health care in recent years. Chapter 4 provides a detailed description of how to build teams and ensure that they operate most effectively to improve quality in health care.

KOTTER'S CHANGE MODEL

A traditional model that is used to define a culture of change and in particular the role of vision and leadership is the eight-stage change model developed by John Kotter (1996), which is outlined in **Table 2–1**. The discussion of leadership, organizational culture, and teamwork presented previously described "what is" the type of culture that is needed to implement successful CQI initiatives; Kotter's model describes "how to" implement major change and also provides guidance on traditional errors to avoid. These two approaches are closely related. There is clear overlap between Kotter's model and the factors defined in Figure 2–1, which describe the culture of excellence. These common elements include empowerment, communication, feedback loops to produce more change, and, most important, the central role of vision and anchoring change in the culture.

TABLE 2-1 Kotter's Eight-Stage Process of Creating Major Change

---

1. Establishing a sense of urgency
2. Creating the guiding coalition
3. Developing a vision and strategy
4. Communicating the change vision
5. Empowering broad-based action
6. Generating short-term wins
7. Consolidating gains and producing more change
8. Anchoring new approaches in the culture

Source: Adapted from Kotter, 1996.

One key point of Kotter's model that is worthy of a bit more discussion here is his first point: "Establishing a sense of urgency." This effort relates to an earlier point about how long it takes, or should take, to implement CQI concepts. The emphasis is not that decisions should be rushed, but that complacency is to be avoided. Complacency may be due to many reasons that can be associated with the need for CQI in health care. These include, according to Kotter, "too much past success, lack of visible crises, low performance standards, [and] insufficient feedback from external constituencies. . . . Without a sense of urgency, people won't give that extra effort that is essential. They won't make needed sacrifices. Instead they cling to the status quo and resist initiatives from above" (1996, p. 5). This point directly relates to CQI in health care; the importance of ensuring safety and quality in health care requires a sense of urgency.

See Kotter's text for a comprehensive description of the elements in Table 2–1 and the broader subject of how to implement organizational change.

CONCLUSIONS

The factors that are associated with successful CQI applications have been clearly identified, from its earliest applications in industry and throughout its evolution into health care. Most notable among these factors are leadership and teamwork and their synergistic role in developing a vision that leads to a culture of excellence, embracing CQI. This has led to widespread use of CQI in health care and the emergence of a new set of leaders who lead by example, teach others, and continue to develop and expand both the philosophy and processes of CQI.

Despite the widespread use of CQI methods and a good understanding of the leadership and teamwork processes that make it work, its effectiveness and its further adoption in health care remain subjects of ongoing research and continue to meet challenges; most notably, there has been lack of documentation of substantial progress in improving quality of health care and, most importantly, reducing harm to patients (Landrigan et al., 2010; Wachter, 2010). The literature on diffusion of innovation suggests some guidelines to understand factors that influence the adoption of CQI. Most notable is the fact that complexity inhibits further adoption, just as it does for other forms of innovation. Understanding the factors that enable or influence adoption of CQI, as well as the factors that present barriers, is particularly important as more countries around the world are utilizing CQI to solve health challenges, including resource-poor countries (see Chapter 19), and as national health plans are being modified or introduced around the world, including in the United States.

While CQI implementation is slowing down in some health care sectors after the impact of early adopters may have worn off, other sectors of health care, such as public health (see Chapter 16) and nursing (see Chapter 17), are embracing and expanding CQI concepts and methods. Likewise, the increasingly successful use of CQI in QIOs (see Chapter 15) is having a significant impact on quality of care for large populations of Medicare and Medicaid patients in the United States. The impact of accreditation across multiple sectors continues to be noteworthy (see Chapter 18) as a broad global force for the greater adoption of quality improvement methods. These experiences and those that led to them provide a rich source of knowledge for how to diffuse CQI more widely in health care; the challenge is to understand how to accomplish this in the face of declining health quality in many places.

With challenges come opportunities. One example is the use of novel approaches such as social marketing to further the adoption of new CQI tools and processes. Social marketing is an example of a planned, central approach that has been shown to be effective in promoting the spread of innovations in health services and for analyzing the impact or lack of impact of innovations (Greenhalgh et al., 2005). As described in Chapter 8, it may be useful for understanding and promoting compliance with CQI initiatives, such as the surgical safety checklist. This is one of several areas of needed research to better understand how to encourage wider adoption of proven CQI ideas.

Overall, despite the need for wider diffusion of CQI in health care, current trends indicate a continuation of cross-disciplinary learning and significant interprofessional spread of CQI. So while it is important to understand the factors that inhibit the broader use of CQI and the problems affecting the improvement in health care overall, it is more important to review what works so that others may learn. These factors and approaches illustrate how the new sectors within health care that are enthusiastically adopting the CQI philosophy and processes may improve their performance within the health care system.

Cross-References to the Companion Casebook

(McLaughlin, C. P., Johnson, J. K., and Sollecito, W. A. [Eds.]. 2012. *Implementing Continuous Quality Improvement in Health Care: A Global Casebook.* Sudbury, MA: Jones & Bartlett Learning.)

Case Study Number	Case Study Title	Case Study Authors
6	Planning a Transition	*Gwenn E. McLaughlin*
8	Dr. Charles Bethe, DO, Network Medical Director	*William Q. Judge and Curtis P. McLaughlin*
9	Forthright Medical Center: Social Marketing and the Surgical Checklist	*Carol E. Breland*
20	The Houston Medical Center Bed Tower: Quality and the Built Environment	*Debajyoti Pati, Thomas E. Harvey Jr., and Paul Barach*

REFERENCES

AHRQ Patient Safety Network. 2011. Glossary: Safety culture. Retrieved January 1, 2011, from http://psnet.ahrq.gov/popup_glossary.aspx?name=safetyculture

Arndt, M., and Bigelow, B. 1995. The implementation of total quality management in hospitals. *Health Care Manage Rev*, 20: 3–14.

Balestracci, D. 2009. *Data Sanity: A Quantum Leap to Unprecedented Results.* Englewood, CO: Medical Group Management Association.

Berwick, D. M. 2003. Disseminating innovations in health care. *JAMA*, 289: 1969–1975.

Bigelow, B., and Arndt, M. 1995. Total quality management: Field of dreams? *Health Care Manage Rev*, 20: 15–25.

Bosk, C. L., Dixon-Woods, M., Goeschel, C. A., et al. 2009. The art of medicine—Reality check for checklists. *Lancet*, 374: 444–445.

Brook, R. H. 2010. The end of the quality improvement movement: Long live improving value. *JAMA*, 304(16): 1831–1832.

Byham, J. C., and Cox, J. 1998. *Zapp! The Lightning of Empowerment—How to Improve Quality, Productivity and Employee Satisfaction*. New York: Fawcett Ballantine, The Ballantine Publishing Group.

Byrne, J. 1993. The virtual corporation. *Business Week*, 3304: 98–102.

Chassin, M. R., Loeb, J. M., Schmaltz, S. P., et al. 2010. Accountability measures: Using measurement to promote quality improvement. *N Eng J Med*, 363: 683–688.

Deming, W. E. 1986. *Out of the Crisis*. Cambridge: Massachusetts Institute of Technology Center for Advanced Engineering Study.

Deming, W. E. 1993. *The New Economics for Industry, Government, Education*. Cambridge: Massachusetts Institute of Technology Center for Advanced Engineering Study.

de Vries, E. N., Prins, H. A., Crolla, R. M., et al. 2010. Effect of a comprehensive surgical safety system on patient outcomes. *N Engl J Med*, 363: 1928–1937.

Foy, R., MacLennan, G., Grimshaw, J., et al. 2002. Attributes of clinical recommendations that influence change in practice following audit and feedback. *J Clin Epidem*, 55: 717–722.

Galbraith, J. 1973. *Designing Complex Organizations*. Reading, MA: Addison-Wesley.

Gawande, A. 2009. *The Checklist Manifesto*. New York: Metropolitan Books.

Goldberg, H. I., Wagner, E. H., and Finh, S. D. 1998. A randomized controlled trial of CQI teams and academic detailing: Can they alter compliance with guidelines? *Joint Commission J Quality Improve*, 24: 130–142.

Greenhalgh, T. E., Robert, G., Macfarlane, F., et al. 2005. *Diffusion of Innovations in Health Services Organizations: A Systematic Review of the Literature*. Oxford, UK: Blackwell Publishing.

Grove, A. S. 1995. *High Output Management*. New York: Vintage Books.

Haynes, A. B., Weiser, T. G., and Berry, W. R. 2009. A surgery safety checklist to reduce morbidity and mortality in a global population. *N Eng J Med*, 360: 491–499.

Institute of Medicine. 2000. *To Err Is Human: Building a Safer Health System*. Washington, DC: National Academies Press.

Institute of Medicine. 2001. *Crossing the Quality Chasm: A New Health Paradigm for the 21st Century*. Washington, DC: National Academies Press.

Kaluzny, A., Veney, J. A., Gentry, J. T. 1974. Innovation of health services: A comparative study of hospitals and health departments. *Millbank Memorial Fund Q: Health Soc*, 52: 51–82.

Kelly, D. L. 2007. *Applying Quality Management in Healthcare: A Systems Approach* (2nd ed.). Chicago: Health Administration Press.

Kilo, C. M. 1998. A framework for collaborative improvement: Lessons from the Institute for Healthcare Improvement's Breakthrough series. *Q Manage Health Care*, 6: 1–13.

Kotter, J. P. 1996. *Leading Change*. Boston: Harvard Business School Press.

Landrigan, C. P., Parry, G. J., Bones, C. B., et al. 2010. Temporal trends in rates of patient harm resulting from medical care. *N Engl J Med*, 363(22): 2124–2134.

Lawrence, P. R., and Lorsch, J. W. 1967. *Organization and Environment*. Boston: Harvard University Press.

Leape, L. L., Kabcenell, A. I., Gandhi, T. K., et al. 2000. Reducing adverse drug events: Lessons from a breakthrough series collaborative. *Joint Commission J Quality Improve*, 26: 321–331.

Leatherman, S. *et al.* 2003. The busines case for quality: Case studies and an analysis. *Health Affairs*, 22(2): 17–30.

Leonhardt, D. 2009. Making health care better. *New York Times*, November 24, 1–14.

McGlynn, E. A., Asch, S. M., and Adams, J. 2003. The quality of health care delivered to adults in the United States. *N Engl J Med*, 348: 2635–2645.

McLaughlin, C. P., Johnson, J. K., and Sollecito, W. A. (Eds.). 2012. *Implementing Continuous Quality Improvement in Health Care: A Global Casebook*. Sudbury, MA: Jones & Bartlett Learning.

Mehta, R. H., Das, S., Tsai, T. T., et al. 2000. Quality improvement initiative and its impact on the management of patients with acute myocardial infarction. *Arch Intern Med*, 160: 3057–3062.

Melum, M. M., and Sinioris, M. K. 1993. *Total Quality Management—The Health Care Pioneers*. Chicago: American Hospital Publishing.

Plsek, P., and Greenhalgh, T. 2001. The challenge of complexity in health care. *Br Med J*, 323(7313): 625–628.

Pronovost, P., Needham, D., Berenholtz, S., et al. 2006. An intervention to reduce catheter-related bloodstream infections in the ICU. *N Engl J Med*, 355: 2725–2732.

Rogers, E. 1995. *Diffusion of Innovations*. New York: Free Press.

Rouse, W. B. 2008. Health care as a complex adaptive system. *Bridge*, 38: 17–25.

Schein, E. H. 1991. *Organizational Culture and Leadership*. San Francisco: Jossey-Bass.

Senge, P. 1990. *The Fifth Discipline: The Art and Practice of a Learning Organization*. New York: Doubleday.

Shortell, S. M., Bennett, C. L., and Byck, G. R. 1998. Assessing the impact of continuous quality improvement on clinical practice: What will it take to accelerate programs. *Millbank Q*, 76: 593–624.

Solberg, L. 1993. *Improving Disease Prevention in Primary Care.* Washington, DC: AHCPR Working Paper.

Swensen, S. J., Meyer, G. S., Nelson, E. C., et al. 2010. Cottage industry to postindustrial care: The revolution in health care delivery. *N Engl J Med,* 362: e12(1)–e12(4).

Tichy, N. M. 1997. *The Leadership Engine.* New York: Harper Business.

Tichy, N. M., and Devanna, M. A. 1986. *The Transformational Leader.* New York: John Wiley and Sons.

Wachter, R. M. 2010. Patient safety at ten: Unmistakable progress, troubling gaps. *Health Affairs,* 29: 165–173.

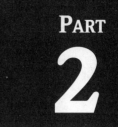

Basics of Quality and Safety

CHAPTER 3

Measurement, Variation, and CQI Tools

Diane L. Kelly, Susan Paul Johnson, and William A. Sollecito

"Statistical thinking will one day be as necessary for efficient citizenship as the ability to read and write."

—H. G. Wells

Measurement is a central element of any continuous quality improvement (CQI) effort. Health care institutions are full of data, but they are also full of factoids, opinions, and anecdotes masquerading as facts and as data. An analytical approach requires using data to evaluate the current situation, analyze and improve processes, and track progress.

As shown in Chapter 1, the quality evolution from industry to health care has been ongoing and encompasses all aspects of CQI. In line with that evolution, industrial statistical tools may be transferable and meaningful to quality improvement efforts in health care, and health care organizations have increasingly adopted these tools. The methods presented in this chapter to analyze health care data include both those originally developed for industrial models of quality management and those developed in the specialties of biostatistics, economics, epidemiology, and health services research. It is important to understand that analytical tools must not be isolated according to their source; rather, tools from these various disciplines should be considered as an integrated portfolio to draw from, depending on the needs of the problem at hand.

Many valuable "how to" texts are available that explain the mechanics of CQI approaches, methods, and tools (Balestracci, 2009; Bialek et al., 2009; Brassard, 1996; Breyfogle, 2003; Carey and Lloyd, 2001; Kelly,

2003; Langley et al., 2009; Lighter and Fair, 2004; Streibel et al., 2003). This chapter will not duplicate the information provided in those texts. Rather, the purpose of this chapter is to assist in understanding the role of variation in quality improvement, why measurement and statistical analysis are vital to quality improvement efforts, and how several fundamental CQI tools are used to enhance our learning about process changes and facilitate improvement in health care. Particularly in regard to these classic CQI tools, a sufficient amount of detail will be provided to enhance understanding and enable the reader to develop and apply these tools.

LEARNING FROM MEASUREMENT

Although this chapter will present an array of tools and techniques, before reviewing these useful methods, it is important to pause and reflect on the primary purpose of measurement in any quality improvement initiative—to make improvements. This sounds very simple, but in our modern age of high-speed computing, it is all too easy to apply statistical methods and focus on results without the necessary step of thinking critically and understanding what our data tell us about the system we are trying to improve. This point was emphasized in 1996 by Dr. Donald Berwick, among others, when he noted that "measurement is only a handmaiden to improvement but improvement cannot act without it. We speak here not of measurement for the purpose of judgment (for deciding whether or not to buy, accept, or reject) but for the purpose of learning" (p. 621). Not only is this view consistent with the guidelines for improvement spelled out in the earliest applications of CQI—for example, by W. Edwards Deming in his well-known 14 points (1986)—this view is also well understood and espoused in recent statistical literature (Balestracci, 2009). With this cautionary note in mind, we will proceed in this chapter to address the important concepts of understanding variation and describing the use of quality improvement tools.

THE ROLE OF VARIATION IN QUALITY IMPROVEMENT

It has long been established that a starting point for any quality improvement effort is understanding the type and causes of system variation (Deming, 1993; Nolan and Provost, 1990). It was Shewhart's idea (1931) that statistical control (also called statistical process control) of stable, or "in control," processes is the foundation of all empirical CQI activities. Determining variation and understanding its causes is one primary function of total quality management (TQM), and later CQI.

One of the key elements of the system of profound knowledge proposed by Deming is knowledge about variation and how it interacts with other elements to lead to system improvements (1993). As quality improvement has evolved over the years from business applications to health care, the business concepts related to understanding variation have also been extended specifically to health care with many examples of the causes and types of variation that can occur in health systems (Carey and Lloyd, 2001; McLaughlin and Kaluzny, 2006; Nelson et al., 1998).

This section introduces the general concept of variation, discusses variation in relation to organizational processes, and begins to describe why measurement and analysis are vital to understanding and monitoring process variation. Its emphasis is on health care applications, with numerous examples presented.

Variation: What Is It and Why Study It?

Variation is the extent to which a process differs from the norm. It is related to the statistical concepts of variance and standard deviation, familiar to most health care professionals. One can think of variation as a band of output around the central measure of a process. For example, on average, it may take 10 minutes to complete an X-ray exam on a patient; however, the exam may take as few as 8 minutes or as long as 15 minutes. This range indicates the extent of the variation of the process.

The concept of variation in health care may be viewed from several different levels. Studying variation at the national level highlights health care quality issues relative to access, medical errors, patient outcomes, and resource allocation and may best be summed up by Leatherman and McCarthy (2002):

> The unique organization and financing of health care in America explains why the World Health Organization (WHO) rates the United States as having the most individually responsive health care system in the world, while it ranks the U.S. in 37th place overall (among 191 countries) because of the significant disparities that exist between those who have predictable access to health care when needed and those who do not. . . . In the U.S., studies published in leading medical journals consistently report findings that people

with acute and chronic medical conditions receive only about two-thirds of the health care that they need while 20 percent to 30 percent of the tests and procedures provided to patients are not needed or beneficial. . . . The last several decades have produced a large amount of evidence that there are significant variations in the use of medical treatments and procedures, even for patients whose . . . symptoms and illness are similar. . . . This quality problem of unjustified variation reflects a failure to consistently practice in accordance with the scientific evidence and professional expert consensus, as well as a lack of clear evidence in some situations on what approach works best. Unjustified variation not only has potential implications for patient outcomes, but also constitutes mismanagement of resources. (pp. 11–12)

Studying variation from the organizational management perspective provides insights on the links between variation and organization effectiveness and results. Health care organizations are increasingly facing the need to meet requirements for regulatory, public, and payer reporting; to remain competitive through demonstrated improvements in organizational outcomes; and to reduce medical errors through creating a culture free from blame and fear. However, without a clear understanding of variation and its implications, managers may unintentionally undermine their ability to meet these requirements. Attempting improvement efforts in the absence of an understanding of variation puts the manager at risk of the following (Carey and Lloyd, 2001):

1. Seeing trends where there are not trends

2. Blaming or giving credit to others for things over which they have no control

3. Building barriers, decreasing morale, and creating an atmosphere of fear

4. Never being able to fully understand past performance, make predictions about the future, or make significant improvements in the processes

Studying variation from the individual perspective may be considered from practitioner, employee, and customer points of view. With respect to medical management of patients, Dr. Brent James (1989) notes the role of individual practitioner variation relative to productivity, risk management, cost-effectiveness, and professional competency:

Variation that increases costs but does not lead to improved medical outcomes is a hallmark of low productivity. When differences in the processes that lead to apparently identical medical outcomes are identified, three possibilities exist: (1) some practitioners are under-utilizing and run an increased risk of quality failures, (2) some practitioners are over-utilizing and use resources that aren't really required, or (3) there are differences in skills and clinical acumen among the practitioners. (p. 22)

To ensure quality outcomes, care providers and other employees must be able to effectively, efficiently, and safely execute their responsibilities. Berwick (1991) describes the role of variation in processes carried out daily in health care organizations:

Those who prepare [patients] for [cardiac] surgery rely . . . upon the predictability of the systems . . . that affect [their] care and outcome. The surgeon knows that coagulation test reports will be returned within 20 and 25 minutes of their being sent; the anesthesiologist knows that blood gas values will be back in 4 to 8 minutes; the pump technician knows that tubing connections will tolerate pressures within a certain range. Each makes plans in accordance with those predictions, and each bases those predictions on prior experience, which is judged to be informative. Sudden, unpredicted variation is experienced as trouble. (p. 1217)

The influence of variation on patients' clinical outcomes may not be discernable to them; however, predictability and consistency in the care they receive will be reflected in their perceptions about their experiences with the health care system. Patients are often asked to rate their experiences in areas that reflect predictability and consistency; the following examples are taken from two widely used patient satisfaction instruments:

- Sometimes in a hospital, one staff member will say one thing and another will say something quite different. Did this happen to you? (Picker Institute Europe, 2003)
- Following arrival at the hospital, how long did you wait before admission to a room or ward and bed? (Picker Institute Europe, 2003)
- How well did the staff work together to care for you? (Press Ganey Associates, 2001)
- How long did the admissions process take? (Press Ganey Associates, 2001)
- How long was your wait for tests or treatments? (Press Ganey Associates, 2001)

From the national, organizational, or individual perspective, one cannot escape the role and influence of variation on health care quality (Gold, 2004). Identifying, managing, and reducing variation where appropriate is the goal of CQI.

Nature of Process Variation

The innate nature of variation in processes makes us distinguish between two general categories of variation, which were first described by Deming (1986). Arraying data in various ways to facilitate its analysis, Deming sought to identify two types of sources of improvement in processes. The first was elimination of "special" causes of process variation: unnecessary variation associated with specific material(s), machine(s), or individual(s). The second was elimination of "common" causes of variation: those associated with aspects of the system itself such as design, training, materials, machines, or working conditions. Special causes of variation can be addressed by those people who are working directly with the process, whereas common causes of problems are the responsibility of management to correct, according to Deming, since these are system problems, and as Deming is well known for saying, management is responsible for correcting and preventing system problems (1986).

Common cause variation is that inherent variance in the process that is a result of how the process is performed. It is often referred to as systemic or internal variation. Special cause (or externally caused) variations are those that can be attributed to a particular source. While special cause variation may be traced to the source and eliminated, common cause variation can only be reduced by improving the underlying process or system.

As mentioned in the previous examples, one way to think about variation is to think about the predictability of a process. Can anyone tell a patient entering a health care process what to expect with a high degree of certainty? Can anyone tell the patient how long it will take, whom they are likely to see, or how much it will cost? These are the questions that managers will increasingly be expected to answer with a "yes." The amount of certainty in the answer will depend on the amount of variation that has been observed in a process. The less variation that exists, the more certain management can be about answers and vice versa. Reducing inappropriate variation in the process increases the certainty with which managers may expect or predict performance results.

An important characteristic in the health care environment is that no two patients—a key input to the health care system—are exactly alike. Any approach to quality in health care must accept and deal with this variability in the human condition. While managers and clinicians may have little influence on the human variation, they have much influence on the variation in the clinical and work processes. Though variation exists in every process and always will, understanding and managing variation helps managers and clinicians to better align the capability of health care and organizational processes with desired results (McLaughlin, 1996).

MEASUREMENT AND STATISTICAL ANALYSIS

Measurement and statistical analysis are used to assess the impact of an improvement effort. In addition, measurement and statistical analysis are used to measure the capability of an existing process to define the need for improvement. This section explores how to interpret and use the information about process capability.

Process Capability

To understand the expected output of a process, or the behavior of the process, a process capability study may be used. In such a study, the variable or attribute to be studied is measured and characterized. Plotting outputs from the process on a histogram can provide the first clues to the question "Is the process inherently predictable or dependable?" For example, **Figure 3–1** shows a histogram plotting the turnaround time for 223 STAT blood tests during a 24-hour period at one large hospital. The x-axis represents the number of minutes from the time the test was ordered until the time the test results were reported to the provider. The y-axis reflects the number of tests. Another way of phrasing the question "Is the process inherently predictable or dependable?" is "How likely is it that the results of a laboratory test will be reported to the provider within 15 minutes of when it was ordered?" The chances are 18 in 223. This type of performance demonstrated by the laboratory process may be considered not predictable or not dependable.

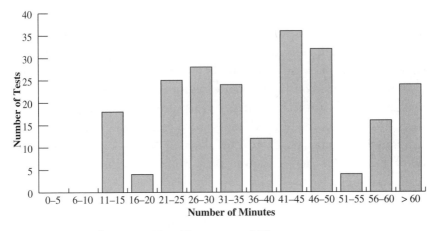

FIGURE 3–1 Laboratory Test Turnaround Time

Figure 3–2 shows a histogram of time spent in the dentist's waiting room before being led to the dental chair for the exam to begin. This graph shows data collected for the 35 patients scheduled on a particular date. For this example, the generalized question "Is the process inherently predictable or dependable?" is answered by "How likely is it that the patient will be seen within 10 minutes of arrival?" The chances are 29 in 35. This type of performance demonstrated by the dentist's process may be considered predictable or dependable. A process that displays little special cause variation or variation only under predictable circumstances is said to be *under control.*

The shape of the curve formed by the histogram (normal or non-normal), a measure of central tendency (mean, median, or mode), and its standard deviation all provide valuable information about how the

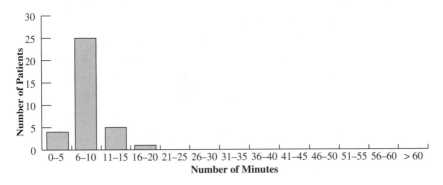

FIGURE 3–2 Waiting Time at the Dentist

process is performing. The shape of the curve suggests which type of tools should be used for further analysis. (Note: This chapter will focus on the normal distribution.) The measure of central tendency provides information about the average level of performance, while the standard deviation shows the range of performance that may be expected.

In these two examples, the time period was a single day. However, the average daily or monthly performance may also be plotted on a chart over time. By plotting the variables over time, managers may begin to see patterns or trends in the data that can signal that there is a problem with the process, indicating that it is time to identify the source of the problem, to prompt action to resolve the problem, and to monitor the impact of the solution.

Interpreting Process Performance

Variation exists in every process and always will. It is the manager's job to determine if the average level of performance and amount of common cause variation is acceptable. But what is "acceptable"? In both the laboratory and the dentist's office examples, it is impossible to determine the acceptable level of performance without first understanding the expectations or requirements for the process. A provider working in the emergency department (ED) would require more rapid turnaround time (TAT) of laboratory results than a provider working in a primary care office. A 30-minute TAT in the ED may be unacceptable, whereas a 24-hour TAT may be acceptable for a primary care office. There may also be specific requirements for analyzing the laboratory specimen. Technology used for one type of test may require 30 minutes to be processed, while a different type of test can be completed within seconds. Customer and technical requirements must both be taken into account in order to interpret whether the performance of the process is acceptable or whether the process needs to be improved.

Process Requirements

Process requirements may be thought of as the criteria from which the effectiveness of a process may be evaluated. They function as both inputs to designing a process and outputs from executing a process. In health care organizations, requirements may be considered from three perspectives: the customer, other stakeholders, and the market in general. **Figure 3–3** illustrates the sequence of questions that should be asked to interpret process performance.

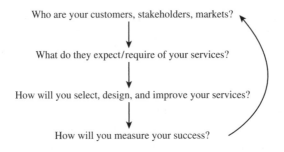

FIGURE 3–3 Process Requirement Determination: Sequence of questions

It is essential to first identify the customers, stakeholders, or markets for a process. Chapter 6 provides an in-depth discussion of customers of health care organizations. Brief definitions are provided here. A customer is defined as anyone who has expectations regarding a process operation or outputs. In health care delivery organizations, the primary customer is the patient, while the community may be the primary customer for a public health agency. Internal customers are those within the organizations and are sometimes thought of as those departments or coworkers "downstream" from the process. For example, the recovery room or post-anesthesia care unit may be thought of as the customer of the operating room. Patient care units may be thought of as customers of diagnostic departments (i.e., laboratory, radiology). Payers may be considered as external customers—that is, those outside the provider organization. A stakeholder is anyone with an interest in or affected by the work you do. Regulatory bodies such as The Joint Commission (TJC), formerly known as the Joint Commission on Accreditation of Healthcare Organizations, or the National Commission on Quality Assurance (NCQA) would be considered stakeholders for hospitals and health insurance companies, respectively. Professional societies that define practice standards may also be thought of as stakeholders. The market refers to the environment in which you operate and do business and may include socioeconomic, demographic, geographic, and competitive considerations.

Once customers, stakeholders, and markets have been identified, it is essential to identify and understand what they require of your services. For example, patients may require access and competent, courteous providers; payers may require a certain level of clinical results delivered in a cost-effective manner; regulatory bodies require compliance; and markets may require a culturally diverse approach to delivering services.

These requirements are vital to determining how services should be specified and how the processes comprising the services are designed and improved. These requirements also provide the basis for selecting variables or attributes that will measure the process performance. The outputs of the process are then evaluated against these requirements to determine if the process performance is acceptable. Because the health care industry is a dynamic one with customers, stakeholders, markets, and requirements changing over time, the feedback loop in Figure 3-3 illustrates the ongoing nature of this process.

Tables 3–1 and **3–2** illustrate how one health services organization operationalizes the links between customer requirements, process design, and measurement. The first column in Table 3–1 summarizes requirements from important stakeholder groups (e.g., regulatory, accreditation). The next column lists the key organizational processes that address the requirements of these groups. The third column lists the attributes or variables that the organization measures to understand the degree to which its processes are meeting stakeholder requirements, and the fourth column indicates the related performance goals. Note that if the process capability is not aligned with organizational goals as derived from the stakeholder requirements, then the process must be improved.

Table 3–2 illustrates the core processes for each phase of the continuum of inpatient care. The patients' interface with this organization follows the following path:

Admission → Assessment → Care Delivery/Treatment → Discharge

The core process(es) for each phase of care are shown in the first column. The second column lists the key requirements for the process, derived from a variety of methods targeted toward understanding requirements of patients, internal customers, stakeholders, and the market in which the organization operates. The third column lists the attributes or variables that the organization measures to understand the degree to which its processes are meeting stakeholder requirements.

It is management's job to ensure that the process requirements (also referred to as the Voice of the Customer) and the process performance (also referred to as the Voice of the Process) are aligned (Carey and Lloyd, 2001; Wheeler, 2000). If the two are not in alignment, then the process must be studied and then changed to improve the process capability.

TABLE 3-1 Links Between Customer Requirements, Process Design, and Measurement

Requirements	Key Processes	Measures	Goals
Regulatory–legal	• Corporate responsibility process	• Number of government investigations	• 0
	• Contract review	• Turnaround time	• 24–48 hours
	• Licensure	• Licensure	• Licensure
Accreditation	• TJC survey	• Scores	• 100%
Risk management	• Public safety	• Infection rates	• 0
		• Dangerous abbreviations	• 0
		• Restraints	• 0
		• Patient falls	• 0
Community health	• Charity care	• Cost of charity care	• 25% prior year's operating margin
	• Healthy communities programs	• Health status in selected populations for individual projects	• Project specific

TABLE 3-2 Links Between Process Stages, Requirements, and Measures

Process	Key Requirements	Key Measures
Admit		
Admitting–registration	Timeliness	• Time to admit patients to the setting of care • Timeliness in admitting–registration rate on patient satisfaction survey questions
Assess		
Patient assessment	Timeliness	• Percentage of histories and physicals charted within 24 hours and/or prior to surgery • Pain assessed at appropriate intervals per hospital policy
Clinical laboratory & radiology services	Accuracy and timeliness	• Quality control results–repeat rates • Turnaround time • Response rate on medical staff satisfaction survey
Care delivery–treatment		
Provision of clinical care	Nurse responsiveness, pain management, successful clinical outcomes	• Response rate on patient satisfaction and medical staff survey questions • Wait time for pain medications • Percentage of CHF patients received medication instruction–weighing • Percentage of ischemic heart patients discharged on proven therapies • Unplanned readmissions–return to ER or operating room mortality

(continues)

TABLE 3–2 Links Between Process Stages, Requirements, and Measures (*continued*)

Process	Key Requirements	Key Measures
Pharmacy–medication use	Accuracy	• Use of dangerous abbreviations in medication orders • Medication error rate of adverse drug events resulting from medication errors
Surgical services–anesthesia	Professional skill, competences, communication	• Clear documentation of informed surgical and anesthesia consent • Peri-operative mortality • Surgical site infection rates
Discharge Case management	Appropriate utilization	• Average length of stay (ALOS) • Payment denials • Unplanned re-admits
Discharge from setting of care	Assistance and clear directions	• Discharge instructions documented and provided to patient • Response rate on patient satisfaction survey

Figure 3–4 illustrates ways to assess process capabilities. Segment (a) provides a graphical description of overall process performance, with measures of central tendency (mean, μ) and variability displayed; it describes a highly predictable process. Segment (b) describes a less predictable process; it illustrates a way of identifying outliers by highlighting the areas out of specification in the shaded areas.

The graphs in Figure 3–4 are examples of process performance charts, also known as statistical process control charts. A process performance chart is the most effective way to measure, document, analyze, and understand the capability of a process.

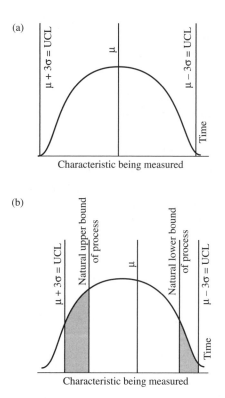

FIGURE 3–4 Process Performance vs. Process Limits: (a) A process that does not have difficulty maintaining quality will have normally distributed observations over time. (b) A process that has difficulty maintaining quality may have symmetrically distributed observations over time but may have control limits outside the natural bounds of the process and a mean that is not at the center of the distribution. The shaded areas in this diagram represent the areas out of specification.

QUALITY IMPROVEMENT TOOLS

In order to improve a process capability to deliver desired performance results, a systematic, fact-based approach that enables you to implement permanent solutions to root causes of problems should be used. In Chapter 1, Shewhart's Plan, Do, Study, Act (PDSA) cycle was introduced, with an emphasis on its broad applicability as a framework in which many other CQI processes can be applied. Many organizations, including health care organizations, have adopted the Shewhart cycle or a tailored version of it as their overall framework for CQI. Different tools, techniques, and methods may be used to accomplish the purpose of each phase of the PDSA cycle.

There is not one specified point in the CQI process where one needs to use a given method of measurement and analysis. It should be used on a continuous basis. In the context of the PDSA cycle, data and analytical tools may be used throughout the entire cycle. Different tools will be more helpful in different stages of each improvement project, from the initial analysis to monitoring changes that have already been instituted. Reemphasizing the point made earlier in this chapter about using data to learn about improvement, Berwick (1996) notes that it is critical at the studying stage of a PDSA cycle to take the time to reflect and learn about the impact of improvements that have already been made. This should include evaluating whether these changes have actually been improvements and then deciding on what further improvements to make.

There are numerous tools and techniques available to assist managers, clinicians, and organizational teams in improving processes to deliver desired results. These tools include activity network diagrams; affinity diagrams; brainstorming; cause-and-effect diagrams; check sheets; concentration diagrams; control charts; failure mode and effects analysis (FMEA); flowcharts (process, deployment, top-down, opportunity); force field analysis; frequency plots; histograms; interrelationship digraphs; matrix diagrams; Pareto charts; prioritization matrices; process capability charts; radar charts; run charts; scatter diagrams; Suppliers, Process steps, Inputs, Outputs, Customers (SPIOC) diagrams; time plots; tree diagrams; and workflow diagrams.

While space does not permit detailed description of this list of tools, we explain seven fundamental tools that provide a basis for CQI efforts in health care. These tools are the process flowchart, cause-and-effect diagram, histogram, Pareto chart, regression analysis, run chart, and control chart.

These tools are suitable for any stage of the quality improvement process. However, one can visualize a life cycle of the improvement team's efforts showing how these tools might be applied sequentially at various project stages. How these tools might be utilized over a project life cycle is outlined in **Table 3–3**.

TABLE 3–3 CQI Process Stages and Quality Tools

CQI Process Stages				
Tools	**Describe Process and Identify Sources of Variation**	**Conduct In-Depth Analyses to Clarify Knowledge and Present Results**	**Weigh Alternatives and Make Choices**	**Measure Improvements and Monitor Progress**
Flow diagrams or charts	Key tool here	Revisit and update		Keep current
Cause-and-effect diagrams	Key tool here, especially after brain-storming	Stratify for detail		
Pareto diagrams or charts		Key tool here to stratify causes	Key to deciding on vital few	Use to show change
Frequency distribution (histograms)		Helpful in presentation	Assess patterns	Helpful in monitoring
Run charts		Important to relate data temporally to changes		Key to knowing whether improvement has been associated with change
Control charts		Important to relate data temporally to changes		Key to seeing whether the process is or remains under control
Regression analysis			Assess strength of association and test hypotheses	

Process Flowchart

One of the most powerful improvement tools is the flowchart. Flowcharts are pictorial representations of how a process works. Simply put, they trace the steps that the "object" of a process goes through from start to finish. The object may be a specimen in laboratory tests, a piece of paper in medical records, or a patient in a specialty clinic. Flowcharts are also used to describe the sequence of actions that must be carried out in order to complete a particular task.

To develop a flowchart, one may proceed as follows:

1. Define the basic stages of a process.

2. Further define the process, breaking down each stage into specific steps needed to complete the process.

3. Follow the object through the process a number of times to verify the process by observation.

4. Discuss the process with the project team or other employees to clarify the process and include any steps that might be missing.

As the steps of a process are described, they may be documented with the symbols customarily used, which we illustrated in **Figure 3–5**. An activity or action step is represented by a rectangle, a decision step by

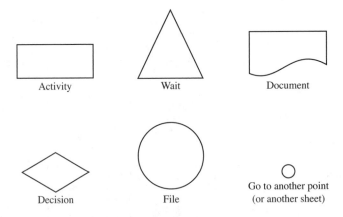

FIGURE 3–5 Flowchart Symbols: Arrows are used to connect the symbols indicating sequencing and interrelationship.

a diamond, a wait or inventory by a triangle, a document by a symbol that looks like a rectangle with a curve at the bottom, a file by a large circle, and the continuation of the flowchart to another sheet of paper by a small circle.

Flow diagrams may be as simple or as complex as you wish. It is important to agree on what level of detail is suitable for the purpose. For example, very detailed flow diagrams may be used in standard operating procedures (SOPs) for highly technical procedures. A high-level flow diagram may be used to describe a general overview of how the process is carried out. **Figure 3–6** shows a high-level flowchart of the medication administration process for the inpatient setting. Once the general process is described, more detail may be added, depending on the purpose of the analysis.

Figure 3–7 shows a more detailed flowchart of a similar process. As more detail has been added, the process has evolved from "medication administration" to "medication management" to include additional

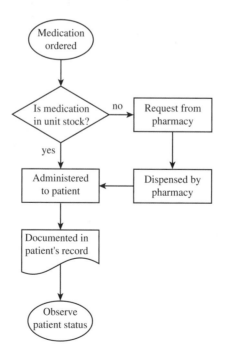

FIGURE 3–6 Simple Flowchart of Medication Administration Process

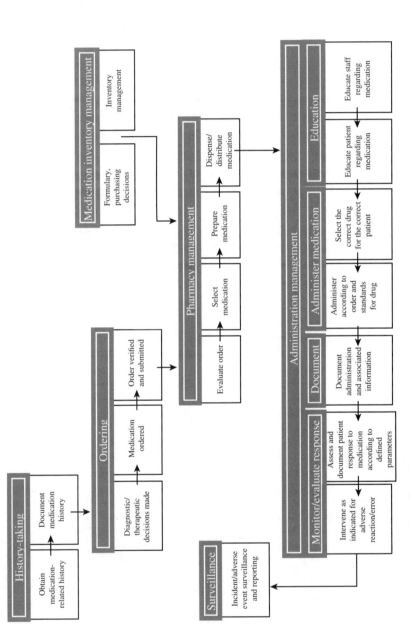

FIGURE 3-7 Flowchart of Medication Management

Source: Reprinted with permission by VHA and First Consulting Group from the VHA 2002 Research Series publication, *Surveillance for Adverse Drug Events: History, Methods and Current Issues* by Peter Kilbridge, MD, and David Classen, MD. First Consulting Group.

process stages involving medication inventory management, pharmacy management, and surveillance for adverse drug events. Each step of this process may in turn be charted with a finer level of detail.

Members of a work team or improvement project team are likely to find that there is not a common understanding of how the current process or system works, especially if multiple providers or departments are responsible for carrying out different steps of the process. The development of flowcharts, with input from all team members, allows the team to achieve a common understanding of their work processes. With an accurate, shared representation of how the process works, the team is then able to consider how to improve it.

Once agreement is reached on the representation of the current process, the team may begin to ask questions about that process, including:

1. How effective is the process in meeting customer requirements?

2. Are there performance gaps or perceived opportunities for improvement?

3. Have the relevant stages of the process been represented? Are "owners" of each stage represented on the team? If not, what needs to be done to gather their feedback and ideas?

4. What are the inputs required for the process, and where do they come from? Are the inputs constraining the process or not? Which ones?

5. Are there equipment or regulatory constraints forcing this approach?

6. Is this the right problem process to be working on? To continue working on?

The potential benefits of flowcharting are considerable. Staff come to know the process much better. The results can be used as a training aid. People begin to take ownership of the process by participating in this activity, and most importantly, the possibilities for improvement become clear almost immediately.

Cause-and-Effect Diagram

Cause-and-effect diagrams, also called Ishikawa or fishbone diagrams, are one of the most widely used tools of CQI. This tool was developed by Kaoru Ishikawa (University of Tokyo) for use at Kawasaki Steel Works in 1943 to sort and interrelate the multiple causes of process variation (Ishikawa, 1987).

Cause-and-effect diagrams are most useful to begin to identify sources of variation once the process has already been described and documented using a process flowchart. There is likely to be evidence of variation in the identified problem (either real or anticipated). Additional causes may be revealed either through the flowcharting process or during brainstorming discussions.

Cause-and-effect diagrams are a schematic means of relating the causes of variation to the effect of variation on the process. Another way of thinking about a cause-and-effect diagram is as a schematic drawing to organize the contributing causes to a problem to prioritize, select, and improve the source of the problem. The diagram is also referred to as a "fishbone" diagram because the shape resembles the skeleton of a fish.

This tool is especially suited for team situations and is quite useful for focusing a discussion and organizing large amounts of information resulting from a brainstorming session. It can be taught easily and quickly, allowing the group to sort ideas into useful categories for further investigation.

Figure 3–8 shows the multilayered process of making a fishbone diagram. Step 1 of the diagram shows the identified performance gap or problem at the right and a big arrow leading to it that represents the overall causation. Step 2 involves drawing spines from that big arrow to represent main classifications or categories of causes, such as labor, materials, and equipment. Step 3 adds the specific causes along each major spine, which also may occur at multiple levels. Sometimes it is useful to draw the diagram in two stages—one showing the main causes and a separate chart with a spine representing the main cause and its associated levels.

The first pass at a cause-and-effect diagram may not be enough to understand the process, identify the specific cause of an error, and quantify it. Therefore, it may be necessary to stratify cause-and-effect diagrams further to achieve finer gradations of error causes. Increasing the level of detail about causes can help with identifying specific corrective action.

Figure 3–9 illustrates a fishbone diagram that may be used to describe root causes of adverse drug events in a hospital setting. The problem is

Step 1: Draw spine

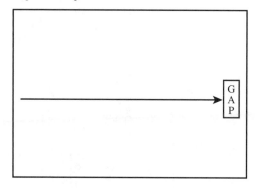

Step 2: Add main causes

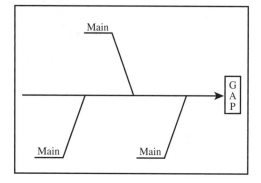

Step 3: Add specific causes

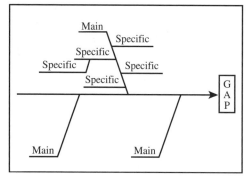

FIGURE 3–8 Multilayered Process of Developing a Fishbone Diagram

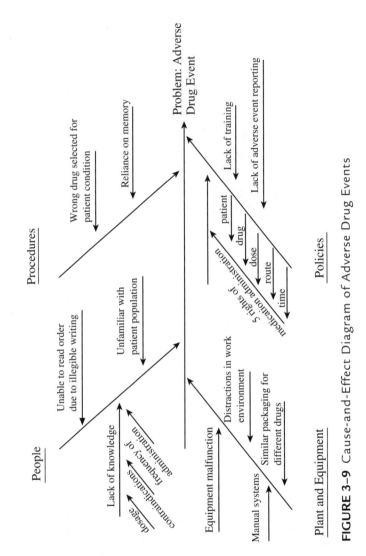

FIGURE 3–9 Cause-and-Effect Diagram of Adverse Drug Events

"adverse drug events." The main classifications in this example are people, policies, procedures, and plant and equipment, each showing a variety of levels of causes.

Histogram and Pareto Diagram

Once a cause-and-effect diagram is generated, data are collected to quantify how often the different causes occur. These data must then be presented to the study team and later to others. The simplest display is a histogram, a vertical bar chart representing the frequency distribution of a set of data; it was introduced earlier as a tool to describe process capability. The bars are arrayed on the *x*-axis representing equal or adjacent data intervals or discrete events. The length of the bar against the *y*-axis shows the number of observations falling on that interval or event classification. The histogram displays the nature of the underlying statistical distribution. Successive histograms can be used to indicate whether there has been a change in the variability of a process. **Figure 3–10** shows a histogram of the frequency and causes for the discarding of hospital linens.

A Pareto diagram is a vertical bar chart with the bars arranged from the longest first on the left and moving successively toward the shortest. The arrangement of the vertical bars gives a visual indication of the relative frequency of the contributing causes of the problem, with each bar representing one cause.

The diagram is named after the 17th-century Italian economist, Vilfredo Pareto. When he studied the distribution of wealth, he observed that the

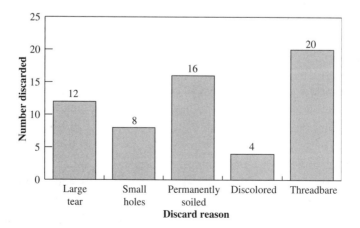

FIGURE 3–10 Histogram of Linen Discard Causes

majority of the wealth had been distributed among a small proportion of the population (Pareto's law). Juran (1988) applied this concept to quality causes, observing that the "vital few" causes account for most of the defects, while others, the "useful many," account for a much smaller proportion of the defects. He noted that these vital few causes are likely to constitute the areas of highest payback to management. Concentrating on the high-volume causes should have the largest potential for reducing process variation.

On the same Pareto diagram, one also develops a cumulative probability distribution incorporating all the proportions of the observations to the left of and including the bar. It is common to display the frequency scale on the left-hand side of the *y*-axis and the cumulative percentage scale on the right-hand edge. Segregating the causes that have large frequencies can help identify potential improvements. However, just because a cause is identified as having the greatest frequency does not necessarily mean it should be worked on first. It must also be tractable and not cost more to change than it is worth. It is likely, however, that the first cause to be studied in detail will be among the left-most group. It is important to remember that even though a cause may not be among the most frequent, if it has a devastating result such as causing a patient death, it must be addressed in the course of the improvement effort.

Once the cause-and-effect diagram, such as the one in Figure 3–9, has been described, data would be collected on the frequency of the causes. **Figure 3–11** illustrates how a Pareto chart can be developed to analyze the frequency of causes identified in the cause-and-effect diagram. For example, Figure 3–11 displays how often the "five rights of medication administration" contributed to an adverse drug event (ADE). Of 100 ADEs investigated, the Pareto chart shows that "wrong time" occurred most frequently, with "wrong patient" next, and so on.

Through these examples, one can begin to see how the tools fit together both to describe the problem and to promote identifying solutions. Since the Institute of Medicine report *To Err Is Human* (2000) was published, the topic of medical errors and adverse events has become a priority area for customers and stakeholders of health care organizations. TJC's review process now includes accreditation standards addressing patient safety, medical errors, and adverse events. As illustrated by the preceding examples, various CQI tools, alone and in combination, can be used to address this critical area of concern.

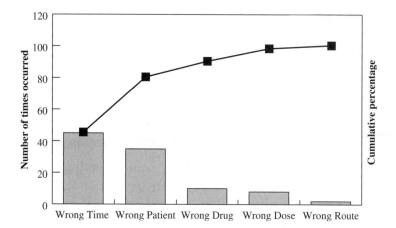

FIGURE 3-11 Pareto Chart: Five Rights of Medication Administration: Cause of Adverse Drug Events

Regression Analysis

In seeking causes of problems or ideas for improvement, it may be important to determine whether one event is temporally or causally related to another. Although direct causality cannot be proven statistically, the degree of association or correlation among variables can be analyzed, and hypotheses regarding the strength of associations can be tested using regression analysis and its closely associated descriptive counterpart, the bivariate scatter plot. A bivariate scatter plot is very useful as a CQI tool to describe pairwise associations between variables. Pairs of values of two continuous variables (e.g., caloric intake and weight) are plotted on horizontal (x) and vertical (y) axes to assess whether they are correlated with one another. For example, is lower caloric intake correlated with lower weight? Although a simple and useful tool, the scatter diagram is limited to analyzing the relationship between only two measures. Many processes that are the subject of CQI efforts in health care are more complex in nature and often include multiple variables that may be interrelated. Therefore, these efforts may require additional, more complex analyses (e.g., considering or controlling for other variables, including temporal factors).

In addition to information from descriptive analyses, such as scatter plots, quality improvement teams or managers may have a priori ideas about what associations exist that influence process improvements. However, individuals may assume associations where they do not exist, so hypotheses suggested by expert opinions, or by observation of the distribution of the data, including scatter plots, should be tested statistically by some form of statistical modeling, such as regression analysis (Kleinbaum et al., 2008). For example, in 1980, Gardner and McLaughlin developed a regression model to forecast the utilization of perishable blood products in a large teaching hospital. Their forecasting model predicted demand quite effectively based on hospital census and some seasonal patterns. The staff reported, however, that one of the attending (faculty) physicians utilized these products much more than the other three attending physicians on that service. Since the attending physicians rotated on a monthly basis, it was important to include variables in the regression analysis to account for the physician who was on duty during a given month. The model that was augmented to include the physicians indicated that there was not a significant difference in utilization among the four physicians. What the staff assumed about the one physician was not borne out by the data analysis.

Negative findings about causal relationships are not a bad outcome in CQI. They help reduce the complexity of the set of hypotheses to be studied and focus on other alternative sources of variability. Teams report that they frequently started with erroneous impressions about the causes of poor performance. This is not surprising—otherwise, they might already have corrected it. If the CQI team had not conducted experiments and analyses to check those hypotheses early, they would have continued to work in unfruitful areas. This is one advantage of the CQI approach. The team is empowered to use scientific methods of analysis to verify and support any changes they would like to make, instead of guessing what to do next. Regression analyses or other statistical techniques provide a way of quantifying suspected associations and can help to focus improvement efforts on the (statistically) most likely causes of errors or variation.

Run Charts and Control Charts

CQI requires that performance data be monitored on an ongoing basis to identify trends or other characteristics of the phenomenon being observed that change over time. This allows the experienced observer (1) to see the temporal behavior of the process and (2) to establish the time of process performance changes so that they can be linked to the time of other possibly related events.

Two of the most powerful tools that are often used to answer these questions are run charts and control charts, which were first developed by Shewhart in the 1920s (Deming, 1993). The run chart is a simple plot of a measurement over time with a line drawn at the median. The run chart allows for an assessment of data trends that may be indicative of special cause variation, which would be indicated, for example, by multiple values in sequence (a run) below (or above) the median. A run length of eight or more is used by many authors to define the potential presence of a special cause (Balestracci, 2009).

Control charts are similar in concept to run charts as well as to process performance charts that were presented earlier in Figure 3–4. Control charts also plot measurement over time and allow for an assessment of trends, but in addition they provide a determination of whether measurements are within control limits (defined as a measure of central tendency, such as a mean, plus or minus three standard deviations). Values outside control limits may be an indicator of special cause variation. **Figure 3–12** shows a series of control charts and some diagnostic interpretations of those data.

Run charts and control charts are very easy to generate using spreadsheet software. However, their interpretation can be very complex, as one tries to distinguish special cause and common cause variation and also make the distinction between control limits and specification limits (Balestracci, 2009; Deming, 1993). In general, a process that is stable or under statistical control will be described by a control chart that exhibits all values randomly distributed above and below the mean (with no runs of eight or more in either direction) and that has no points outside the control limits.

Run charts and control charts are frequently used in the quality improvement process to answer the questions "How are we doing?" and "Are we doing better since implementing the improvement intervention?"

Two types of measures can be used to develop run charts and control charts. Measures can be either attributes or continuous variables.

> Attribute data arise from (1) classification of items, such as products or services, into categories; from (2) counts of the number of items or the proportion in a given category; and from (3) counts of the number of occurrences per unit. . . . Important attributes [are] fraction defective, number of defects, number of defects per unit. (Gitlow et al. 1989, pp. 78, 79, 144)

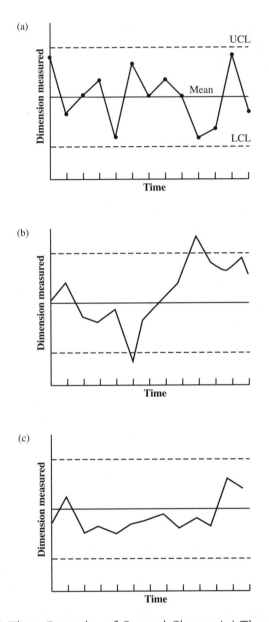

FIGURE 3–12 Three Examples of Control Charts: (a) The data are considered to be under control; the points are apparently randomly distributed on either side of the mean and do not go outside of the control limits. (b) There are extreme values (outside the control limits); thus, the process is not in control. Another thing to beware of is too many observations on one side of the mean. (c) There are too many values in a row (>8) below the mean.

Continuous variables, which have an interval scale (e.g., height, weight, blood pressure), are measured directly or based on direct measures only and do not result from a classification scheme. Run charts and control charts of continuous variables use a median or mean, respectively, as the measure of central tendency to define the centerline. These types of control charts are also referred to as X-bar charts. Attribute data may have a centerline based on the proportion of events to describe the process being observed or improved (e.g., proportion of adverse events). These are also referred to as p-charts. For both types of measures, control limits can be defined based on a standard deviation computed using simple statistical formulas available in statistical and spreadsheet software, and in many handheld calculators.

The following example of a continuous variable that might be analyzed via a control chart is derived from the Centers for Medicare and Medicaid Services (CMS), which has defined required quality indicators for the key inpatient diagnoses of acute myocardial infarction, heart failure, stroke, pneumonia, breast cancer, and diabetes (Jencks et al., 2000; Jencks et al., 2003). One of the quality indicators for acute myocardial infarction (AMI) is the time to thrombolytic therapy, measured in minutes from time of admission, sometimes referred to as "door-to-needle time." Control charts can be used to plot average door-to-needle time to track performance around the care of patients admitted to the emergency department (ED) with the diagnosis of AMI. Since this is a continuous measure, an X-bar chart would be used. **Figure 3–13** presents an example of an X-bar chart of door to needle time.

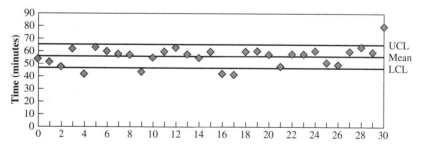

FIGURE 3–13 X-Bar Chart: Door to needle time

Source: Johnson, S. P., Alemi, F., and Neuhauser, D. 1998. Rapid improvement teams. *Joint Commission J Quality Improve*, 24(3): 119–129. Reprinted with permission.

To obtain the data needed for this chart, suppose that each day for one month, the hospital observed five randomly selected cases of AMI. The "door-to-needle" time would represent the difference between the time the medication was administered and the time the patient was admitted. The data would include the mean time for each of the 30 days that were sampled and the range of times for each day.

For our example, the mean is 56.1 minutes, the upper control limit (UCL) is 65.56 minutes, and the lower control limit (LCL) is 45.70 minutes. The X-bar chart is created by plotting the UCL, the centerline, the LCL, and the mean of each group of samples on the chart. The completed control chart is given in Figure 3–13; it indicates evidence of special cause variation as several points fall below the LCL and the last point falls substantially above the UCL.

For an example of a control chart based on attribute data, we consider how one hospital investigated sedation during surgery, an area that plays an important role in both clinical outcomes and patient satisfaction. Pain management and comfort have been identified as an important patient expectation in the hospital setting (Gerteis et al., 1993). In this hospital, a grading scheme was used by the clinicians to record their impressions of the effect of the conscious sedation intervention on the patient (5 = *in pain*, 4 = *talking*, 3 = *awake*, 2 = *asleep*, 1 = *not breathing*). They determined that levels 1, 4, and 5 were not acceptable and that they could and should be avoided. One way to monitor the effect of sedation management is to use a p-chart that combines the adequate sedation levels (2 and 3) and the inadequate levels (1, 4, and 5) into two groups. Then the proportion of inadequate sedation could be monitored and assessed using control charts.

As an example, consider that they recorded the sedation levels of nine persons each day for 30 days. On average, inadequate sedation was seen in 4.8% of patients. This is all the information that is needed to create the control chart. The distribution of p, the proportion defective, is binomial, and the corresponding control charts are easy to develop using widely available statistical formulas. The UCL, centerline, LCL, and the individual data points are plotted to create the control chart. **Figure 3–14** shows such a p-chart; it exhibits a stable process with all values randomly distributed above and below the centerline and none outside of the control limits (UCL and LCL).

The major difference between the p-chart and the others is that the plot is done using attribute data rather than continuous variables (and

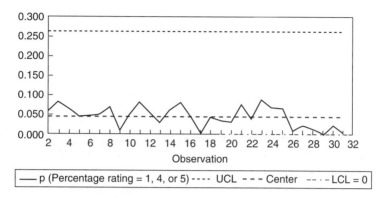

FIGURE 3–14 P-Chart: Sedation during surgery

thus simple statistics cannot be calculated, only proportions). It is important in setting up p-charts to start with a historical proportion, such as the previous mortality rates. Then you can keep track of the proportion dying over the intervention period and after and compare results.

The p-chart plots the proportion that is measured for each group of observations on the *y*-axis with a midline indicating the historical proportion. At the very least, the proportion may be monitored for patterns and trends over time.

The goals of improvement efforts are to improve the level of performance and reduce variation. Run and control charts are valuable tools that are useful in meeting these goals.

Procedures for computing control charts are found in the texts cited at the beginning of this chapter and online at Web sites such as StatSoft (http://www.statsoft.com/textbook/quality-control-charts/). Run and control charts can also be developed directly using spreadsheet software.

RECENT TRENDS IN CQI TOOLS

In addition to the traditional CQI tools described in this chapter, progress has been made in developing new tools that have specific applications to health care. These range from measurement tools to analysis tools and are the result of rigorous research and, in some cases, the availability of recent advancements in computing technology. (See Chapter 12 for a more complete discussion of the impact on CQI of advances in information technology.) In the final section of this chapter, we will present a brief overview of some tools that are new or that have recently received attention as being particularly useful in health care.

Measuring Medical Errors

Quality and safety and the impact of medical errors are discussed throughout this text, with extra focus in Chapters 9, 11, and 13 as well as in the companion casebook (McLaughlin et al., 2012). Due to the importance of these issues, there is value in learning about any new tools that help to measure and reduce safety problems. For example, in addressing the prevalence of medical errors, progress has been made in methods for measuring and classifying actual or potential errors. As noted earlier in this chapter, measurement is the first step in our ability to understand causes of variation and means for improvement; critical to this step is the use of reliable measurement tools.

One useful measurement tool in medical care is the Global Trigger Tool for Measuring Adverse Events developed by the Institute for Healthcare Improvement. This tool can be used for tracking rates of adverse events and medical errors in hospital records over time (Griffin and Resar, 2007). "Triggers" are defined as clues in patient records that indicate adverse events or medically induced harm. As with any data measurement instrument, it is most important that it produce reliable data, which has been found to be the case with the trigger tool (Office of the Inspector General, 2010; Sharek et al., 2010). Its large-scale use and feasibility has been demonstrated to produce high-quality results. One recent example of the use of the trigger tool is a 6-year study of more than 2,300 medical admissions in 10 hospitals in North Carolina; it was used to measure rates of harm to patients from medical care. The trigger tool was found to have very high specificity, reliability, and sensitivity. The authors of this study note that although the manual use of the tool can be labor intensive, as the use of electronic medical records becomes more common, automation will lead to more efficient use of this tool. The published report of this large study (Landrigan et al., 2010) in the *New England Journal of Medicine* provides a good starting point for understanding the steps needed to implement this useful tool.

Checklists

The next example of a new tool also focuses on patient safety. As with other CQI examples presented in this text, the evolution of business applications to health care has continued, with new tools included in that evolutionary process. Although it is neither a statistical tool nor a completely new tool in quality improvement, one that is getting greater use and attention in regard to health care safety is the checklist.

Checklists have been used for many years in other industries, such as the airline industry, and they have long been an important component of the project manager's tool kit in many different industrial and health care settings. Their role in improving airline safety is well documented and is an important reason that they have now seen an accelerated evolution into medical care, which has had a greater focus on safety issues in the early part of the 21st century (Gawande, 2009; Pronovost et al., 2009). The first 10 years of this century have yielded mounting evidence about the value of checklists as an effective safety tool in surgery (de Vries et al., 2010; Haynes et al., 2009) and other medical specialties (Gawande, 2009; Pronovost et al., 2006). Although not without controversy regarding their effectiveness (Bosk et al., 2009), their adoption as a medical safety tool, to be used in conjunction with other well-established evidence-based practices, continues as we have entered the second decade of this century.

In addition to the references cited in the preceding paragraph, Chapters 1 and 2 of this text provide further discussion of the use of checklists in health care. Case 9 in the companion casebook describes how to overcome some of the difficulties surrounding checklist implementation through the use of a social marketing approach (McLaughlin et al., 2012).

Six Sigma

Similarly, the evolution from industry to health care CQI has included new statistical analysis tools and techniques that can be applied in health care. One notable addition to the collection of business statistics methodologies that are currently being applied to health care CQI is the Six Sigma methodology, which is well known for its use at the Motorola Corporation, where it was developed in the 1980s (Brue, 2002; Pande et al., 2000).

Although it is more than a statistical methodology, Six Sigma, as its name implies (sigma being the Greek symbol used in statistics to measure variation), utilizes statistical methods to identify and remove errors and minimize variability in processes. It can be called a set of practices or strategies, and despite being criticized by some as not being innovative (Paton, 2002), its application increased in the first decade of the 21st century.

Six Sigma is widely used in traditional business and in health care organizations, with increasing numbers of managers and leaders being trained and recognized for their proficiency using a system of colored belts (e.g., green belts) similar to those awarded in the martial arts (Taylor, 2008).

Six Sigma has been applied in several areas of health care, including public health (Duffy et al., 2009). As described by Duffy et al., Six Sigma starts with process mapping to identify elements critical to quality and then focuses on changes to these elements through the DMAIC (define, measure, analyze, improve, control) methodology.

Often used in conjunction with Six Sigma is the "lean" methodology, which is defined as a systematic approach to identifying and eliminating waste, where waste is defined as any nonvalued tasks. Lean methods are not new; in fact, they have their roots in the 1950s work of W. Edwards Deming and Joseph Juran.

"Lean Six Sigma" adoption in health care and public health represents an evolution resulting in part from alliances and interchanges with corporate and government partners, which is another mechanism for promoting the evolution of CQI across industries (Duffy et al., 2009). The combination of lean methodology and Six Sigma is now being used in a wide range of health care applications, providing a synergistic methodology for analyzing and reducing or eliminating waste in health care processes.

Lean and Six Sigma methods are parallel to, and can also be used in conjunction with, umbrella approaches like the PDSA cycle, as part of one or more of the four broad steps of the change and improvement cycle (e.g., as part of the "do" stage, in PDSA), as well as in conjunction with collaborative improvement strategies. These combined methods and approaches have also been applied in various global health settings and are described in greater detail later in this text with examples of applications in resource-poor countries (see Chapter 19). The citations given in the preceding paragraphs offer further information about these methods and the joint application of lean and Six Sigma, as does the Juran Institute's Web site (http://www.juran.com/solutions_improve_quality_of_products_and_services_lean_six_sigma.html).

Likewise, there are Web sites that provide tutorials and software to facilitate the understanding and use of other methodologies discussed in this chapter, including the seven traditional CQI tools (e.g., http://asq.org/learn-about-quality/seven-basic-quality-tools/overview/overview

.html; http://www.qualityamerica.com/spcsoftwareproducts.html; http://www.statsoft.com/textbook/).

CONCLUSIONS

This chapter has described the importance of measurement concepts in CQI. Most important is understanding variation and, in particular, causes of variability, and the distinction between special and common causes of variation.

Also described are the tools typically used to identify, measure, and interpret processes, problems, and improvements by CQI teams. The value of these tools as aids in the overall improvement process and their use in conjunction with other improvement strategies, such as the PDSA cycle, is also addressed. Used appropriately they will help teams (1) implement the CQI philosophy and processes with maximum effectiveness and provide valuable information that will aid in the ultimate goal of learning how to make system improvements and (2) assess the impact of improvements that have been made to increase the knowledge gained and motivate further improvements.

Cross-References to the Companion Casebook

(McLaughlin, C. P., Johnson, J. K., and Sollecito, W. A. [Eds.]. 2012. *Implementing Continuous Quality Improvement in Health Care: A Global Casebook*. Sudbury, MA: Jones & Bartlett Learning.)

Case Study Number	Case Study Title	Case Study Authors
7	Dawn Valley Hospital: Selecting Quality Measures for the Hospital Board	*Joseph G. Van Matre, Karen E. Koch, and Curtis P. McLaughlin*
9	Forthright Medical Center: Social Marketing and the Surgical Checklist	*Carol E. Breland*
14	Continuing Improvement for the National Health Service Quality and Outcomes Framework	*Curtis P. McLaughlin*
19	Cal Mason, COO, Metro Children's Hospital: Planned Experimentation in CQI	*Lloyd P. Provost*

REFERENCES

Balestracci, D. 2009. *Data Sanity: A Quantum Leap to Unprecedented Results.* Englewood, CO: Medical Group Management Association.

Berwick, D. M. 1991. Controlling variation in health care: A consultation from Walter Shewhart. *Medical Care*, 29: 1212–1225.

Berwick, D. M. 1996. A primer on leading the improvement of systems. *BMJ*, 312: 619–622.

Bialek, R., Duffy, G. L., and Moran, J. W. 2009. *The Public Health Quality Improvement Handbook.* Milwaukee, WI: ASQ Quality Press.

Bosk, C. L., Dixon-Woods, M., Goeschel, C. A., et al. 2009. The art of medicine— Reality check for checklists. *Lancet*, 374: 444–445.

Brassard, M. 1996. *The Memory Jogger Plus Featuring the Seven Management and Planning Tools.* Salem, NH: Goal/QPC.

Breyfogle, F. W. 2003. *Implementing Six Sigma: Smarter Solutions Using Statistical Methods* (2nd ed.). Hoboken, NJ: Wiley.

Brue, G. 2002. *Six Sigma for Managers.* New York: McGraw Hill.

Carey, R. G., and Lloyd, R. C. 2001. *Measuring Quality Improvement in Healthcare: A Guide to Statistical Control Applications.* Milwaukee, WI: American Society for Quality Press.

Deming, W. E. 1986. *Out of the Crisis.* Cambridge: Massachusetts Institute of Technology Center for Advanced Engineering Study.

Deming, W. E. 1993. *The New Economics for Industry, Government, Education.* Cambridge: Massachusetts Institute of Technology Center for Advanced Engineering Study.

de Vries, E. N., Prins, H. A., Crolla, R. M., et al. 2010. Effect of a comprehensive surgical safety system on patient outcomes. *N Engl J Med*, 363: 1928–1937.

Duffy, G. L., Farmer, E., and Moran, J. W. 2009. Applying Lean Six Sigma in public health. In Bialek, R., Duffy, G. L., and Moran, J. W. (Eds.), *The Public Health Quality Improvement Handbook.* Milwaukee, WI: ASQ Quality Press.

Gardner, E. S., Jr., and McLaughlin, C. P. 1980. Forecasting—A cost control tool for health care managers. *Health Care Manage Rev*, 5(3): 31–38.

Gawande, A. 2009. *The Checklist Manifesto.* New York: Metropolitan Books.

Gerteis, M., Edgman-Levitan, S., Daley, J., et al. (Eds.). 1993. *Through the Patient's Eyes: Understanding and Promoting Patient-Centered Care.* San Francisco: Jossey-Bass.

Gitlow, H., Gitlow, S., Oppenheim, A., et al. 1989. *Tools and Methods for the Improvement of Quality.* Homewood, IL: Irwin.

Gold, M. 2004. Geographic variation in Medicare per capita spending: Should policymakers be concerned? *Reseach Synthesis Report No. 6.* Princeton, NJ: The Robert Wood Johnson Foundation.

Griffin, F. A., and Resar, R. K. 2007. Trigger tool for measuring adverse events: IHI Innovation Series white paper. Cambridge, MA: Instiute for Healthcare Improvement. As cited in Landrigan, C. P., et al. 2010. *N Engl J Med*, 363(22): 2124–2134.

Haynes, A. B., Weiser, T. G., Berry, W. R., et al. 2009. A surgery safety checklist to reduce morbidity and mortality in a global population. *N Engl J Med*, 360: 491–499.

Institute of Medicine. 2000. *To Err Is Human: Building a Safer Health System.* Washington, DC: National Academies Press.

Ishikawa, K. 1987. *Guide to Quality Control* (trans. Asian Productivity Organization). White Plains, NY: Kraus International Publications.

James, B. 1989. *Quality Management for Healthcare Delivery.* Chicago: The Health Research and Educational Trust of the American Hospital Association.

Jencks, S. Cuerdon, T., Burwen, D. R., et al. 2000. Quality of medical care delivered to Medicare beneficiaries: A profile at state and national levels. *JAMA*, 284: 1670–1676.

Jencks, S., Huff, E. D., and Cuerdon, T. 2003. Change in the quality of care delivered to Medicare beneficiaries, 1998–1999 to 2000–2001. *JAMA*, 289: 305–312.

Johnson, S. P., Alemi, F., and Neuhauser, D. 1998. Rapid improvement teams. *Joint Commission J Quality Improve*, 24(3): 119–129.

Juran, J. 1988. *Juran on Planning for Quality.* New York: Free Press.

Kelly, D. L. 2003. *Applying Quality Management in Healthcare: A Process for Improvement.* Chicago: Health Administration Press.

Kilbridge, P., and Classen, D. 2002. Surveillance for Adverse Drug Events: History, Methods, and Current Issues. VHA Research Series.

Kleinbaum, D. G., Kupper, L., Nizam, A., and Mueller, K. E. 2008. *Applied Regression Analysis and Other Multivariable Methods* (4th ed.). Belmont, CA: Thomson/Cole.

Landrigan, C. P., Parry, G. J., Bones, C. B., et al. 2010. Temporal trends in rates of patient harm resulting from medical care. *N Engl J Med*, 363(22): 2124–2134.

Langley, G. J., Nolan, K. M., Nolan, T. W., et al. 2009. *Improvement Guide: A Practical Approach to Enhancing Organizational Performance* (2nd ed.). San Francisco: Jossey-Bass.

Leatherman, S., and McCarthy, D. 2002. *Quality of Care in the United States: A Chartbook.* New York: The Commonwealth Fund.

Lighter, D. E., and Fair, D. C. 2004. *Principles and Methods of Quality Management in Health Care.* Sudbury, MA: Jones and Bartlett Publishers.

McLaughlin, C. P. 1996. Why variation reduction is not everything: A new paradigm for service operations. *Int J Serv Ind Manage*, 7(3): 17–30.

McLaughlin, C. P., Johnson, J. K., and Sollecito, W. A. 2012. *Implementing Continuous Quality Improvement in Health Care: A Global Casebook.* Sudbury, MA: Jones & Bartlett Learning.

McLaughlin, C. P., and Kaluzny A. D. (Eds.). 2006. *Continuous Quality Improvement in Health Care* (3rd ed.). Sudbury, MA: Jones and Bartlett Publishers.

Nelson, E. C., Splaine, M. E., Batalden, P. B., et al. 1998. Building measurement and data collection into medical practice. *Ann Internal Med*, 128: 460–466.

Nolan, T. W., and Provost, L. P. 1990. Understanding variation. *Quality Progress*, 23(5): 70–78.

Office of the Inspector General. 2010. Adverse events in hospitals: Methods for identifying events. Washington, DC: Department of Health and Human Services, OEI-06-08-00221. As cited in Landrigan, C. P., et al. 2010. *N Engl J Med*, 363(22): 2124–2134.

Pande, P. S., Neuman, R. P., and Cavanagh, R. R. 2000. *The Six Sigma Way: How GE, Motorola and Other Top Companies Are Honoring Their Performance.* New York: McGraw–Hill.

Paton, S. M. 2002. Juran: A lifetime of quality. *Quality Digest*, August. Retrieved February 19, 2011, from http://www.qualitydigest.com/aug02/articles/01_article.shtml

Picker Institute Europe. 2003. Picker NHS Inpatient Questionnaire. Retrieved February 27, 2011, from http://www.pickereurope.org

Press Ganey Associates, Inc. 2001. Inpatient Survey, 2001. Retrieved February 27, 2011, from http://www.pressganey.com

Pronovost, P. J., Goeschel, C. A., Olsen, K. L., et al. 2009. Reducing health care hazards: Lessons from the commercial aviation safety team. *Health Affairs*, 283: w479–w489.

Pronovost, P. J., Needham, D., Berenholtz, S., et al. 2006. An intervention to reduce catheter-related bloodstream infections in the ICU. *N Engl J Med*, 355: 2725–2732.

Sharek P. J., Parry, G., Goldmann, D. A., et al. 2010. Performance characteristics of a methodology to quantify adverse events over time in hospitalized patients. *Health Serv Res.* August 16, 2010. Epub. As cited in Landrigan, C. P., et al. 2010. *N Engl J Med*, 363(22): 2124–2134.

Shewhart, W. A. 1931. *Economic Control of Quality of Manufactured Product.* New York: D. Van Nostrand Company.

Streibel, B. J., Sholtes, P. R., and Joiner, B. L. 2003. *The Team Handbook* (3rd ed.). Madison, WI: Joiner/Oriel, Inc.

Taylor, G. 2008. *Lean Six Sigma Service Excellence: A Guide to Green Belt Certification and Bottom Line Improvement.* New York: J. Ross Publishing.

Wheeler, D. J. 2000. *Understanding Variation: The Key to Managing Chaos.* Knoxville, TN: SPC Press.

CHAPTER 4

Understanding and Improving Team Effectiveness in Quality Improvement

Bruce Fried and William R. Carpenter

"There is no substitute for teamwork and good leaders of teams to bring consistency of effort along with knowledge."

—W. Edwards Deming (1986, p. 19)

Teams play a major part in all aspects of health care. In the area of quality improvement, the team is the primary vehicle through which problems are analyzed, solutions are generated, and change is evaluated. As introduced in Chapter 2, effective teamwork is a key factor influencing the diffusion and successful implementation of continuous quality improvement (CQI) in health care.

In this chapter, brief In-Practice cases are used to illustrate the potential of teams for fostering improvement in organizations, and the problems encountered when teams are poorly organized. **In-Practice 4–1** illustrates both the positive and negative potential of teams. State University Hospital (SUH) sought to assemble an integrated, multidepartmental team to address a complex problem involving many organizational components that rarely interacted in a concerted, coordinated manner.

Each department had developed systems addressing end-of-life records and documentation for its own processes, but because these were not integrated with the other departments' systems, all departments—indeed, the organization as a whole—experienced problems that were badly compounded by an unpredicted environmental change brought to light by State Donor Services (SDS). In its initial attempt to address the organ donation problem, the team was given inadequate time to get organized, leading to a production schedule that was unrealistic. The tight time frame did not provide adequate time to determine the composition of the team. Several members were inexperienced, and while they were supportive of the team's goals, they could not contribute in a significant way to the team's work. Senior management provided inadequate support to the team, neglecting to extend the authority of organization leaders to the team and its chair. This led some key team members to dismiss the team as inconsequential and to an overall lack of commitment.

IN-PRACTICE 4-1

State University Hospital and State Donor Services

State Donor Services (SDS) centrally manages the state's organ procurement and donation process. There had been a trend of declining organ availability for transplant, despite efforts to increase awareness and success in registering donors through the Division of Motor Vehicles. To help solve the problem, SDS approached State University Hospital (SUH), one of the biggest sources of and utilizers of donated organs through its renowned organ transplant programs. Initial exploration of the problem quickly indicated a consistent demand for organs, but organ donations at SUH were down, matching the pattern seen by SDS.

Chris Carter—the new administrator for SUH's emergency department—was asked to build a team to solve this problem for SUH. The hospital's Chief Operating Officer (COO) told Chris that this was a top priority because of the high visibility of the transplant programs, the revenues it brought to the institution,

(continues)

In-Practice 4–1

and the fact that the Chairman of Surgery had just threatened to leave the institution if SUH "didn't fix this problem it had obviously created." The COO gave Chris 2 weeks to get a team together and develop a solution, which Chris would present at SUH's monthly Executive Committee meeting. Chris asked the COO for advice regarding whom to have on the team, and the COO referred him to the Chief Nursing Officer (CNO).

Chris went immediately to the CNO, but the first available meeting time she had was in 3 days. In the meantime, Chris gathered as much information as possible. On the third day, the CNO's secretary called to cancel the meeting but suggested that he talk with the Nursing Division Director for Medicine. She met with Chris that afternoon, and together they formulated a list of people they thought would be able to address the issue. SUH was a functionally structured organization, so they built a team with nursing directors from each of the transplant services and the emergency department, the Director of Patient Care Services, a clerk and a physician from the emergency room, the State Medical Examiner—whose office was located at SUH and who was responsible for autopsies—and a clerk from his office.

The earliest possible meeting time for this group was in 3 weeks—well beyond the COO's deadline. Nonetheless, Chris set up a meeting with as many team members as possible and met with the others individually. Members from this team would be able to meet only once, or perhaps twice at most, given the aggressive deadline and members' schedules.

Fearing the approaching deadline and wanting to waste no time, Chris got right to business when the group met. He told the group his goals and invited an open discussion of each team member's experiences with organ procurement. It quickly became evident that several members of the team were too new or too junior to be helpful, with a few of Chris's invitees having asked more junior colleagues to be a part of the team in their stead. The Medical Examiner immediately called into question the validity of the group and the authority by which he had been called to this meeting. When Chris told

(continues)

In-Practice 4–1

him this was a high-priority project for the COO and CNO—stating only their names and not their titles—the Medical Examiner indignantly replied that he had never heard of these people and that this was a waste of his time. When Chris clarified their titles, the Medical Examiner became less vocal, but remained indignant. He had been focused on solving a problem of declining autopsies, which placed SUH at risk of violating a state regulation. He was angry to have been diverted from this pressing problem and felt that Chris's group would draw organizational focus and energies away from his own needs. His sourness spread to others in the group, which, coupled with their inexperience and a lack of appropriate representation, rendered the meeting—and the group—effectively useless.

In an effort to avoid a public display of this disaster, Chris reported his lack of success to the COO prior to the Executive Committee meeting. The COO realized the impossibility of the goals he had set for Chris. He extended the deadline 3 months and also extended the weight of his authority by agreeing to attend the next team meeting. These two key factors allowed Chris to rebuild a more appropriate, representative, and experienced team.

Ultimately, the organ donation problem was traced to a series of new federal regulations and SUH's fragmented approach to processing end-of-life paperwork. In summary, each operational unit had set in place its own processes for responding to the regulatory requirements, none of which were integrated with the other operational units, thus creating hours of work for the clinical staff, most of whom gave up trying to secure organ donations. Interestingly, the Medical Examiner's problem of a declining autopsy rate was also a result of this same disjointed method of paperwork processing.

These events at SUH exemplify the violation of many of the central tenets of building a successful, high-performing team. The situation was improved, however, as senior management became more involved, setting an appropriate timeline, changing membership, and articulating the importance of the team to the organization. As team composition and size were restructured to include the proper participants, senior management also granted the team visible and legitimate authority to undertake its tasks, and an environment of psychological safety was created where open communication was encouraged and individual team members could contribute with no risk of rebuke by others.

Teams exist everywhere in health care. Teams are used for virtually every activity carried out in health care organizations, including both clinical and management-focused activities. While medical knowledge is growing exponentially, the application of that knowledge to clinical service delivery is limited by the effectiveness and efficiency of teams charged with putting that knowledge into practice. Similarly, as new management techniques and technologies are developed, including quality improvement methods, successful use of these approaches is dependent upon appropriately staffed, well-functioning teams. Clearly, we have moved well beyond the era of the autonomous heroic clinician (or manager, for that matter). Behind every successful clinician or manager is a high-functioning team. And given what we know about the effectiveness of teams in most organizations, it can safely be said that the performance of virtually all clinicians and managers could be markedly improved by improvements in team effectiveness.

Teams also play a critical role in improving the performance of health care systems, whether a medical group practice, a hospital inpatient unit, a long-term care facility, or local public health departments. While effective patient care certainly requires that physicians possess current clinical knowledge, patient outcomes are dependent upon how well a patient care team works—whether team members understand and agree on patient care goals, how members communicate with each other, and the effectiveness of team leadership. In sum, teams are the building blocks of health care organizations and are absolutely essential to implementing an organizational strategy, caring for individual patients, designing and implementing a new information system, or identifying and solving quality problems. Teams are not an option but a necessity. As such, it makes great sense to examine these building blocks and see how they can be strengthened.

In this chapter, we use the concept of *team* very broadly, and borrow from the concept of the *microsystem* (Nelson et al., 2002). A microsystem is one of several subsystems of a larger system that is integral to system performance. This perspective, drawn from systems theory, is not a new concept but clearly helps us understand how the human body, an automobile, or an organization operates. When examining the performance or health of any system, it is essential to examine (among other factors) the effectiveness of each component subsystem (e.g., the respiratory system), how these subsystems communicate with each other and work together (e.g., the nature and adequacy of coordination between a hospital pharmacy and an inpatient unit), and the adequacy of information about system and subsystem performance (e.g., the extent to which the driver of an automobile is provided with information about the automobile's performance).

According to this view, a health system is composed of many subsystems. In the patient care arena, these may be referred to as *clinical microsystems* or *frontline systems,* referring to teams charged with meeting the needs of the patient population. It is these smaller microsystems that actually provide those services that result in positive patient outcomes, provider and patient safety, system efficiency, and patient satisfaction. And as is true with any large system, the effectiveness of any large health care system can be no better than the microsystems of which it is composed (Nelson et al., 2002).

Using the terminology of the microsystem, it is apparent how a microsystem is in fact one type of team, as defined by Nelson et al. (2002):

> A clinical microsystem is a small group of people who work together on a regular basis to provide care to discrete subpopulations of patients. It has clinical and business aims, linked processes, and a shared information environment, and it produces performance outcomes. Microsystems evolve over time and are often embedded in larger organizations. They are complex adaptive systems, and as such they must do the primary work associated with core aims, meet the needs of internal staff, and maintain themselves over time as clinical units. (p. 474)

This definition may be slightly altered to apply to all other types of teams in health care. The key concepts in relation to teams are as follows:

- People work together toward specific goals.
- They use multiple interconnected processes.
- They produce performance outcomes.
- They have access to information about the team's performance.

In addition, such teams must adapt to changing circumstances, ensure the satisfaction of team members, and maintain and improve their performance over time.

In this chapter, we bring together classical research and theory about teams with recent work on clinical microsystems. We demonstrate how our knowledge of teams informs our understanding of team performance and the role of teams in quality improvement efforts. Chapters 9 and 13 provide further in-depth discussion of clinical microsystems, emphasizing their role in improving quality and safety.

TEAMS IN HEALTH CARE

As medical knowledge grows increasingly complex and the medical specialties continue to develop around specific focus areas of that knowledge, there is a risk that health care organizations will lose their patient-centered orientation. There is a paradox in relation to the adoption of new medical technologies and procedures. On the one hand, increasingly specific diagnostic and treatment procedures imply a narrowing of focus. This is desirable because we all support the discovery and implementation of procedures to improve the accuracy and specificity of diagnoses and the development of pharmaceuticals, technology, and procedures that treat a disease in a manner that is most specific to the individual and the disease state. However, to diagnose, treat, and follow up with a patient requires information from multiple sources and, very often, the involvement of multiple individuals. For example, psychopharmacology is becoming increasingly specific and sophisticated. However, better utilization of new pharmaceuticals for the benefit of the patient requires that psychiatrists have an understanding of patients' home environments. Moreover, a team of individuals (e.g., social worker, psychiatric nurse) is likely required to ensure that patients are compliant and that home support and respite services are available to caregivers. Thus, the need for patient-centered multispecialty teams becomes ever more important as health care providers and organizations strive to deliver the best care possible.

Health care system complexity extends beyond the clinical care arena and into administrative areas. Teams fill an organizational need of helping to identify and respond to such changes, as health care organizations continue to operate in environments with increased regulation and oversight, ever more complex payer contracts, and increasing pressure for cost-effective and efficient operations.

At the most basic level, clinical health care teams are comprised of health care providers—and, in some cases, nonclinical personnel—from multiple disciplines, focusing on a patient or a group of patients with similar health care needs. This patient-centeredness has extended upward and outward to all aspects of many health care organizations. Indeed, the industry has seen a trend away from organizational structures based on functional areas of technical expertise (e.g., nursing, environmental services, registration, medicine, surgery) and toward functionally integrated organizational structures with clinical care teams based on patient needs (e.g., children's services, women's services, cancer care services). The individual clinical specialists serving on these teams report not only to their disciplinary head (e.g., chief of nursing, chair of medicine), but also to team leaders associated with specific patient-centered service areas. This "dual reporting" format is described in organizational management literature as a matrix structure (Grove, 1995; Shortell and Kaluzny, 2006).

While the multidisciplinary team model has been adopted by patient-centered health care organizations, these teams and supporting organizational structures do not spontaneously form, nor are they easily managed. Given the functional nature of most health care organizations, there are clear forces working against the formation and maintenance of teams. As discussed later in this chapter, reward systems are typically designed around performance of one's particular discipline, rather than a team focus. Where teams do exist, performance is, more often than not, suboptimal. A substantial body of research demonstrates that key elements are necessary for teams to perform to their maximum potential (Hackman, 2002). If these elements are not attended to, teams can easily exhibit poor communication, member dissatisfaction, patient dissatisfaction, disjointed care provision, and inefficient and ineffective operations nested in a cumbersome bureaucracy.

HIGH-PERFORMANCE TEAMS AND QUALITY IMPROVEMENT

The focus of this chapter is on the importance of high-performing teams to quality improvement efforts and on approaches to improve the outcomes produced by teams. The value of teams was established in the earliest applications of quality improvement as a way to improve input and output at any stage and as a means of ensuring multidisciplinary sharing of knowledge and ideas for improvement (Deming, 1986). In modern health care, teams are critical to success in quality improvement for a number of reasons.

1. Quality problems are often not visible to individuals at senior management levels, but the impact of problems can be experienced by the entire organization, as seen in the organ donation case (In-Practice 4–1). Hospital staff nurses, for example, may see repeated examples of poor communications between shifts that result in a myriad of problems for patients and families, physicians, and other hospital staff. Each occurrence of a problem may be dealt with, but in aggregate, communication problems become costly in terms of time, quality, and continuity of care. It is the individuals doing the work, or those within the clinical microsystem, who are most aware of problems that have become systemic in nature and that require systematic solutions. The farther one is from the front line of care, the more removed one is from seeing day-to-day problems. Thus, if we wish to identify quality problems, we need individuals on our teams who are close to the problem and understand its manifestation and nuances.

2. Individuals involved in a dysfunctional process are usually those who are most knowledgeable about the process and its context. Much of quality improvement involves process analysis and process improvement. To understand a process, it is essential to have participation from individuals who have the best, most detailed understanding of the process. What appears on paper as a theoretical process flowchart may be quite inaccurate when compared to how a process actually operates.

3. Individuals at the front lines often have the most feasible suggestions for improvement. It has long been known that individuals at relatively low levels of the organization often acquire considerable expertise and, in some cases, power. A receptionist in a pediatric group practice, for example, may have a very clear understanding of why waiting times are unacceptably long at certain times. Because of this individual's many years of experience in this position, he or she may also have developed an understanding of how the practice operates and may have valuable suggestions about how scheduling and staffing may be altered to help ameliorate the waiting time problem.

If we are interested in solving such a problem, it is important to have individuals on a team who both understand the problem and can suggest interventions that are both effective and feasible.

4. Addressing quality problems requires the support of all individuals in the organization, not simply those at a senior level. Identifying and proposing solutions to quality problems is key to quality improvement efforts, but unless those involved in solution implementation understand fully the rationale for the effort, implementation is likely to fall short. Quality improvement initiatives cannot simply be handed off to a team for implementation. Those involved in implementing the solution must be involved so that they understand the quality improvement strategy and can identify possible obstacles to effective implementation.

5. High-functioning teams empower people by providing opportunities for meaningful participation in problem identification and problem solving. Participants feel they are contributing in a positive way to the success of the organization, and more than simply through their particular discipline. Among the consequences of empowerment is that people feel greater commitment to the organization and exhibit a sense of ownership. Together, these consequences promote in people a greater willingness to identify quality problems and participate in developing and implementing solutions.

As seen in the introductory organ donation example, the well-intentioned manager tasked with solving an institution-wide problem was unable to compose his team of the most appropriate members; thus, the team was unable to realize these benefits, was unable to become a high-performing team, and was unable to reach its goals. The manager's inability to build an appropriate team was, in turn, a function of an unrealistic timeline and a lack of initial support by senior management. Given a second chance, and provided with a more appropriate timeline and sufficient authority, the manager built a team of individuals with appropriate experience and organizational diversity; this team was able to develop, perform, and reach its goals. Such well-designed and well-managed teams can maximize communication, collaboration, patient and staff satisfaction, and effective and efficient clinical care provision in an organization that is continually able to adapt and improve in the changing environment.

How do we develop and sustain high-performing quality improvement teams? There is much that we know about successful teams, and while there is no guarantee that using all of the concepts and recommendations in this chapter will bring success, the chapter provides a framework to use to assess the likelihood of team success and guide intervention in specific areas to improve performance.

UNDERSTANDING AND IMPROVING THE PERFORMANCE OF QUALITY IMPROVEMENT TEAMS

In this section, we present information about teams and their management, relate the information specifically to the area of quality improvement teams, and use our case examples to illustrate selective concepts and principles.

The Task

The particular task given a group affects many other aspects of team management, such as team size and team composition, and the manner in which decisions are made. Most quality improvement teams are faced with the task, generally speaking, of engaging in the PDCA cycle: Planning, Doing, Checking, Acting (see Chapter 1). They are typically also involved in problem analysis and often in identifying alternative courses of action. The clarity of the task as well as the authority of the team to carry out the PDCA cycle is very important. Related to this, the team must have a shared understanding of the goals of the team.

Although certain types of teams have clear and self-evident goals, quality improvement teams may face ambiguity. Most commonly, teams are unclear about their authority to implement change. Does a team have the authority to make decisions about change or simply to make recommendations? There is no magic answer to this question; many highly variable factors ranging from organizational priorities to intraorganizational dynamics to environmental changes may drive such a decision. What is most important is that teams have a clear understanding of their goals and their authority, whatever those goals and that authority may be. It is disheartening and demotivating for a team to think it has the authority to implement a change only to face the reality that the team is intended simply to suggest or recommend. Goals do sometimes change in quality improvement efforts, particularly as more fundamental problems are identified that underlie the presenting problems.

As illustrated in the Greenwood Family Medicine example (see **In-Practice 4–2**), goal definition presents a problem. The initial goal in this situation was to improve the provision of preventive services. However, little analytic effort was spent trying to understand the important causes of this problem. The team adopted a premature solution, and the goal drifted away from improving preventive service rates to constructing and implementing a preventive services chart. While such a chart may have been useful as part of the solution to the performance gap in preventive services, the team became fixated on this as the solution, at the expense of generating other additional alternatives. Implementing a solution became the goal, losing the initial focus on the problem of low preventive services rates. Team member time was spent constructing a tool instead of trying to understand the fundamental causes of the problem. Basically, a "solution" presented itself, and the solution became the goal in itself. A key problem faced as a result of this is that the team did not work on what seemed to be a very major problem facing the practice, namely, the variation in protocols for preventive services. The team also did not sufficiently examine the problem of record keeping and never did come to an understanding of whether their rates were really low or whether the problem was an artifact of poor record keeping. The use of a cause- and-effect diagram (see Chapter 3) may have helped, and most importantly, effective leadership may have kept the team on task and focused on its primary goal.

Team Characteristics

Team characteristics refer to basic physical and psychological aspects of a team and include team composition and size, team relationships and status differences, psychological safety, team norms, and the stage of team development. Each characteristic is discussed next.

Team Composition and Size

What is the optimal team size? This answer obviously depends upon the nature of the team, its goals, and tasks. In some cases, team size and composition are mandated. Examples of this include sports teams and accreditation teams. Teams must be sufficiently large to have the requisite

IN-PRACTICE 4-2

Preventive Services at Greenwood Family Medicine

Greenwood Family Medicine is a five-clinician family medicine practice serving a largely middle-class suburban population. In addition to the medical staff, the practice employs four nurses, one receptionist, and three medical records and insurance technicians.

The practice recently identified two priority areas: attention to family concerns and greater emphasis on ensuring the provision of timely preventive services. The latter effort was prompted by one of the physicians, who had recently attended a continuing medical education program on preventive services. Upon her return, she decided to assess the practice's provision of preventive services.

With a nurse and one of the medical records technicians, she reviewed a sample of children's patient charts. She and the other physicians were surprised when she distributed the results:

- Half of the children were behind schedule in at least one immunization.
- Vision screening was noted on no patient charts.
- Fifty percent of children had had anemia screening.
- Twenty-five percent of children had their blood pressure recorded in the chart.
- Fifteen percent had had tuberculosis screening.
- Thirteen percent of children had been screened for lead.

The medical staff was surprised by these findings, but medical records personnel and nursing staff found this information consistent with their impressions. The review indicated that even children who were seen for an annual physical were often not updated on preventive services—or this information was not recorded in the patient chart. It was felt that high patient volume made it impossible to ensure that appropriate preventive services were provided to all children. In addition, the practice saw many drop-in patients. The nurses felt that while these drop-ins caused added tension

(continues)

In-Practice 4–2

from the increased workload, they also presented an opportunity to check on preventive services needs.

The findings were discussed at the monthly meeting for all staff, and it was decided to form a team to address the problem. A medical records technician was asked to schedule a meeting. It was decided that two nurses and four physicians would participate on this team.

The first meeting was scheduled over the noon hour (12:00 PM to 1:00 PM). One physician arrived at 12:20, while another had to leave early, at 12:45. Virtually the entire meeting was spent attempting to find an appropriate date and time for follow-up meetings.

At the next meeting, the physicians stated that during an acute visit, physicians simply do not have time to go through the chart to determine if a patient needs updating on preventive services. It was decided, therefore, that the nurses would review each chart for the day's patients and fasten a form listing all preventive services. Services needing updating would be circled. The medical records staff was asked to design this form.

When the physicians saw the resulting form, they felt it was poorly designed. Some services were not included, and immunization schedule information was not included. The physicians asked the medical records technician to redesign the form. The technician and a nurse added the immunization schedule and other information. When presented to the physicians, they discovered disagreements in several areas. Immunization schedules differed, and practices varied on lead and TB screening. They decided that the form should include separate columns for each physician, each column specifying a physician's preventive services preferences. A form was created reflecting each physician's preventive service preferences.

After the new preventive services chart was developed, the nurses expressed concern about the lack of time available to record preventive services needs but agreed reluctantly to start reviewing charts and entering preventive service information on

(continues)

In-Practice 4–2

each chart. After 6 weeks of working with this system, the following events unfolded:

- Nurses complained that medical records staff were not making charts available in time to do the preventive services review.
- Physicians complained among themselves that preventive service information was incomplete or inaccurate in more than 50% of the cases.
- Nurses were spending an additional 1 to 2 hours in the office preparing the next day's files and complained that the charts were very hard to decipher. The nurses requested, and were denied, overtime pay. One nurse left the practice.
- Confusion was rampant when charts were prepared for one physician but another physician actually saw the patient. This caused increased patient waiting time. An even more difficult problem was caused by drop-ins for whom the record review was not prepared. Nurses spent up to 30 minutes reviewing drop-in charts and recording relevant information. Backlogs resulted, and nurses neglected their other roles.
- The system was eliminated, and physicians decided to independently deal with preventive services.

expertise, but not so large that they are cumbersome and difficult to manage. A team size of seven is a general rule of thumb, although this number is derived from experience rather than scientific evidence. In the Greenwood Family Medicine example, the team faced multiple problems because of its large size: scheduling meetings, keeping order during meetings, establishing a protocol for discussion, and decision making.

Interestingly, although the team was too large, it in fact did not have all of the expertise required to address the preventive services problem. Specifically, the medical records staff, who foresaw the difficulties with the new system, were not included on the team—even to selectively provide input or react to proposed solutions. When deciding upon team composition, one needs to consider the tasks facing the team. For example, if information is required about information technology, it would naturally be helpful to have someone knowledgeable in this area. In the Greenwood Family Medicine case, abstracting information from medical records was a key aspect of the intervention. Medical records staff familiar with the structure of the medical record could have contributed substantially to the design of this intervention.

Team size therefore goes hand-in-hand with group composition. The team must have adequate diversity and expertise to inform all necessary aspects of the team's tasks and goals. Yet the team must not be so large that reaching consensus or following an appropriate timeline is impossible. In Greenwood Family Medicine, it would have been advisable to cut the team size by 50% and ask team members to consult and obtain input from their constituencies about the team's work.

Team Relationships and Status

A central tenet of quality improvement is participation of all team members. We often learn of quality problems and solutions from individuals without formal authority in the team or organization. In fact, it is often those on the front lines—people working within the clinical microsystem—who have a unique perspective on a situation. Involving appropriate people is only the first step, however. In any team, people bring with them their roles and status from regular organizational life. Physicians working on a team with nurses bring with them their higher professional status and authority. The physician–nurse relationship is thus "imported" into the team. These preformed relationships and status systems influence the effectiveness of a team. The most obvious example is that of status differences stifling participation. Individuals from a lower status group are less likely to contribute than those of higher status. They may feel condescended to or intimidated, or they may simply feel that their input is not valued. For quality improvement teams, such status differences are dysfunctional. Quality improvement team leaders need to find a way to diminish the impact of status differences.

As discussed in Chapter 17, the important role of nurses as equals on quality improvement teams should not be underestimated. For example, this recognition has contributed to the important leadership role of nurses in the implementation of surgical safety checklists (Gawande, 2009).

Team members also bring with them other aspects of interrelationships from outside the team. We may find two individuals with a history of interpersonal problems serving on the same team. Unfortunately, relationship problems and dysfunctional status differences can dramatically affect the work of a team. It is truly the remarkable team that can dispose of status differences and interpersonal animosities in the interest of team goals. At the very least, team leaders need to be aware of the presence of status differences and the impact of those differences on communication and team effectiveness. One way to avoid the problems of status difference and interpersonal conflict is to have a team leader with sufficient authority and respect act as moderator, encouraging lower status members to participate, keeping higher status members in check, and defusing tension driven by team member conflict.

Quality improvement teams often come together amidst great enthusiasm about tackling a difficult problem. However, the work of a group may create frictions and bring to the surface latent conflicts or reignite old disputes. Interprofessional rivalries may also surface in quality improvement teams, and multidisciplinary teams should explicitly agree to put aside such conflicts. Otherwise, a substantial amount of work time will likely be spent managing these conflicts. Quality improvement teams, like other teams, are also prone to personality clashes that may be very destructive to the work of a team. Health care is particularly prone to difficulties posed by status differences because of the traditional professional hierarchy that is still maintained in most organizations.

In Greenwood Family Medicine, status differences were destructive to the work of the group. First, medical records staff were not included, likely because they were considered nonprofessional staff and their perspectives and opinions were therefore discounted. Status differences, with likely elements of intimidation, also prevented both nurses and medical records staff from voicing their reservations about the use of the preventive services chart. There was also tension and status differences between the two "high-volume" physicians and others in the practice. These differences were not beneficial to the work of the team.

Psychological Safety

Team psychological safety is defined as a shared belief that the team is safe for interpersonal risk taking (Edmonson, 1999). A central tenet of quality improvement is the belief that people must be forthcoming and honest about quality problems. Individuals involved in improvement efforts must feel that their suggestions will be heard without fear of intimidation, condescension, or castigation (Deming, 1986). Where people feel this safety, there is a greater likelihood of their participating effectively in quality improvement efforts. Furthermore, psychological safety is an important prerequisite for implementing organizational change. People need to feel psychologically safe if they are to feel secure and capable of changing (Schein and Bennis, 1965).

Status differences certainly affect psychological safety. Where status differences have an oppressive presence, it is very unlikely that team participants will feel the willingness to participate in discussions of quality. In the Greenwood Family Medicine case, the medical records staff had a clear sense that the preventive services chart plan was doomed to failure, but felt uninvited. Although they voiced reservations about the plan privately, they did not feel psychologically safe to voice their concerns. More than likely, they would have been criticized by others in the practice for being negative, resistant to change, or perhaps lazy. This is similar to the Donor Services case (In-Practice 4–1), where many of the lower status team members were reluctant to participate actively or positively given the negative and highly vocal nature of the Medical Examiner, a higher status individual with whom many of the team members had to work on a daily basis. They felt that if they didn't follow his lead in the team meetings, they would incur repercussions later.

Team leaders need to consider questions of psychological safety: Do participants feel safe in making recommendations, participating in discussions, and perhaps of greatest importance, expressing skepticism and disagreement? It is only by creating such a climate that team members will not become "yes-men" and "yes-women."

Team Norms

A norm is a standard of behavior that is shared by team members. Norms have a strong impact on individuals in organizations, essentially establishing the "rules" under which people function. Norms set expectations and establish standards of behavior and performance. Behavioral norms consist of the rules that govern the work of individuals. In a team context, behavioral norms might designate how people are expected to participate on a team, attendance at meetings, the type of language and dress that are acceptable, and the use of formal procedures (e.g., Robert's

Rules of Order). Norms are different in every team. In Greenwood Family Medicine, we see the interaction between status differences and norms. Although there was likely a superficial belief in the desirability of a democratic and participative climate, it was clear that among the behavioral norms of the team was that of hierarchy. For example, nurses were directed to produce a form (and then several versions), and physicians declared the termination of the quality improvement initiative. Norms about attendance at meetings were very loose—at least for the medical staff. One meeting, in which arguments ensued about whether the preventive services issue was officewide or specific to the physicians, ended with no conclusion, summary, or future plans. Evidently, norms were never established for how meetings would be conducted or expectations for attendance. Collectively, these were dysfunctional norms. Participation was inhibited, full discussion of issues was repressed, and meetings were inefficient and ineffective.

In contrast to behavioral norms, performance norms govern the amount and quality of work expected of team members. In the Greenwood Family Medicine case, performance norms were broken, leading to difficulties for the practice. While there were expectations about working hours for nurses, the new preventive services chart system caused them to work up to 3 hours after regular working hours. This change in work demand was not anticipated, and breaking this performance norm caused morale problems and the departure of at least one nurse.

Stage of Team Development

Teams go through various life cycle stages, and different tasks and levels of productivity characterize each stage. We can conveniently think of teams going through four stages: forming, storming, norming, and performing. A team begins in the forming stage when goals and tasks are established. It is characterized by generally polite behavior among team members, which may mask underlying conflicts. Individuals often do not feel psychologically safe at this time and may be reluctant to contribute and unlikely to disagree. Team members, still unclear about the norms of the team, may stand back until they get a sense of the team.

When team members begin to feel more comfortable, there is usually a period of "storming," which may be mild or severe. Team members may compete for roles, may argue about team goals and processes, or may simply attempt to stake their ground.

If the team resolves its storming stage (which does not always happen), a norming stage emerges in which there is agreement on team norms and expectations. Team member roles are clarified, although these may change during the life of a team.

Following the norming stage is a performing stage in which the team is in the best position to accomplish its goals. Conflicts have been resolved, roles are clear, norms are established, and team time can be spent on the substantive work of the team rather than on resolving issues of process.

Teams can function at all stages of their development. However, at earlier stages, much energy is lost to "process loss"—that is, focusing the team's energies and time on team maintenance functions rather than on the substantive work of the team. Teams are most effective when they have matured, meaning they have successfully progressed through the first three stages and are able to focus on team goals and tasks.

What stage of development did the Greenwood Family Medicine team reach? The team assembled for the preventive services improvement project included virtually all members of the practice. This team did not show evidence of maturity. Norms of behavior were unclear (for example, attendance at meetings), decision making and rules for discussion were not well developed, and perhaps most importantly, role relationships among participants still reflected their roles in the practice. Physicians assumed a rather superior role in the practice, which may or may not have been appropriate. On the improvement team, however, such a role was clearly inappropriate and blocked the team from accessing information needed to address the preventive services problem. It is likely that the events that transpired in this case could have been predicted from observing the team in its normal operations.

RESOURCES AND SUPPORT

As open systems, teams require resources in order to survive and flourish. Resources come in a number of forms, including financial resources; intellectual resources; information; people with the necessary knowledge, skills, and abilities; equipment; communication systems; and moral support and credibility. Furthermore, individual team members require support, including recognition for their work on the team and rewards for their performance. At the most fundamental level, a team functions best when ensconced within an organization that supports the concept of teamwork and, more specifically, respects the work done by the team. We begin our discussion of resources and support at this level, which we refer to as organizational culture.

Organizational Culture

Many definitions have been suggested for organizational culture. Broadly speaking, organizational culture refers to the fabric of values, beliefs, assumptions, myths, norms, goals, and visions that are widely shared in the organization (French, 1998). An organization can have a single culture, although there are often subcultures within the organization. Among health care organizations, for example, we would expect to see cultural differences between a large teaching hospital and a small rural medical practice. Within an organization, teams themselves can develop their own culture; as with ethnic cultures, these organizational cultures may include rituals, a specific language, particular modes of communication, and unique systems of rewards and sanctions.

Organizational culture has a number of implications for teams. First, effective teams are usually characterized by strong cultures that are supportive of the work of the team. In a quality improvement team, for example, we would hope to see a culture characterized by interdisciplinary respect, open communication, and a collective spirit. It would be very difficult to imagine a successful quality improvement team that does not share these and other cultural characteristics. As described in Chapter 2, these same characteristics, in addition to others, such as systems thinking, contribute to an overall "culture of excellence" that will sustain ongoing quality improvement at the larger organizational level. However, a team can have an appropriate culture but be enmeshed within an organization with a contrary culture. Kiassi et al. (2004) report that organizations select those quality improvement programs that fit with their existing cultures.

Consider an organization characterized by intense and dysfunctional competition, low staff participation in decision making, and interprofessional rivalries and antagonism. We can consider this type of organization as having a dissonant culture (Fleeger, 1993). Notwithstanding the skills of an effective team leader, can we really expect team members drawn from such an environment to perform effectively on a multidisciplinary team? More than likely, team member attitudes would mirror their attitudes and behaviors outside the team. Team members would probably exhibit distrust, a "them vs. us" norm, and skepticism about their role in decision making. Consider the behavior and attitudes of team members drawn from a positive or consonant culture. We would expect team members to bring with them the very supportive cultural attributes of the larger organization; this would contribute to team growth and performance. We can see how the larger organizational culture can be viewed as a resource: The larger culture can be highly supportive, unsupportive, or in fact destructive to the work of the team.

Cultures are very difficult to change, so team leaders and participants must understand the impact of the culture of the larger organization on the work and culture of the team. Team members' negative or dysfunctional attitudes may simply reflect how they are treated in the larger organization. Team leaders should acknowledge the difficulty of leading a participative improvement team within a larger organizational culture that is nonparticipative and autocratic. Staff who work in a rigid, overbearing culture are likely to become skeptical when suddenly asked to participate in decision making, wondering whether their opinions will be valued, and so forth. CQI efforts in health care often confront this contradictory culture issue, experiencing the difficulties of attempting to introduce a culture that is inconsistent with the dominant organizational culture.

In the state regulatory agency case (see **In-Practice 4–3**), there was a culture that stressed the importance of customer relations. Great value was placed on the need to provide accurate and timely information. The team that was formed to analyze and make recommendations about the problem of providing inaccurate information was motivated by the same belief in the importance of its service mission. Complaints from customers about poor information were greeted with sincere concern. In no case were attempts made to discount the truthfulness of these complaints.

Material and Nonmaterial Support and Recognition

Regardless of their function, effective teams require material resources. As noted previously, material resources come in a number of forms and vary depending on the purposes and needs of the team. Provision of necessary material and nonmaterial support to a team is a reflection of the moral support and encouragement given a team by the larger organization and, in particular, senior management or other authority. Consider a team that is given appropriate space and time to meet, where senior managers

IN-PRACTICE 4–3

Erroneous Information at a State Regulatory Agency

The Department of Health and Emergency Services is a state regulatory agency dealing with a variety of health care professional issues. Its roles include credentialing emergency medical service (EMS) personnel, providers, and educational institutions; developing and enforcing administrative code; and serving as a primary collection point for statewide EMS data. Among its most important roles is responding to requests for information about credentialing requirements for health and EMS personnel. These requests come from physicians, hospitals, EMS providers, city and county governments, and other organizations.

The agency has one main office and three regional offices. The main office has 30 staff members; each regional office is staffed by 5 to 7 people. Each regional office has a regional manager reporting to the Operations Section Chief. Since each regional office serves approximately one-third of the state, the volume of requests can be overwhelming. Each staff member is responsible for serving as primary contact for 8 to 14 counties.

The agency recently learned that a significant amount of inaccurate information has been distributed by regional staff. The agency learned about this problem from complaints that inaccurate and contradictory information had been given out. For example, a hospital requested information about how nurses could challenge the EMS exam. The hospital was informed that nurses could challenge the EMS exam when in fact agency policy prohibits any health care provider from challenging a credentialing exam.

In response to this problem, the agency director formed an education/credentialing team with one liaison in each regional office and the team leader in the main office. The team's goals included improving consistency among the three regional offices, ensuring accurate information distribution, and educating regional staff on agency policy. In addition to the team leader and regional office liaisons, the team also included members representing each specialty within the agency. These specialists would provide

(continues)

In-Practice 4–3

technical information about their particular specialty and serve as the primary contact for regional offices in their area of expertise.

The team met monthly for 12 months to discuss issues and develop policy. One of its first tasks was to determine the underlying reason(s) for its information dissemination problem. The team obtained information from its membership and through discussions with other staff in the state and regional offices, EMS providers, physicians, and educational institutions. Information was obtained through formal and informal discussions, surveys, and a Web-based forum.

Among the team's discoveries was that staff did not have clear channels of communication with senior management and were not informed about changes in regulatory requirements. The team also learned that regional office staff were trying to be "experts" in too many different fields.

The team suggested a number of changes, including the following:

- Each regional staff member will be assigned an area of specialization; thus, each member will serve the entire region instead of 8 to 14 counties. For example, one provider specialist would be the primary point of contact for all provider issues for the entire regional office.
- Each of these specialists will serve as the regional office representative on all statewide and intra-agency committees that focus on that area of specialization.
- Each regional manager will serve on a committee with senior management that will meet monthly to ensure that up-to-date information is distributed to each regional office.

These changes were implemented at the state and regional offices. Mandatory committee attendance was difficult because of statewide travel restrictions and budget shortfalls. These obstacles were overcome by using advanced computer technology and telecommunications. Other obstacles included changes in job descriptions

(continues)

In-Practice 4–3

that were resisted by several "old timers." Their fears were eased by giving them an opportunity to assist with writing their job description.

Six months after these changes were put in place, the distribution of incorrect credentialing information dramatically decreased. Specialists in the regional offices actively consulted other specialists to learn about current policy in their area. An informal telephone survey found consistent information dissemination from each regional office. Among the most successful strategies was formation of teams. This promoted consistency in information exchange and developed interagency communication between all regional offices and the main office. It was also felt that success was attributed in large part to the manner in which team members were selected and how the teams functioned.

The team concept has continued to grow within the agency, and currently every staff member within the agency serves on at least one team. Some members serve on several teams and have taken on additional work responsibilities because the team approach has provided them the opportunity to have a strong voice within the agency. Senior leadership was careful not to push the team approach too fast and did not force anyone to join a team right away. Since the education team was formed first, management emphasized the work that team performed and allowed the education team to provide monthly updates to staff. This helped show that voice is important within the agency and that if staff members work together as a team, the team will have a significant influence on agency policy as well as administrative code.

on occasion voluntarily drop in on team meetings to provide information or simply to reinforce the importance of a team's task, and where support staff are assigned to the team to assist in its work. Furthermore, while the team is given a specific mandate and set of goals, the team decides the manner in which it carries out most of its work. Finally, upon presenting a preliminary report, detailed feedback and questions are provided the team. In all likelihood, team members will feel as if their work is valued and that the team's work is indeed making a contribution to the larger organization. Consistent with the motivational and satisfying qualities of jobs defined in the Job Characteristics Model, such a team provides members with autonomy, feedback, a sense of meaningfulness, and a belief that their work is having a broad impact (Hackman and Oldham, 1980). In sum, giving teams appropriate support can be highly motivating. Where this support is absent or ambiguous, teams will be starved for support and will be unlikely to produce at an optimal level.

The state regulatory agency case (In-Practice 4–3) provides a good example of how a team was provided with adequate support. Perhaps the most important resource provided was the time and energy of various individuals internal and external to the agency. Time was provided for team meetings, and team members felt that the work they were doing was worthwhile and valued by others in the larger organization. Where travel restrictions posed obstacles to team members meeting, computer technology—telecommunications and teleconferencing—was used. This again reinforced the importance not only of the team's work but also of the importance of each team member's contributions.

Rewards

Related to support and recognition is the need for team and individual rewards. From the perspective of the team, rewards typically come in the form of recognition and commendation for the team's work. In quality improvement, team rewards usually consist of the intrinsic satisfaction of achieving results. Rewards may also consist of the positive feelings created by a successful team effort.

In addition to team rewards, individuals on teams need to be rewarded. Participation on teams is often thought of as something of a voluntary effort, that it is not a part of a staff member's "real job." Job descriptions themselves may indicate little about team participation. Performance appraisals may not include team participation criteria, and compensation and promotion decisions may not take into consideration a staff member's contribution to the work of a team.

A team-oriented organization will be more likely to recognize individual contributions on teams. Performance appraisal and incentive pay programs will explicitly consider team member contributions. Such systems may actually elicit performance feedback from team members and leaders. If team meetings are to be held after normal work hours, appropriate compensation is provided.

Rewards are therefore important from the perspective of both the team and its individual members. Like individuals, teams are motivated by appropriate recognition and rewards. Individuals working on teams should receive the message that their participation on teams is important, necessary, and a key part of their jobs.

Members of the state regulatory agency team from In-Practice 4–3 were able to see the consequences of their work, namely, a substantial decrease in the amount of erroneous information provided and better relations with their customers. Team members also saw their recommendations put into action, which communicated to team members the value of the team's work. This set the stage for a more team-focused agency and the likelihood that future team efforts would meet with success.

TEAM PROCESSES

Team processes refer to those aspects of the team dealing with leadership, communication, decision making, and member and team learning. Each of these factors can have an important impact on the effectiveness of a team.

Team Leadership

Leadership in teams refers to the ability of individuals to influence other members toward the achievement of the team's goals. Note the use of the word *individuals* rather than *leader*; as will be discussed, an individual with no formal authority may emerge as a leader and influence member behavior. This concept was first introduced in Chapter 2, where it was noted that leaders within a team can include scientific experts but also well-respected opinion leaders and champions for change and improvement.

There is no single model of leadership that is appropriate for all teams. Depending on the team's purpose, leadership may be focused on one individual or it may be shared or rotated among team members. Teams also have formal and informal leaders. A sports team, for example, may have a coach or manager, but there clearly can be informal leaders, usually not specifically appointed as such, but nevertheless assuming a leadership function. A multidisciplinary health care team may have a nominal team leader, but typically power and authority flow to that person (or persons) with specialized expertise. There are therefore numerous sources of leadership and power.

Consider the case of Jones Hospital (see **In-Practice 4–4**), which has many different, unique programs and program leaders with specific clinical expertise. These providers sometimes work independently, but more often than not work in concert to collaboratively provide multidisciplinary care for a heterogeneous oncology patient population. While these individuals guide their individual programs' operations on a daily basis, these program leaders are unified under the constructs of the Strategic Governance Council and the Program Meeting, where the roles and influence of each are formalized, and they are each able to communicate in a fairly respectful and egalitarian environment. These forums provide information to the Oncology Leadership Group, which distills the information of the larger forums into guiding principles and strategies for oncology services as a whole. While the Leadership Group has a physician head who holds authority within the group, it is not possible to say that this position holds unilaterally directive authority over all the programs. The position and indeed the group serve to integrate the perspectives and needs of the multidisciplinary programs and as such provide continuity and uniformity of vision, strategy, and upward and outward communication for oncology services as they seek to continuously improve clinical care and the health care experience for the oncology patient population.

Where a team task is clear and unambiguous, a top-down leadership style may be justified, although even in such settings, input from team members may be valuable. In essence, the role of a leader in such a situation is to see that the job is done and that team members communicate and coordinate their work. In the quality improvement area, however, leadership must take on a different look. Quality improvement is by definition ambiguous and is largely a problem-solving process. Team members participate on a quality improvement team because they have expertise relevant to the problem. Team members do not need to be told what to do, but rather to participate actively in identifying problems, analyzing causation, developing interventions, evaluating the impact of change, and so forth. Team members are brought onto a quality improvement team because no single person has the expertise to solve a particular problem. Team member passivity is most definitely not an appropriate strategy.

So we can see that the style of leadership most appropriate in quality improvement is one that emphasizes participation and that builds trust

IN-PRACTICE 4-4

Formation of a Medical Center Service Line to Address Needs for Communication and Quality Improvement

In 1998, Jones Hospital decided to develop service lines in an effort to better coordinate administrative, clinical, and business development needs of the institution. Jones Hospital is an academic medical center with 850 beds and an operating budget of more than $1 billion. The objectives of this initiative were to integrate hospital and physician practice operations and bring together support services in an effort to develop more efficient and effective operational planning, market development, and patient care quality improvement. To accomplish this, the hospital divided all functional areas into 13 service lines, one of which was the Oncology Clinical Service Unit (CSU). This CSU encompassed, among others, inpatient medical oncology units, radiation oncology, and the adult bone marrow transplant program.

A few of the organization's goals were realized in the first 4 years after the creation of the CSU structure: communication among functional areas was enhanced, identification of strategic opportunities was improved, and day-to-day management was stronger. However, expectations were not met regarding strategic plan development, collaborative business plan development, resource allocation, and revenue management. It was noted that the challenges of meeting organizational goals were in part due to the continuing decentralized management of several critical areas. Even with the creation of the CSU, other oncology areas remained independent of the service line: the Jones Oncology Network, the NCI-designated Comprehensive Cancer Center, the Tumor Registry, the Cancer Protocol Coordination Team, the medical school clinical departments, and the faculty practice plan's outpatient clinics. These, in addition to various support functions such as Management Engineering and Medical Center Finance, were critical to success with oncology strategy and operations. Yet there was no structure that pulled the various constituencies together to work toward improving cancer patient care.

(continues)

In-Practice 4–4

To address this problem, the medical center conducted a review of all oncology service areas and related support functions, including an assessment of specific challenges attributable to the current infrastructure. The review and assessment revealed operational fragmentation due to a lack of coordination and communication, independent priority setting among areas, few change-implementation efforts, and a misalignment of incentives regarding both compensation and patient flow. Furthermore, the review pointed to the near impossibility of developing strategic and business plans for growing patient populations since there was not an agreed-upon process for developing and approving such plans among the many stakeholders.

To address these difficulties, the CSU developed an internal program model to enhance efficiency and effectiveness by taking a patient-centered, quality improvement approach. Based on the major cancer patient populations, specific programs were created inside the CSU, including the Adult Bone Marrow Transplant Program, the Breast Oncology Program, the GI Oncology Program, and the GYN Oncology Program, among others. Each program operated using a matrix model centered on the cancer patient experience. This structure allowed the CSU and others to focus on the needs of specific patient populations regardless of location or type of service. It reduced the organizational unit to a more manageable size in which problems could be more easily identified, analyzed, and solved by the people who were (1) the most familiar with the specific needs of each type of patient and (2) the most capable of developing a solution.

Two groups provided the leadership for this new structure: the Strategic Governance Council and the Program Meeting. These groups comprised representatives from all areas of oncology. The Strategic Governance Council addressed issues of strategic direction and included the most senior physician from each of the major areas of oncology in addition to the senior administrator from the service line, physician practice plan, oncology clinics,

(continues)

In-Practice 4–4

and oncology outreach program. This council set the strategic direction and approved all plans in a well-defined planning process. The Program Meeting led the operational implementation of the strategies and plans created by the Strategic Governance Council and further served as the central forum for communication of strategic priorities and progress reports on major projects and issues for all oncology operations, health system–wide.

Critical factors contributing to the successful creation of this new structure included agreement on planning processes and sufficient resourcing by centralized services such as informatics, finance, clinical laboratories, pharmacy, and radiology. The creation of the new model resulted in significant improvements in communication, planning, and resource management; cooperation among the many stakeholders; shared decision making regarding strategic and operational plans; expedited operational problem resolution; and a dramatic financial improvement in the service line overall.

among team members. It is a style that encourages members to express their views and to take risks, and that develops the team and helps it to become mature and more effective. All of these traits can be seen in the Jones Hospital oncology service line. Leadership must also focus on keeping people engaged, motivated, and stimulated to create and innovate. Quality improvement teams are, if not voluntary, dependent upon the goodwill of participants for their success. Some successful teams encourage shared leadership by allowing specific individuals on a team to take on leadership roles for particular phases of the quality improvement process. The overall leader therefore also assumes a training role, helping to develop team members' skills in team leadership and project management.

This participative style is appropriate not because it is humane and fosters a happy workforce (although it is likely to do so), but because team members' active participation is absolutely essential to success. Because quality improvement teams often do not exist within the formal hierarchical structure of the organization, leaders must certainly attend to issues of motivation and commitment as well.

Communication Networks and Interaction Patterns

A key maintenance task in any team is the exchange of information. Methods of communication are essential and central in any team activity, whether it is an operating room team, a string quartet, a sports team, or a quality improvement team. Communication is necessary not only within the team but also between the team and the larger external environment, including other teams. Communication is critical and cannot be left to chance. Consider the consequences, for example, of there being no formal means of communication between attending physicians and nursing staff in a hospital—or if there were no forum for communication among the 30 or more oncology programs at Jones Hospital. This was actually what drove Jones Hospital to completely restructure its organization to a service line format. Communication and coordination deficiencies were identified as the underpinning factors contributing to less than optimal performance, declining patient care coordination and patient satisfaction, and a perception of reduced quality of care.

In any team, information must be conveyed, and a key question is how? And how effectively and accurately is the information being exchanged? Like all other teams, quality improvement teams require a communication structure. Interestingly, a substantial proportion of health care quality problems reside in communication structure problems in the organization.

Communication networks come in several varieties, and each situation demands a different type of communication structure. Where the team task is simple, it may be most efficient to use a centralized structure in which information passes from the team leader to other team members. Alternatively, information can be passed from the team leader to another team member who, in a hierarchical manner, passes it down to the next individual. Neither of these models allows for upward communication. In other teams, one individual assumes the role of network hub and communicates with other members. Information from team members must pass through the hub in order to reach other team members. An all-channel communication structure is dense; communication lines are open and encouraged between all members of the team. Such a structure is most useful for complex situations where the work of each team member is interdependent with others' work. In such situations, formal lines of authority are blurred or meaningless. In teams focused on patient care, quality improvement, research, or management, it is important for team members to have ready access to other team members, as is seen in the service line of Jones Hospital, which provides such access through formalized communication forums. Information is passed not only from the team leader but also among team members, making centralized models inappropriate. Similarly, going through an intermediary is inefficient and may use up valuable time.

Quality improvement teams typify teams requiring such a rich communication structure. The work of a quality improvement team is complex, and communication lines must be open between all members. For example, an intervention aimed at decreasing waiting time in a clinic requires interaction between clinicians on the team, support staff within the clinic, those involved in data collection, and so forth. The leader of such a team would assume the important role of ensuring that communication networks are in fact open and that team members are able to communicate with each other.

Communication between a team and its external environment is also important. As an open system, teams are often dependent upon other individuals and other teams inside or outside the organization. Leaders here assume boundary-spanning roles, in which they ensure that relationships with critical outside groups are workable. This is particularly important in a hospital setting in which a particular work unit's operations are highly dependent upon interactions with other units (for example, patient care units are highly dependent upon the pharmacy, dietary department, and so forth). The Oncology Leadership Group fills this role within the oncology service line at Jones Hospital. The Leadership Group is the broker between the oncology department and the medical center's senior administration for such needs as major redeployments of resources to support oncology's strategic priorities, redesign and reallocation of clinical space, or needs for changes in the operational interface with independent departments such as Pharmacy Services, which, to fit strategic and political needs, maintains an independent departmental structure in the organization. A quality improvement team likely relies on information and resources from outside the immediate team, and just as communication networks among team members are critical, so are strong and reliable networks between the team and other units and teams.

An isolated team that neglects its external relations is likely to perform poorly because key relationships will not be well managed.

Decision Making

Decision making is a task of all teams, and the manner in which decisions are made is critical to team success. Teams may reach decisions by consensus or voting, or team members may simply advise the team leader, leaving the final decision to the leader. There is no single best way for a team to make decisions, and the mode of decision making is often dependent upon the circumstances and goals of the team. The president of a hospital, for example, may charge a team with the task of analyzing an acquisition possibility. The team may return with recommendations and options, but the final decision remains with the president. In a multidisciplinary mental health treatment team, it is likely that decisions will be based on team consensus, although the team leader (who may be the psychiatrist) may reserve the right to override the team's recommendations. In still other teams, particularly those where there is no single person in a position of formal authority, the team as a whole may make decisions. In such situations, team members should discuss how decisions are to be made—by voting, by working toward consensus and compromise, or perhaps by deferring to the individual most knowledgeable about a particular issue to be decided.

In the Jones Hospital example, the decision-making process and the people who make the decisions are highly dependent on the decisions themselves. Depending on the nature and criticality of the issue at hand, there are decisions made by formal vote in the Strategic Governance Council, by informal consensus in the Program Meeting, and by mandate in the Leadership Group. The success of such decision making is dependent upon open communication among the members of these groups; all information is shared, and a record of decisions made is kept through meeting minutes of all bodies. When an individual has a problem with a decision made by the Leadership Group, for example, the forum for discussion of such concerns is formally built in to the service line structure via the other two groups.

Regardless of the mode of decision making, it is critical that team members understand their role in decision making. Assuming an advising rather than decision-making role is acceptable to team members as long as they do not expect to be in the position of making decisions.

The decisional authority of the team and that of team members needs to be specific and clear.

Teams often strive for cohesion, and in general cohesion is a positive force. Efforts should be made to develop a team such that members understand each other, are at ease communicating with each other, and feel a unified sense of purpose and solidarity. Taken to an extreme, however, cohesion can develop into conformity and "group think"; in such a case, team members become so cohesive that they lose their independence as free thinkers and may fear expressing views opposed to what they consider to be the team consensus.

Member and Team Learning

Peter Senge popularized the idea of the learning organization in his book *The Fifth Discipline* (1990). A specific application of learning organization concepts to health care quality improvement is presented in Chapter 10. Briefly, a learning organization is one that proactively creates, acquires, and transfers knowledge and changes its behavior on the basis of new knowledge and insights (Garvin, 1993). The implication of this definition for teams is clear. First, effective teams continuously look for new information to improve their performance, whether new technology, new organizational processes, or new concepts. They are open to new ideas and in fact seek them out. They do this by including people on teams with new expertise and alternative perspectives, and by ensuring that team members are engaged in continuous training and learning. Effective teams then attempt to use new information, ensuring that new knowledge is transferred to the team. This new knowledge is then used to change the team's behavior in pursuit of higher levels of achievement. Teams may enhance their ability to learn and apply new knowledge through the use of a number of facilitating factors, including scanning the environment for new information; identifying performance gaps within the team; adopting an "experimental mindset," such that team members are open to new approaches; and having leadership supportive of change. (See Moingeon and Edmondson, 1996, for a more in-depth discussion of facilitating factors.)

Team and organizational learning are key aspects of CQI, and it is no surprise that the capacity to learn is a hallmark of effective teams. A quality improvement team is faced not only with enhancing the learning of the organization, or the organizational subunit with which it is working, but also with improving the learning and performance of itself as a team. Effective quality improvement teams review their own performance and the satisfaction of members and seek to develop strategies and new team management techniques that will enhance their performance. Some teams "debrief" after each meeting to review the progress of their work and the manner in which they worked and seek to learn from this and improve their capabilities. Learning from experience and learning from the broader external environment are trademarks of effective organizations and teams.

CONCLUSIONS

In this chapter, we have reviewed the importance of teams and effective teamwork in health care and most importantly in regard to the successful implementation of quality improvement efforts. Steps in team development and team processes were reviewed; these include development of balanced team relationships and equal status to ensure participation of all team members, and open communication and feedback, which will ensure efficient team performance through empowerment and high levels of motivation. Critical to the success of any team effort is the role of team leaders, who can come from within the team or from traditional leadership positions; also critical to success is developing a team's culture. Finally, ongoing team learning was described as one of the most important aspects of teamwork in CQI; it provides a means for sharing knowledge and improving performance of a team as well as the larger organization in which the team exists.

Cross-References to the Companion Casebook

(McLaughlin, C. P., Johnson, J. K., and Sollecito, W. A. [Eds.]. 2012. *Implementing Continuous Quality Improvement in Health Care: A Global Casebook.* Sudbury, MA: Jones & Bartlett Learning).

Case Study Number	Case Study Title	Case Study Author
1	West Florida Regional Medical Center	*Curtis P. McLaughlin*
2	Holtz Children's Hospital: Reducing Central Line Infections	*Gwenn E. McLaughlin*

REFERENCES

Deming, W. E. 1986. *Out of the Crisis.* Cambridge: Massachusetts Institute of Technology Center for Advanced Engineering Study.

Edmonson A. 1999. Psychological safety and learning behavior in work teams. *Administrative Science Quarterly*, 44(4): 350–383.

Fleeger, M. E. 1993. Assessing organizational culture: A planning strategy. *Nurs Manage*, 24(2): 40.

French, W. L. 1998. *Human Resources Management* (4th ed.). Boston: Houghton Mifflin.

Garvin, D. A. 1993. Building a learning organization. *Harvard Bus Rev*, 71(4): 78–91.

Gawande, A. 2009. *The Checklist Manifesto.* New York: Metropolitan Books.

Grove, A. S. 1995. *High Output Management.* New York: Vintage Books.

Hackman, J. R. 2002. *Leading Teams: Setting the Stage for Great Performances.* Boston: Harvard Business School Press.

Hackman, J. R. & G. R. Oldham. 1980. *Work Redesign.* Reading, MA: Addison-Wesley.

Kiassi, A., Kralewski, J., Curoe, A., et al. 2004. How does the culture of medical group practices influence the types of programs used to assure quality of care? *Health Care Manage Rev*, 29(2): 129–138.

Moingeon, B., and Edmondson, A. 1996. *Organizational Learning and Competitive Advantage.* Thousand Oaks, CA: Sage.

Nelson, E. C., Batalden, P. B., Huber, T. P., et al. 2002. Microsystems in health care: Part 1. Learning from high-performing front-line clinical units. *Joint Commission J Qual Improve*, 28(9): 472–493.

Schein, E. H. and W. Bennis. 1965. *Personal and Organizational Change via Group Methods.* New York: Wiley.

Senge, P. M. 1990. *The Fifth Discipline: The Art and Practice of the Learning Organization.* New York: Doubleday.

Shortell, S. M., and Kaluzny, A. D. 2006. *Health Care Management— Organization Design and Behavior* (5th ed). Clifton Park, NY: Thomson Delmar Learning.

CHAPTER 5

The Outcome Model of Quality

Susan I. DesHarnais

"Quality is never an accident. It is always the result of intelligent effort."

—John Ruskin

A critical question facing most health care quality improvement efforts is how to evaluate clinical performance. The objectives of this chapter are to:

- Present a conceptual framework for measuring the quality of health care
- Provide a definition of quality that focuses on the outcomes of care
- Present a brief historical overview of outcome measurement in the United States
- Examine the data requirements and risk-adjustment techniques for comparing health outcomes across providers and/or over time

A CONCEPTUAL FRAMEWORK AND DEFINITIONS OF QUALITY

Quality may be defined in many ways and from many perspectives. Dr. Avedis Donabedian (1980, 1982, 1986) observed that definitions of quality ordinarily reflect the values and goals of the current medical care system, as well as those of the larger society of which it is part. In 1980, Donabedian presented his model for categorizing the different ways that one might measure the quality of health care in a given setting. His model has provided an excellent framework for conceptualizing quality in a broad manner and then classifying the measures that one can use to assess different aspects of the quality of care.

Donabedian began by differentiating three aspects of care:

- *Structure*: The resources available to provide adequate health care. Resources include facilities, equipment, and trained personnel.
- *Process*: The activities of giving and receiving care (the patient's activities in seeking care as well as the practitioner's activities).
- *Outcomes*: Primarily, changes in the patient's condition following treatment; outcomes also include patient knowledge and satisfaction.

In addition, Donabedian broadened the definition of quality to include not just the technical management of the patient but also the management of interpersonal relationships, as well as access to care and continuity of care. The conceptual framework shown in **Table 5–1** allows us to appreciate the complexity of defining and measuring the quality of health care and provides guidance in what aspects of care we might wish to measure. One could then fill in this matrix to apply to a particular setting. For example, in **Table 5–2**, the matrix is applied to the care provided at a cancer center. This approach is important in that it gives a broad definition to quality of care that goes well beyond simply looking at technical management.

In 1988, the U.S. Office of Technology Assessment (OTA) defined quality of care as "the degree to which the process of care increases the

---

TABLE 5-1 Donabedian's Matrix for the Classification of Quality Measures

	Structure	Process	Outcome
Accessibility			
Technical management			
Management of interpersonal relationships			
Continuity			

Source: Donabedian, A. 1980. The definition of quality and approaches to its assessment. In *Explorations in Quality Assessment and Monitoring* (Vol. 1, pp. 95–99). Ann Arbor, MI: Health Administration Press.

TABLE 5-2 Donabedian's Matrix for the Classification of Quality Measures Applied to Cancer Care

	Structure	Process	Outcome
Accessibility	Hours of operation of mammogram facility	Waiting time for mammogram appointment	Satisfaction with various aspects of accessibility
Technical management	Certification of nurses in oncology nursing; availability of various pieces of up-to-date radiation equipment	Systematic use of evidence-based practices	5-year survival rates for stage 1 breast cancer patients ages 50-70 at the time of diagnosis
Management of interpersonal relationships	Physicians and nurses trained in cultural competency techniques	Involving the patient in treatment decisions	Patient satisfaction with whether they were able to participate in treatment decisions
Continuity	Presence of a trained nurse navigator	Number of contacts per patient with the nurse navigator	Patient satisfaction with continuity of care

probability of outcomes desired by the patient, and reduces the probability of undesired outcomes, given the state of medical knowledge." This is a useful definition because it emphasizes the patient's role and perspective in choosing among possible treatments. This definition also makes an explicit connection between the processes of treatment that are used and the resulting outcomes, thus demanding that evidence-based medicine be the standard of care. One is therefore forced to focus on evidence of the effectiveness of various treatments from the patient's point of view. This definition also implies that there are no meaningful or useful measures of quality if there is no effective treatment known for a given condition. Thus, one can use quality measures only for those conditions where the technology is reasonably effective and also acceptable to the patient.

More recently, the Institute of Medicine (IOM) discussed quality of care in a series of reports. *To Err Is Human: Building a Safer Health System* was released in 2000, and *Crossing the Quality Chasm: A New Health System for the 21st Century* was released in 2001. These two reports documented the scope of quality and safety problems in the United States and offered an analysis of these problems. These committees stressed that quality health care must be all of the following (IOM, 2001, pp. 5–6):

- *Safe*—avoiding injuries to patients from the care that is intended to help them
- *Effective*—providing services based on scientific knowledge to all who could benefit and refraining from providing services to those not likely to benefit
- *Patient centered*—providing care that is respectful of and responsive to individual patient preferences, needs, and values and ensuring that patient values guide all clinical decisions
- *Timely*—reducing waits and sometimes harmful delays for both those who receive and those who give care
- *Efficient*—avoiding waste, including waste of equipment, supplies, ideas, and energy
- *Equitable*—providing care that does not vary in quality because of personal characteristics such as gender, ethnicity, geographic location, and socioeconomic status

This definition of quality broadens the earlier definitions of quality to recognize that high-quality care must not only focus on the processes of care (timeliness), patient outcomes (safety and effectiveness), and the patient's perspective (patient centered), but must also focus on some of the broader requirements of the social and economic system within which health care is provided (efficiency and equity). While recognizing this broader perspective, this chapter will concentrate on the measurement of health outcomes, a difficult enough task in itself.

Why might one choose to use outcome measures, when it is much easier to measure or monitor structure or processes of care? Structure measures are relatively simple to use. In many cases, one can simply do an "inventory" of structural measures by using a checklist of those resources that are thought to be necessary to ensure the capacity for providing a given type of care. The Joint Commission (TJC) took this approach in its early days because there was some agreement that certain structural elements were needed as minimal standards to ensure an environment in which good care was possible. However, it should be evident that adequate inputs alone do not ensure good outcomes. All the structural measures can do is indicate whether a facility has the capacity to provide good care.

Then why not focus on process measures, which take into account professional performance? It is often easier to measure provider performance than it is to measure patient outcomes. Processes of care are generally documented in patient records, and also in billing or claims data sets, since the procedures that are done usually determine the payment that the professional receives. However, there are several problems with using process measures to look at the quality of care. For a process measure to be valid, there must be good evidence regarding what a professional should do under defined circumstances. This means that a particular process must be strongly linked to better patient outcomes, compared with alternative processes.

While it is sometimes possible to use evidence from clinical trials and published studies, and to translate these studies into treatment guidelines, often this is not possible. Clinical trials are often done on carefully selected people/subjects, and compliance is carefully monitored. Once the treatment goes into general use, it does not work in the same way. The people who actually get the treatment may be older, may have comorbid conditions, and may be noncompliant with various aspects of the treatment protocol. Therefore the evidence from clinical trials may not be generalizable to the population for which the treatment is intended.

Because of this problem, it is often necessary for a group (or groups) of experts to translate evidence from clinical trials into treatment guidelines. It is very difficult to develop consensus among relevant professional groups on treatment guidelines and then to develop explicit process criteria that state under what circumstances one should or should not follow the guidelines, due to certain combinations of comorbid conditions, the advanced age of the patient, patient preferences, or other valid reasons. Another difficulty of using process measures is that the provider may do the "right thing in the right way," but the patient may be dissatisfied, may be noncompliant, or may respond poorly to the treatment. The process, though done correctly, may not always produce the desired outcome.

Using a process measure, rather than an outcome measure, to evaluate the quality of care is valid if and only if there is solid evidence that supports doing so. This means that there is strong evidence that there is a very high correlation between "doing the right thing in the right way" and getting good outcomes. This criterion will be met for some conditions, but not for all. For example, if a certain type of treatment is very effective and has few side effects, then the process of doing that treatment can be used as a valid and useful quality measure, rather than trying to monitor the effects of the treatment on patients' health status. Unfortunately, not many treatments fall into this category.

Outcome Measures

Outcome measures are what we really would like to use, since the whole point of treating the patient is to increase the probability of outcomes desired by the patient and reduce the probability of undesired outcomes, given the state of medical knowledge, according to the OTA definition of quality previously cited. Outcome measures are, in effect, the "gold standard" for measuring the quality of care.

However, it is much more difficult to gather and analyze outcome data than it is to measure structure or process. Ideally one would like to have data on each patient's health status before and after treatment for a large national sample of patients treated for each common condition. Instead, the only information available in most of our databases is information on what procedures were done and, to some extent, what adverse events occurred. Data on patient outcomes are usually missing.

There are many reasons why useful health status information is often lacking. In most cases, there is a time delay until one can really assess the effect of a treatment on a patient. One must wait until the patient has recovered from the treatment. It is expensive to try to follow up on patients once they have completed treatment and recovery, and it is difficult to systematically measure the health status of each patient after treatment. Moreover, health status following treatment is often not a direct result of the care provided, since outcomes are not determined solely by professional performance. Other patient-related factors, such as comorbid conditions, patient age, patient compliance, and financial resources, also enter into the equation. Unless one can adequately account for these factors, one cannot validly compare the performance of different providers by looking at patient outcomes. Outcomes attained by a provider treating higher risk patients cannot really be compared with outcomes attained by a provider treating lower risk patients unless one can adequately adjust for the impacts of the risks when comparing the providers.

Because of these difficulties in measuring outcomes, we are often forced to measure negative outcomes rather than positive outcomes. Since the purpose of care is to produce the positive outcomes while minimizing the negative outcomes, this is a real problem. Some examples of the type of positive outcomes we would like to measure include the proportion of patients who have the following outcomes:

- A better score on a depression scale 3 months after a specific drug treatment
- A given level of improvement in range of movement of a joint 1 year following joint replacement
- Greater time between hospitalizations for acute episodes for patients with a chronic disease, such as diabetes or alcohol/drug problems
- Return to work within 60 days after a given type of heart surgery
- A given level of improvement in quality of life after back surgery

Instead, we often end up using available data, and thus measuring negative outcomes, such as the proportion of patients who have the following outcomes:

- Death during their hospital stay
- Unscheduled readmission to the hospital within 30 days of discharge
- Complications of surgery during their hospital stay
- Preventable adverse events, including medication errors, wrong site surgery, and so on, during their hospital stay

While the information on negative outcomes is useful, it is only part of the picture when we are measuring patient outcomes. Instead, we would like to measure quality using data on both positive and negative outcomes of care.

What do we do when we find unacceptably high rates of negative outcomes? The general approach is to go back and see what went wrong with the processes of care the patient received. Sometimes a good process has been described, but the health care professionals are not using it. In that case, we need to understand why they are not willing to use the process. More often, we will discover that we may have to redesign the processes to attain better outcomes. As described in *Crossing the Quality Chasm*:

> Health care has safety and quality problems because it relies on outmoded systems of work. Poor designs set the workforce up to fail, regardless of how hard they try. If we want safer, higher-quality care, we will need to have redesigned systems of care, including the use of information technology to support clinical and administrative processes. (IOM, 2001, p. 4)

Risk adjustment is crucial in accurately evaluating providers. In terms of quality, we want to take into account what health outcomes we could reasonably expect from a provider, given the technology available, the severity of the disease treated, and other risk factors of the provider's patients. It is therefore essential to risk-adjust outcome variables to allow for valid comparisons of these outcomes across hospitals.

INFORMATION TECHNOLOGY/DATA AVAILABILITY CHANGES

In the second half of the 20th century, computers and large databases made it much easier to benchmark and monitor the outcomes of hospital care (see Chapter 12). Also, researchers began to develop more sophisticated techniques for modeling risk factors affecting the outcomes of care. The increased availability of data on the use, cost, and outcomes of medical services also enabled consumers, insurance companies, and regulatory agencies to independently analyze trends in the use and costs of health care services and to draw their own conclusions.

In the mid-1980s, the Health Care Financing Administration (HCFA), which is presently known as the Centers for Medicare and Medicaid Services (CMS), began releasing information on hospital mortality rates to the public. Because the methods HCFA used to derive these rates had major flaws, in many cases the findings were invalid. Hospitals needed to defend themselves against such data releases. In some communities, hospitals received negative publicity for having high mortality rates when, in fact, their mortality rates were better than what would have been expected, given the severity and complexity of the cases they treated.

By the late 1980s, several states began to gather mortality data for various types of cardiac surgery. In 1980, the New York State Department of Health and its Cardiac Advisory Committee began an effort to reduce mortality from coronary artery bypass grafts by collecting clinical data on all patients undergoing that procedure. In 1990, the department made public the data on mortality rates, both crude and risk-adjusted. Surgeon-specific data on mortality were released after a lawsuit by a newspaper. Subsequently, other data releases were made, some of which were likely misleading and superficial (Chassin et al., 1996). Understandably, many surgeons and hospitals had unfavorable reactions to these releases. There were concerns with the accuracy of the data, as well as the methods of risk adjustment. Many of these problems have been resolved, and public releases of high-quality mortality data have become more common.

Pennsylvania has had a similar program of reporting hospital performance. In 1986, the Pennsylvania Health Care Cost Containment Council was established by the General Assembly and the state governor to help improve the quality, and restrain the costs, of health care. This council developed a series of "Hospital Performance Reports," covering 28 different conditions that are reasons for hospitalization. Reports are divided into regions and are hospital-specific. These reports have been made available on the Internet for several years.

In addition, various sites on the Internet have had an influence on public awareness of outcome measures, including mortality rates. An example is http://www.HealthGrades.com, which has been publishing hospital ratings since 1999, as well as other Web sites that have focused a great deal of attention on the quality of health care.

By the end of the 1990s and the early 2000s, another type of information about health care quality was put before the public. As mentioned earlier, several important reports were issued by the IOM, which brought serious quality problems to the public eye. These included the Committee on the Quality of Health Care in America IOM report *To Err Is Human: Building a Safer Health System* (2000), which focused on patient safety issues, and the 2001 report *Crossing the Quality Chasm: A New Health System for the 21st Century*, which focused on how the health care delivery system can be designed to improve the quality of care. In addition, the IOM Committee on Understanding and Eliminating Racial and Ethnic Disparities in Health Care published *Unequal Treatment Confronting Racial and Ethnic Disparities in Health Care* in 2003. This report focused on the clinical encounter that minority patients experience and the processes of care that have resulted in poor care for minority patients. Since these reports have been made public, a variety of other books, research reports, and broadcasts have focused on these quality problems.

Data availability has increased further in the 21st century and has been characterized by greater information access by individuals and organizations to complex information sources via the Internet. Employers, unions, consumers, and insurance companies began to demand access to data. This change in data availability was significant, making it possible for both professionals and others to compare the performance of various providers. Organizations that have the mission and the capability to analyze and interpret secondary data sources, such as Quality Improvement

Organizations (QIOs), began to focus more on available outcome data to make recommendations for health improvements based on CMS and other large national databases. A further discussion of the role of QIOs is presented later in this text (Chapter 15) and can be found in associated CMS Web sites (e.g., http://www.cms.gov/QualityImprovementOrgs/).

Interest in evaluating the quality of care had clearly moved from the professional domain to the public domain. Many physicians felt that the medical profession was under attack from the outside as government and consumers sought to measure and evaluate quality. In addition, governmental, consumer, and industry groups were attempting to measure the value received for their money, to evaluate the relative effectiveness of various treatments, and to compare the quality of care provided by different hospitals and physicians. This interest led to, or paralleled, the development of more sophisticated, complex, and useful models of medical decision making, including computerized decision-making systems, complex treatment protocols for various diseases, and risk-adjusted measures of hospital performance (DesHarnais et al., 1988). As a result, there was an increase in the demand for information about the quality of care, and particularly about the outcomes of care. This interest was manifested in many different ways.

Consumers Take a More Active Role

Consumers began to take a much more active role in their own health care. The women's movement in the 1960s and 1970s was a force that was critical of many medical practices. Consumers began to independently analyze trends in the use and costs of health care services. Various consumer interest groups question effectiveness of various practices. Individual consumers, more knowledgeable about health care, get second opinions, review data on providers, and make decisions concerning treatment options. They have become interested in obtaining accurate and useful data on costs in relationship to the outcomes of care.

Hospitals Become Interested in Outcomes

Hospitals became much more interested in measuring patient outcomes as a defense against public release of mortality data. Hospitals also need information on physician performance for appointment and reappointment decisions. Hospitals often lacked the ability to compare physician performance in terms of outcomes produced or resources utilized. As cost-containment pressures increased alongside concerns for quality, many hospitals wanted objective information on physician performance as part of decision making on privileges.

Hospitals also want information on both quality and costs for planning and marketing. Many facilities are developing integrated management information systems that provide data on both inputs and outcomes. These information systems can integrate medical records, risk management, quality management, and financial management systems.

In 2009 and 2010, CMS took several actions to reduce hospital payments for hospitalizations that include various complications and for hospitalizations that are unplanned readmissions. These changes in reimbursement policies make it even more important for hospitals to track such problems, due to the negative financial impact that these events will have on hospital revenue.

Professional Societies Seek Information on Outcomes

Specialty societies and certifying boards for various specialties would like information on the outcomes of care for relevant procedures for several reasons. First, such information could promulgate standards for better practice of medicine within their specialty. Outcome data could be used to help evaluate the relative effectiveness of various ways of treating patients, when different treatments are possible and there are wide variations in practices. Second, the information could help set standards for certifying specialty physicians. Information on outcomes could be analyzed and used in designing certification examinations.

While data on patient outcomes could be useful for these endeavors, the various specialty societies are just beginning to understand that this is a very difficult proposition. To gather and use outcome data effectively, it is necessary to do the following:

1. Standardize data reporting requirements

2. Mandate reporting of outcomes data

3. Develop and maintain a patient registry

4. Risk-adjust the data

5. Develop a reporting and benchmarking mechanism

The American College of Surgeons has, in fact, been able to develop such a registry, the National Cancer Data Base, because cancer is reportable by law and because they have had the authority to certify cancer programs. They have made data reporting one of the requirements of their approval. Most other specialty societies are not currently in a position to take such actions to gather outcomes data from their members.

Insurance Companies Want Outcome Measures

HMOs and preferred provider organizations (PPOs) were prevalent in the 1970s and 1980s. These types of organizations demanded data on costs, use patterns, and practice patterns because such information was crucial in managing care in these systems. It was also essential to evaluate the costs and quality of care given by the providers with whom these insurance organizations contracted. PPO contracts required the contracting agency to exercise care when designing preferred providers. If these providers were producing poor outcomes, marketing of the plan would be impossible, and the PPO could face legal problems. Insurance companies also need such information to market their products successfully in a more competitive environment.

Regulators Seek Data on Outcomes

It also became clear that federal and state programs were paying large amounts of money for treatments and for procedures that might not be the most effective means of caring for patients. By the 1980s, the federal government began to allocate research dollars for "effectiveness research" to learn more about the most effective treatments in areas where great variations in medical practice were discovered. Some outcomes of this federal initiative are as follows:

- Regulatory agencies began independent analyses of trends in the use and costs of health care services.
- Federal initiatives, including some at the Veterans Administration, focused increased attention on quality measurement and improvement, including outcomes.
- Federal regulators became involved. Through the use of peer review organizations, now known as QIOs, the HCFA began to find new uses for data on cost and outcomes of medical care. The federal government used the information for developing changes in payment systems, both for hospitals (Diagnosis Regulated Groups) and for professionals (relative value scales).

- As mentioned earlier, CMS recently has taken several actions that will reduce hospital payments for hospitalizations that include various complications and for hospitalizations that are unplanned readmissions.
- TJC began to examine the possibility of using outcome measurement as part of its accreditation process.
- To provide standardized data sets on costs and outcomes, insurance commissioners and state legislators in many parts of the United States (California, Florida, Iowa, Maine, Massachusetts, New Hampshire, New York, Vermont, Washington, West Virginia, and others) mandated that hospitals report specific data. Several states prescribed the data elements that were required. In many cases, new data elements were mandated beyond the common data set used for billing purposes, at considerable cost to hospitals.

The National Quality Forum (NQF), which functions as a quasi-regulatory agency for certifying quality measures, would like to eventually be able to develop and use patient outcome measures as part of its repertoire. However, due to the difficulty of doing this type of work on developing and certifying patient outcome measures, NQF has tended to focus on process measures.

New requirements for providers to use electronic medical records may eventually make it easier for regulators to gather some of the data they need to measure patient outcomes. If the required data sets include patient assessments and enough patient information to risk-adjust the outcome data, then it may become possible to incorporate outcome measures into the data used by regulators. If this comes about, we may see that the regulators and insurance companies really can begin to "pay for performance."

Individual Employers Want Data on Quality of Care

A broader concern with quality measurement has developed in industry. Many industries in the United States became highly concerned with methods of measuring and controlling the quality of the products and services they produced. There was a growing focus on using scientific methods and harnessing the energy and creativity of all levels of personnel in an organization. Total quality management (TQM) principles were adopted by many U.S. industries. In many communities, industries using

TQM were represented on hospital boards as well. TQM concepts were introduced into hospital management and eventually began to change the way certain hospitals approach quality.

In addition, unions and industry demanded information on cost, quality, and outcomes as they negotiated contracts. As new benefits were added, it was necessary to analyze whether they were worth what they cost. In some cases, it was necessary to evaluate the performance of providers to decide whether to offer certain plans. Companies that self-insured needed to develop information on users, costs, and outcomes in order to better manage their insurance plans. Local providers that used excessive resources or had consistently poor outcomes could pose a real problem for such plans.

Business Groups/Coalitions Become Interested in Outcomes

Several business coalitions also organized to consider ways to improve health care quality and to control costs. Two examples are the Pacific Business Group on Health and the Leapfrog Group. The Pacific Business Group on Health was founded in 1989 and represents more than 50 large purchasers of health care, with coverage for more than 3 million employees. The coalition identifies health care and business trends, assesses the impact of those trends, and recommends practical steps to advance a common agenda. It works closely with payers, providers, researchers, and others to achieve the highest quality and most cost-effective health care. The Pacific Business Group on Health also works collaboratively with all purchasers in California and with other business coalitions throughout the United States (see http://pbgh.org).

The Leapfrog Group is another example. It represents employers, with more than 34 million covered health care consumers in all 50 states. Composed of more than 150 public and private organizations that provide health care benefits, the Leapfrog Group works with medical experts throughout the United States to identify problems and propose solutions that it believes will improve hospital systems that could break down and harm patients. Leapfrog provides important information and solutions for consumers and health care providers (see http://www.leapfroggroup.org).

Table 5–3 illustrates likely uses of performance measures by various stakeholders.

TABLE 5–3 Performance Measures for Improving Quality

Consumers	Using performance as selection criteria for providers and plans
	Using guidelines to evaluate ongoing care
	Taking a more meaningful role in managing own care
Purchasers	Using quality as selection criteria for providers and plans
	Displaying quality information to employees and families
	Devising incentives to get employees to choose quality
	Developing incentive payment systems to reward provider quality
Health plans	Selecting networks based on quality measures
	Showing quality results to enrollees and physicians
	Developing incentive payment systems to reward provider quality
	Submitting quality measures for review by public
Regulators	Using evidence-based data to develop regulations
	Assessing quality impact of proposed regulations
Clinicians	Practicing evidence-based medicine
	Choosing colleagues and services for referrals
	Submitting quality measures for review by public
	Using quality methods to improve safety and outcomes
Care delivery systems	Making quality a strategic factor
	Developing capacity for quality improvement
	Developing information systems to support evidence-based practice and quality improvement efforts
	Enabling a culture and systems to support quality and safety

---

Source: Galvin, R. S., and McGlynn, E. A. 2003. Using performance measurement to drive improvement: A roadmap for change. *Med Care*, 41(1): 148–160.

Although comparisons of mortality rates and measures of adverse events across institutions are potentially useful to providers and patients as one way to measure quality of care, such information might be misleading and potentially damaging if misused. This is particularly important when considering how such "report cards" can be used by the government or the public. Such information must be compiled and interpreted correctly. Several studies have demonstrated that raw death rates, without adjustment for differences in case mix and case complexity, lead to misleading comparisons among hospitals, with those hospitals that treat higher risk patients appearing to provide poorer care (Knaus et al., 1986; Moses and Mosteller, 1968; Pollack et al., 1987; Wagner et al., 1986). Death rates must be risk-adjusted and interpreted carefully along with other indicators of quality.

RISK ADJUSTMENT AND BENCHMARKING OF OUTCOME DATA: DATA REQUIREMENTS AND TECHNIQUES

As explained earlier, differences in outcomes across hospitals (patients' responses to treatment) can be viewed as a result of many different factors that may influence health outcomes (see **Figure 5-1**).

To measure the effect of provider performance on outcomes with accuracy, it is necessary to control for all the other factors. This is clearly not possible, given the existing data sets and measurement tools. However, because "report cards" on providers are going to be produced, it is essential to try to develop as valid an approach as possible for risk adjustment by accounting for as much of the variation that is due to patient characteristics as possible.

Historically, two different approaches have been used to perform risk adjustment of hospital mortality data: hospital-level variables to adjust crude death rates and indirect standardization of patient-level data.

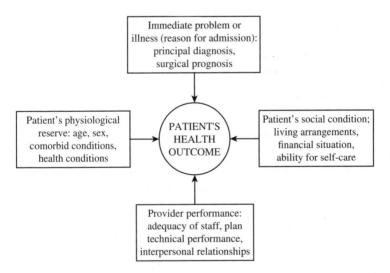

FIGURE 5-1 Schematic Diagram of Some Factors Related to Health Outcomes

Source: Reprinted from DesHarnais, S., Chesney, J. D., Wroblewski, R. T., et al. 1988. The risk-adjusted mortality index: A new measure of hospital performance. *Med Care*, 26(12): 1129–1148, with permission of J.B. Lippincott, © 1988.

Hospital-level data were used in several early studies. In a 1968 study by Roemer et al., hospital-level aggregate measures of patient characteristics (e.g., average age, percentage nonwhite, and percentage of cancer deaths) along with hospital characteristics (e.g., control, occupancy rate, and technology level) were modeled in an attempt to understand whether these proxies for case mix and case complexity were related to the observed differences in crude death rates among hospitals. The authors reasoned that if these hospital-level proxy measures were related to the crude death rates, they could be used to adjust the rates to represent more accurately each hospital's performance.

This early risk adjustment, as the authors acknowledged, was rather crude. They justified the approach by pointing out that detailed patient-level data on diagnosis and severity of illness were not yet available. They acknowledged hospital-level proxy measures to be an indirect approach to estimating case mix and case complexity. The authors stated:

> Ideally, one would like to examine the exact diagnosis of each patient admitted and classify it according to a scale of gravity, which might be based on case fatality rates derived from a general literature of clinical investigation. . . . But it is obvious that such a task of calculating average case severity by such an analytic process could present formidable problems of data collection. (Roemer et al., 1968, p. 98)

It certainly would have been difficult in the 1960s, given the limited availability of computers, to model the risks of death for all types of hospital patients using large data sets, even if such information had been available.

Using Patient-Level Data for Risk Adjustment

Because hospital-level data are of limited use as proxies for differences in case mix and case complexity across hospitals, there is no apparent justification for using such data for risk adjustment today. Discharge-level data are now available and are much more sensitive for measuring differences in case mix and case complexity across hospitals. The techniques of using adjusted discharge-level outcome data are documented in early studies such as the National Halothane Study in the 1960s (Moses and Mosteller, 1968), the Stanford Institutional Differences Study in the 1970s (Flood et al., 1982), and work by Luft and Hunt (1986) on the relationship of surgical volume to mortality.

Risk Adjustment vs. Severity Adjustment

Risk adjustment is an empirical approach, using condition-specific risk factors and outcome-specific models. Severity adjustment is quite different insofar as it makes use of one of any number of standardized indexes to assign a severity score to each case. That score is then used as one of the predictors of the outcome of interest, along with other patient characteristics such as age, gender, and so on. The reason severity adjustment is usually inappropriate for adjusting patient health outcomes is really quite simple: Most of the severity systems are the results of models designed to predict resource use rather than patient outcomes. Since there is little or no correlation between resource use and patient outcomes, it is not helpful to use severity measures for risk adjustment. Instead, risk adjustment should be done when looking at health outcomes. This means using an empirical approach with condition-specific risk factors and outcome-specific models. Severity adjustment can be relevant, however, when adjusting resource use data such as costs for comparison purposes.

What Procedures Are Used for Performing Risk Adjustment?

In an article summarizing many of the methodological issues in the risk adjustment of outcome data, Blumberg (1986) described indirect standardization, the principal technique used for risk adjustment of discharge-level data:

> Indirect standardization is the method most widely used for risk-adjusted outcome studies. It requires estimates of the expected outcome in a study population, based on the outcome experience of a standard population. To estimate expected outcome, the numbers of cases in the study population with risk-related attributes are multiplied by the probability of the outcome in a standard population with matching attributes. These expected outcomes in the study population are then compared with the observed number having that outcome in the same study population. . . . The first step involves the development and testing of a risk-prediction model, while the second step is a study of the residuals of the observed less the expected outcomes in the study population. (p. 384)

Risk-prediction models can be developed using regression methods (see Chapter 3) that allow control for factors, other than provider performance, that may affect patient outcomes (DesHarnais et al., 1991).

USES OF RISK-ADJUSTED DATA: WHAT IS BENCHMARKING, AND WHY MIGHT WE WANT TO DO IT?

Benchmarking is simply the use of external comparisons to understand how one is doing compared to one's peers and/or one's competitors. Usually one benchmarks outcomes at the service level, or even the diagnosis or DRG level, not at the hospital level. To make meaningful comparisons, the data must first be risk-adjusted, since hospitals differ in the "riskiness" of the patients they treat.

External comparisons allow one to identify areas of strength and weakness. These external comparisons are useful when trying to understand how to prioritize problems within one's own hospital (i.e., to decide which quality issues to address first). Benchmarking of risk-adjusted data can also be used to do self-comparisons over time to see if quality improvement efforts are successful.

What Standard Should We Use?

Benchmarking requires a decision regarding the type of standard that should be used when comparing outcomes across facilities or within a facility over time. Such standards may be developed in three different ways:

1. *Absolute (normative)*: In this approach, results are determined by clinical trials and/or consensus conferences. Standards developed in this manner by academic health centers reflect the ideal practice of medicine, or the best possible outcomes that can be achieved under optimal circumstances (i.e., the most skilled surgeon, the best possible equipment, and the best trained team assisting). Although it is useful to know the theoretical "efficacy" of a treatment, or the best possible result one could achieve, such standards may not be realistic under ordinary circumstances of practice. That is why they are often called "best practices." Clinical trials are the basis of "evidence-based" medicine, but they may be better executed than normally because extra resources are put into execution and control. "Consensus conferences" rest on leading expert opinion but still result from a process that one of our colleagues calls GOBSAT, which stands for Good Old Boys Sitting Around Talking.

2. *Empirical*: In this approach, results are assessed relative to other institutions treating similar patients. Standards developed by comparing oneself to other institutions treating similar patients may be useful to help identify problem areas. If, for example, a hospital is experiencing 20% more unanticipated readmissions than other hospitals when treating a specific type of patient, that could be a signal that some correction is needed. On the other hand, it is possible that the "average" care in the community is poor. Such comparisons are only relative to the level of quality in the institutions used for comparison.

3. *Institutional*: In this approach, results are based on self-comparisons over time. Such standards are often used in conjunction with both quality assurance and CQI. One collects observations of the same phenomenon over time to determine if a process is in control (small random variations) or out of control (major fluctuations). This information uses the institution as its own "control" and can be coupled with the goal of continuously raising standards in the institution. Although this approach is useful, some external comparisons are required to understand how to prioritize problems. One needs such external comparisons (benchmarks) to decide which processes to address first.

How to Benchmark Outcomes

To benchmark outcomes, the following steps should be followed:

1. Using the risk-adjustment models, assign the predicted probability of each relevant adverse event to each case. Consider the following examples:

   - An 82-year-old woman is admitted to the hospital with pneumonia, with secondary diagnoses of cancer of the pancreas and type 2 diabetes. Her probability of death is .591. If discharged alive, her probability of readmission within 30 days is .307.
   - A 36-year-old woman is admitted to the hospital with pneumonia with no secondary diagnoses. Her probability of death is .008. If discharged alive, her probability of readmission within 30 days is .001.

TABLE 5-4 Predicted and Actual Mortality and Readmissions, and Ratios, for Hospital A

	Predicted Mortality	Actual Mortality	Ratio (P:A)	Predicted Readmissions	Actual Readmissions	Ratio (P:A)
Pneumonia	23.8	35	0.68	46.9	42	1.12*
All respiratory diseases	70.2	87	0.81	123.3	116	1.06

*Indicates statistical significance at 0.001

2. Add all of the predicted probabilities for each hospital product line; also add all of the actual events for the same product line. Use these numbers to develop reports for each hospital, comparing predicted frequencies for each category of adverse event to the observed frequencies (see **Table 5-4**).

Note that in this example the hospital has mortality that is significantly higher than predicted, both for pneumonia and for all respiratory diseases, given the risk factors of the patients treated. Readmissions within 30 days of discharge, however, are significantly fewer than predicted for the pneumonia patients and lower than predicted (but not significantly) for all respiratory diseases.

3. Perform statistical tests on the differences between predicted and observed frequencies to determine whether the differences are statistically significant or might merely represent random variations.

4. Develop systems profiles, comparing hospitals using these multiple risk-adjusted measures, similar to the example in **Table 5-5**.

We can use these profiles for a "first cut." Hospitals with unusually poor (significant) patterns of adverse occurrences should examine medical records and perform peer reviews to determine whether there are problems with the process of care and, if so, whether administrative actions may be required at a system level. In the preceding example, Hospital A might want to examine why its mortality rates for pneumonia and other respiratory diseases are relatively high; Hospital C might want to look at its readmission rates for respiratory diseases other than pneumonia.

TABLE 5-5 Ratios of Predicted to Actual Values, by Hospital and by Outcome, for Pneumonia and for All Respiratory Diseases in Three Hospitals

	Hospital A	Hospital B	Hospital C
Mortality			
Pneumonia	0.68*	1.09	1.32*
All respiratory diseases	0.81*	0.98	1.03
Readmissions			
Pneumonia	1.12*	1.01	0.99
All respiratory diseases	1.06	1.31*	0.87

*Indicates statistical significance at .001

Recognizing the Limitations of Outcome Measures

Outcome measures derived from discharge abstracts and billing data have inherent limitations because they lack the context provided by the relevant in-depth clinical information. For example, detailed clinical information allows us to determine time sequences; in the preceding example, did pneumonia or another upper respiratory infection develop while the patient was in the hospital, or was it already present at the time of admission? Patient compliance is an obvious factor for predicting readmissions but is not included in billing data. Furthermore, we cannot assume that data quality is good or uniform across hospitals. Problems with data quality will definitely affect hospital scores on these measures. Poor coding of comorbidities can make a hospital look worse; good coding of complications can also make a hospital look worse. There is no evidence that a hospital that does well on one measure is necessarily doing well on the other measures.

Many of these same symptoms are evident in attempting comparisons across cities and countries. Marshall et al. (2003) report that indicators compare reasonably well between the United Kingdom and the United States, but that some caution is needed because of differing practice cultures. Hussey et al. (2004) compared five industrialized countries on the basis of 21 indicators and found that each country performs best and worst in at least one area of care and that all could show improvement.

Problems With the Aggregation of Different Measures of Adverse Events

Are Different Measures Correlated With One Another?

A valid index of hospital performance must encompass the multiple aspects of hospital care. It may not be possible, either conceptually or technically, to construct a single, all-inclusive index of the quality of hospital care. It is possible, however, to construct several indexes that validly measure important aspects of quality and then to examine the relationships among the various measures to see if they are correlated. If the various indicators are highly correlated, we eventually may be able to construct an overall (unidimensional) quality measure. If they are not correlated, we can conclude that the various components measure distinct dimensions of quality and that the separate measures are all necessary in obtaining a valid impression of a hospital's performance.

For example, a 1991 study analyzed the relationships among three measures that seem to be "intrinsically valid," in that they clearly are outcomes to be avoided. The three indicators—mortality, unscheduled readmissions, and complications—were adjusted for some of the clinical factors that are predictive of the occurrence of deaths, readmissions, and complications. Risk factors were established empirically within each disease category for each index. The authors demonstrated that hospitals' rankings on the three indexes were not correlated. This result provides some evidence that these different indexes appear to be measuring different dimensions of hospital performance. Thus the three indexes should not be combined into a unidimensional measure of quality, at least not at the hospital level of analysis. Neither should any one measure be used to represent all three aspects of quality (DesHarnais et al., 1991).

One cannot simply choose one hospital-wide measure such as a "death rate" to validly represent a hospital's performance. Neither can one simply add up occurrences of different types of adverse events and then claim to have a unidimensional measure of hospital performance. Those hospitals that rank well in terms of mortality rates do not necessarily do well on the other measures and may have excessive readmissions or complications.

Can Different Measures of Adverse Events
Be Weighted to Create a Unidimensional Index?

Can these different types of adverse events be weighted in a meaningful way so that they can be combined and used as a tool to rank hospitals? Probably not. Even after careful risk adjustment and data quality control, one is still left with the problem of how to weight a death in importance relative to a return surgery or an unscheduled readmission. Clearly, they are not of the same importance, and it would not make sense to treat them as if they were.

CONCLUSIONS

Quality is something that all health care providers favor, but it is not, as many would like to believe, something that happens without planning and conscientious effort. The outside world is demanding that health care organizations provide care of the highest quality at a reasonable price. Information with which to make assessments of outcome performance in health care is increasingly available. Providers can fight to maintain professional autonomy by trying to push the lay assessors back, or they can take the lead by becoming experts on quality assessment and applying their newfound skills to ongoing operations. They can then educate the public in how to interpret the impact of age, comorbidity, and other risk factors on outcome measures.

The medical profession can educate its members in how to participate in the process of quality improvement, to cooperate with other disciplines and professional groups, to lead the way in analysis and process improvement, and to help develop consensus about what is currently known and what warrants further study. It can go much further in empowering all of its constituents to follow the scientific method at a pragmatic level in all aspects of medicine and in all settings, to the benefit of its consumers. It can move from being on the defensive about consumer-oriented quality and how it is measured toward being its primary advocate.

Cross-References to the Companion Casebook

(McLaughlin, C. P., Johnson, J. K., and Sollecito, W. A. [Eds.]. 2012. *Implementing Continuous Quality Improvement in Health Care: A Global Casebook.* Sudbury, MA: Jones & Bartlett Learning.)

Case Study Number	Case Study Title	Case Study Authors
2	Holtz Children's Hospital: Reducing Central Line Infections	*Gwenn E. McLaughlin*
13	The Folic Acid Fortification Decision Bounces Around the World	*Curtis P. McLaughlin and Craig D. McLaughlin*

REFERENCES

Blumberg, M. 1986. Risk-adjusting health care outcomes: A methodological review. *Med Care Rev*, 43: 351–393.

Chassin, M. R., Hannan, E. L., and DeBuono, B. A. 1996. Benefits and hazards of reporting medical outcomes publicly. *N Eng J Med*, 334: 394–398.

DesHarnais, S., Chesney, J. D., Wroblewski, R. T., et al. 1988. The risk-adjusted mortality index: A new measure of hospital performance. *Med Care*, 26: 1129–1148.

DesHarnais S., McMahon, L. F., Jr., and Wroblewski, R. 1991. Measuring outcomes of hospital care using multiple risk adjusted indexes. *Health Serv Res*, 26: 425–445.

Donabedian, A. 1980. The definition of quality and approaches to its assessment. In *Explorations in Quality Assessment and Monitoring* (Vol. 1, pp 95–99). Ann Arbor, MI: Health Administration Press.

Donabedian, A. 1982. *The Criteria and Standards of Quality*. Ann Arbor, MI: Health Administration Press.

Donabedian, A. 1986. Criteria and standards for quality assessment and monitoring. *Qual Rev Bull*, 14(3): 99–108.

Flood, A., Scott, W. R., Ewy, W., et al. 1982. Effectiveness in professional organizations: The impact of surgeons and surgical staff organizations on the quality of care in hospitals. *Health Serv Res*, 17: 341–366.

Galvin, R. S., and McGlynn, E. A. 2003. Using performance measurement to drive improvement: A roadmap for change. *Med Care*, 41(1): 148–160.

Hussey, P. S., Anderson, G. F., Osborn, R., et al. 2004. How does the quality of care compare in five countries? *Health Aff*, 23(3): 89–99.

Institute of Medicine. 2000. *To Err Is Human: Building a Safer Health System*. Washington, DC: National Academies Press.

Institute of Medicine. 2001. *Crossing the Quality Chasm: A New Health System for the 21st Century*. Washington, DC: National Academies Press.

Institute of Medicine. 2003. *Committee on Understanding and Eliminating Racial and Ethnic Disparities in Health Care: Unequal Treatment Confronting Racial and Ethnic Disparities in Health Care*. Washington, DC: National Academies Press.

Knaus, W., Draper, E. A., Wagner, D. P., et al. 1986. An evaluation of outcome from intensive care in major medical centers. *Ann Intern Med*, 104: 410–418.

Luft, H., and Hunt, S. 1986. Evaluating individual hospital quality through outcome statistics. *JAMA*, 255: 2780–2786.

Marshall, M. N., Shekelle, P. G., McGlynn, E. A., et al. 2003. Can health care indicators be transferred between countries? *Qual Safety Health Care*, 12: 8–12.

Moses, L. E., and Mosteller, F. 1968. Institutional differences in postoperative death rates: Commentary on some of the findings of the National Halothane Study. *JAMA*, 202: 492–494.

Pollack, M., Ruttimann, U. E., Getson, P. R. 1987. Accurate prediction of the outcome of pediatric intensive care: A new quantitative method. *NEJM*, 316: 134–139.

Roemer, A., Moustafa, T., and Hopkins, C. E. 1968. A proposed hospital quality index: Hospital death rates adjusted for case severity. *Health Serv Res*, 3(2): 96–118.

U.S. Office of Technology Assessment (OTA). 1988. The quality of medical care: Information for consumers. OTA-H-386. Washington, DC: U.S. Government Printing Office.

Wagner, D. P., Knaus, W. A., and Draper, E. A. 1986. The case for adjusting hospital death rates for severity of illness. *Health Aff*, 5(2): 148–153.

CHAPTER 6

Measuring Consumer Satisfaction

Shulamit L. Bernard and Lucy A. Savitz

"The key to customer feedback is to ask about the few aspects of the customer experience that matter the most . . . and do something about them!"

—Davis Balestracci (2009)

Measures of consumer satisfaction can serve an important role in monitoring quality and improving health care. Oftentimes overshadowed by measures of clinical process and outcomes in monitoring health care quality, consumer satisfaction has emerged as an important indicator of quality (see Chapter 5). At one time relegated to service improvement efforts by hospitals, measures of patient—or consumer—satisfaction are recognized as the provider's best source of information about "communication, education, and pain-management process, and they (patients) are the only source of information about whether they were treated with dignity and respect" (Cleary, 2003, p. 33). Consumers' experiences can stimulate important insights into how a provider is operating and suggest changes that may "close the chasm between the care provided and that care that should be provided" (Cleary, 2003, p. 33). Furthermore, the marketplace in which the providers operate is demanding that data on patient satisfaction be used to empower consumers and foster provider accountability and consumer choice. Measuring consumer satisfaction provides a comprehensive, systematic, and patient-centered approach for analysis, implementation, monitoring, and improving both the perceived and the clinical quality aspects of care (Ford et al., 1997).

This chapter provides an overview of key issues and methods related to measuring consumer satisfaction. The rationale for measurement is discussed and followed by a series of issues: measurement, data capture, timing, and functional responsibility. An example applying patient satisfaction measures as part of the Balanced Scorecard (a measurement system that adds customer and other dimensions to the customary financial measures [Kaplan and Norton, 1996]) is presented. We conclude with a brief overview of the special issue of case-mix adjustment of reported consumer satisfaction measures.

DEFINING CONSUMER SATISFACTION

Obtaining the views of customers has been a key feature of many modern business practices for many years, and the health care sector has adopted this same view, considering the patient as a consumer, which has led to the application of methods for assessing patient views (Wensing and Elwyn, 2002). The idea of patients as consumers stems from a market perspective on health care in which the providers are assumed to be responsive to competition and in which competition can drive increased quality and lower cost. In the context of satisfaction measures, patients are considered as parties to an exchange of goods and/or services. Health consumers' views can be divided into three types: measures of preferences, evaluations by users, and reports of health care. Preferences are ideas about what should occur in the health care encounter. Evaluations are patients' reactions to their experiences of health care, or whether the process or outcome of their care was good or bad (Pascoe, 1983). Reports are objective observations of an organization or a process of care. They are independent of preferences or evaluations; for example, a report may assess the waiting time for an appointment or response from a nurse (Wensing and Elwyn, 2002, 2003).

The model used to explain postpurchase satisfaction suggests that consumer satisfaction can be defined simply as "the evaluation rendered that the experience was at least as good as it was supposed to be" (Hunt, 1977). Postpurchase satisfaction is classically derived by the relationship between the consumer's expectations and the product's (or service's) perceived performance (LaBarbara and Mazursky, 1983). If the rendered service or product meets or exceeds expectations, then the consumer is satisfied; if the rendered service or product does not meet expectations, then the consumer is dissatisfied. The Buyer-Decision Process (Kotler and Armstrong, 1997) can be summarized in five steps:

1. Recognition of the problem

2. Information search

3. Evaluation of the alternative(s)

4. Choice of the best option

5. Postpurchase behavior

Here postpurchase behavior is directly preceded by four steps that shape expectations against the level of satisfaction that will ultimately be reported. Furthermore, the extent to which consumers spend time moving through these steps is largely associated with the nature of the health care problem being addressed. In the model, the key attributes of the health care concern are complexity, amount of patient discomfort, degree of patient involvement, and urgency. For instance, a mother recognizing that a healthy child is in immediate need of a routine sports physical to comply with a school requirement might skip the information search step and turn to the telephone directory to identify the closest walk-in clinic for a quick appointment. Once the most convenient and timely provider is identified, the purchase decision is made with relatively little investment in the choice. Walking out of the physician's office within 30 minutes and having paid a minimal fee to secure a completed form so that her son could sign up for a team sport may leave both mother and son quite satisfied with the medical encounter. This example can contrast sharply with patients seeking higher-order services or services where the doctor–patient relationship is extended over a protracted time and where the patient perceives a need to make critical choices (e.g., organ transplantation, cancer treatment, prenatal care and delivery, nursing home care).

Application of this marketing model to health care is further complicated by the fact that choices and preferences may be severely limited as a result of health insurance limitations, constraining patient choice and/or physician referral options. The complexity of patients' perceptions and attitudes, together with their sometimes limited cognitive ability to process the nature of their own health care situations, serves to further complicate the decision process beyond attributes of the immediate health concern.

Expectations and preferences are also shaped by a variety of inputs, such as personal experiences, experiences of family and friends, physician recommendations, and directed advertising campaigns.

WHO IS THE CONSUMER?

The consumer, in general, can be viewed as the party using the provided service and/or product of the exchange. From a health care perspective, the consumer is typically assumed to be the patient in a clinical setting or the enrollee in a health plan. The consumer is the recipient of a direct exchange of health care services, and it is this perspective that serves as the basis for the majority of discussion in this chapter. Consumers in health care can include both internal customers (e.g., providers and suppliers) and external customers (e.g., patients and their families as well as communities and government agencies). Thus, measures of consumer satisfaction may broadly target family members, practitioners, staff, and contract service administrators. Examples of other consumers beyond the basic patient–provider exchange are illustrated as follows:

Physicians as consumers:

- Community doctors referring patients to a tertiary care center are consumers of that center.
- Physicians sending specimens to labs for testing and/or ordering scans from radiology centers are consumers of that ancillary service.

Facilities as consumers:

- Hospitals purchasing information systems to monitor the quality process are consumers of these vendors.

Insurers and managed care organizations (MCOs) as consumers:

- Insurers outsourcing claims processing functions are consumers of the third-party service.
- MCOs contracting with physicians, pharmacies, clinics, hospitals, and home health agencies to provide a continuum of care for their health insurance benefits are consumers for the providers and facilities.

Government agencies as consumers:

- Centers for Medicare and Medicaid Services (CMS), by contracting with insurers to provide Medicare and Medicaid risk coverage for eligible beneficiaries, is a consumer for the MCOs.
- State and/or federal prisons, by contracting with health care facilities and providers for services for the incarcerated population, are consumers of these facilities and providers.

Beyond recognizing the roles of these parties in providing a range of health care and health care–related services, it is also important to note the roles of others, such as health care workers, suppliers, communities, and families. In particular, families often act as a key agent in the market exchange for health care services, such as for minors and frail elderly family members, and have often reported either directly or indirectly as proxies concerning patient satisfaction (Schweikhart et al., 1993). However, their perspective, while valuable, must be distinguished from that of the individual experiencing the health care service firsthand. In considering the various consumers of health care, it is important to recognize that patients, providers, and payers all define quality differently. These differences result in different expectations of the health care system and, thus, differing measures of satisfaction in evaluation of quality (McGlynn, 1997).

WHY MEASURE CONSUMER SATISFACTION?

We are in an era when health care consumers want to assert more control over dollars, and many are willing to pay out-of-pocket for quality. Technologically savvy patients and families are surfing the Web and demanding information about health care problems and provider performance. In addition, as hospitals are under pressure to increase the quality of care, ensure the safety of their patients, and lower operating costs, greater attention and scrutiny are being given to the accountability function of consumer satisfaction scores. In this competitive health care environment, consumers want and expect better health care services and hospital systems are concerned about maintaining their overall image. There is also attention to ways in which patient satisfaction measurement can be integrated into an overall measure of clinical quality.

Consumer satisfaction provides a useful outcome measure for quality of care offered by a health care organization.

Ford et al. (1997) review the literature that reports benefits of measuring patient-enrollee satisfaction attributable to the following factors: increased profitability, increased market share, improved patient retention, improved collections, increased patient referrals, improved patient compliance, continuity of care, reduced hospitalization and length of stay, increased willingness to recommend the organization to family and friends, and reduced risk of malpractice. Satisfaction measures, together with clinical outcomes and cost data, are increasingly used by employers as part of their value-based purchasing of health care benefits, by insurers in contracting for network services, and by potential partners in establishing health care alliances and systems (Woodbury et al., 1997).

Quality, loyalty, and satisfaction have important implications for future utilization of hospitals, and all three factors are correlated with the degree of success of overall hospital experience. Expertise in specific illnesses and/or treatment and the history of medical errors have emerged as the most important factors influencing the public's choice of a hospital (Blizzard, 2005). **Table 6–1** shows how respondents to a 2005 Gallup poll panel survey on health care ranked specific factors when choosing a health care facility or hospital. Almost two-thirds of those who responded to the survey indicated that medical expertise "had a great deal of influence in their choice," and more than half said the same of medical errors,

---

TABLE 6–1 Rank of Factors Influencing Choice of Hospital

1. Expertise in specific illness/treatment
2. History of medical errors
3. Doctor referral/doctor's orders
4. Courtesy of staff
5. Hospital location
6. Appearance of hospital/facility
7. Recommendation of family/friends
8. Consumer report cards
9. Insurance coverage
10. Public information (marketing/Web site)
11. Amenities (food, parking, etc.)

Source: Blizzard, 2005.

reflecting growing patient awareness and concern about quality and safety in their choice of hospitals.

Clearly, there is a direct link between patient satisfaction and market share driven by repeat utilization. In addition, positive intermediary influences on compliance and provider change are key with respect to health care behaviors, and loyalty and word-of-mouth advertising are related to reputation. For instance, word-of-mouth advertising has been shown to account for a significant proportion of future encounters whereby satisfied customers tell others about their experiences and refer them accordingly (Davies and Ware, 1988; Kotler and Armstrong, 1997; Savitz, 1994).

External reporting and accreditation requirements made by The Joint Commission and the National Committee on Quality Assurance (NCQA) have heightened the importance of patient satisfaction measures, moving them from internal to external performance monitoring and quality indicators. Patient perspectives on their health care experience have been included in the NCQA annual State of Health Care Quality reports (2003) along with the clinical Healthcare Effectiveness Data Information Set (HEDIS) measures.

Finally, application of continuous quality improvement (CQI) principles in health care organizations has led to the integration of patient-enrollee satisfaction measures that can be used in identifying improvement opportunities in the key components of care—structure, process, and outcome—as described by Donabedian (1982).

Taking Action

In addition to regulatory requirements, the fact that the primary purpose of measuring consumer satisfaction is to improve the quality of care provided should always be kept in mind. This principle should be a guide in what data are collected, how they are collected, and, most importantly, how they are analyzed and reported. As Balestracci warns, "Remember data are a basis for action: vague data with vague objectives yield vague results" (2009, p. 269).

Balestracci goes on to remind us that consumer data should be collected with the idea of identifying trouble areas and not simply validating what we already know; furthermore, taking action includes summarization as well as communication of findings back to the customer (2009). It all starts with understanding the goals of data collection on the front end of the process.

MEASURING SATISFACTION

Zifko-Baliga and Krampf (1997) found that patients used more than 500 criteria to evaluate hospital quality. Personal choice emerged as a significant factor in predicting enrollee satisfaction. In a study done by researchers at Kaiser Permanente, 10,000 adults enrolled in a large group model HMO in northern California in 1995 and 1996 were surveyed. For each of nine satisfaction measures (i.e., time usually spent with physician, explanation of diagnosis and treatment, technical skill of physician, personal manner of physician, use of latest technology, focus on prevention, concern for emotional well-being, patient's overall satisfaction, and recommendation of physician to others), respondents who had chosen their own physician were 16% to 26% more likely than those who had been assigned a personal physician to report their health care as very good or excellent (Schmittdiel et al., 1997). Findings such as these are important to communicate to practitioners an understanding of the exchange process they are involved in and to evaluate appropriate satisfaction measures.

A follow-up study (based on Fletcher et al., 1983) conducted by the American College of Physicians (ACP) in 1993 continues to be relevant today. The study included a series of focus groups with patients and physicians to understand the relative importance of measures of satisfaction in office-based medical care as part of the Patient-Centered Care Project. The critical steps suggested in this study are depicted in **Figure 6–1**.

ACP researchers completed a comparative analysis of physicians' and patients' importance rankings for 125 attributes of the medical care

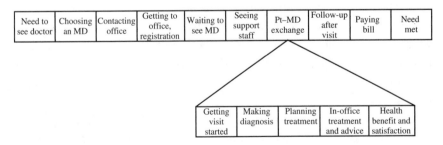

FIGURE 6–1 ACP, The Patient-Centered Care Project: Steps in office-based medical care

encounter. Major discrepancies were found throughout the list, and examples of these are provided in the partial list that follows:

Patient Rank	MD Rank	Difference	Questions How important is it that . . .
26	113	87	the doctor explains the results of any evaluation by a consulting specialist to the patients?
80	10	70	the doctor discusses important information about patients' health in a private place?
12	81	69	the doctor explains the purpose of each medicine prescribed in a way patients understand?
23	79	56	the doctor clearly explains the possible side effects of medicines?
5	58	53	the doctor gives patients solid facts about the likely benefits and risks of treatment?
11	64	53	the doctor tells patients how to take medicines in a way that patients understand?

The ACP study underscores the critical need to measure consumer satisfaction using data from those who utilize the services rather than simply assuming that as providers we understand what patients want and what will ultimately satisfy their expectations. Clearly, practitioner understanding of patient expectations is incomplete. More recent studies confirm that while there is some overlap between clinicians' and patients' expectations in crucial elements of quality, there is also disagreement about the relative importance of elements such as access to care, coordination of care, and provision of information. Patients place greater value on these domains than do physicians (Kaya et al., 2003).

Sitzia (1999) analyzed 195 studies that used instruments to assess the satisfaction levels of health service users and found that, with few exceptions, the survey instruments examined demonstrated little evidence of reliability or validity. An additional problem was that although many hospitals were collecting data about patient experience for their own internal use, these data could not be compared across hospitals because the assessment tools were not standardized. To address this issue, in 2002 CMS partnered with the Agency for Healthcare Research and Quality (AHRQ) to develop and test HCAHPS (Hospital Consumer Assessment of Healthcare Providers and Systems), which is also known as the CAHPS Hospital Survey. This initiative provided a standard for collecting and publicly reporting information about *patient experience* of care, which was gaining leverage with employers, payers, clinicians, and the government (Liang et al., 2002; Scalise, 2003).

After rigorous development and testing, CMS implemented the HCAHPS survey in October 2006. The first public reporting of HCAHPS results occurred in March 2008. Results from hospitals that participate are available at http://www.hospitalcompare.hhs.gov. The HCAHPS survey is 27 questions in length and contains 18 patient perspectives on care and patient rating items that encompass eight key topics:

1. Communication with doctors

2. Communication with nurses

3. Responsiveness of hospital staff

4. Pain management

5. Communication about medicines

6. Discharge information

7. Cleanliness of the hospital environment

8. Quietness of the hospital environment

The survey also includes four screener questions and five demographic items, which are used for adjusting the mix of patients across hospitals and for analytical purposes. More information about HCAHPS, including the survey instruments, is available at http://www.hcahpsonline.org/home.aspx. The survey, its methodology, and the results it produces are in the public domain.

Data Capture

In general, patient-enrollee satisfaction measures are among the most readily available outcome measures. Accreditation requirements and marketing efforts have already been established to collect these measures without the burden of purchasing new and/or reprogramming existing systems to generate such quality measures, as is the experience with clinical quality measures. It is also important, however, to address issues involved in data capture with respect to how the data will be collected, when the data should be collected, and which functional area will be responsible for data capture and reporting.

With the growing use of the Internet and social media, it is very tempting to assume that these modalities are superior to traditional modes of data capture. Web-based technologies have emerged that greatly simplify the process of data collection and analysis (e.g., http://www .surveymonkey.com/and http://www3.formassembly.com/). While we are fast approaching the time when the Internet will be the most appropriate form of communication with consumers, this is not always the case. Care should be taken to understand what tools the consumers being surveyed will be most receptive to and which will produce the highest response rates and, of course, the most reliable information. Also to be considered is the type of information being collected; for example, open-ended information may still be collected most reliably through face-to-face, point-of-service formats or telephone interviews. Likewise, an important consideration is modality of information.

Alternative Modalities

There are multiple modalities available to health service researchers and health care organizations in collecting patient satisfaction data, which can then be translated into information for CQI purposes. Alternative modalities have important advantages and disadvantages that must be considered together with the data needed in determining how to proceed.

Ford et al. (1997) provide a comprehensive comparison of advantages and disadvantages associated with various qualitative and quantitative modalities for measuring consumer satisfaction. While a detailed specification of how to capture satisfaction measures using these alternative modalities exceeds the scope of this particular chapter, an itemized listing of these methods with a brief description is presented. There is an extensive literature on each modality that the reader is encouraged to consult as needed.

Qualitative Modalities

- *Management observation*—formal observation and documentation of the patient care process
- *Employee feedback programs*—formal employee feedback on all aspects of the patient care process

- *Work teams and quality circles*—continuous employee input through teams
- *Focus groups*—input facilitated through an open-ended forum of homogeneous groups of consumers
- *Mystery shoppers*—an observational technique that provides a snapshot of the service experience from a user perspective

Quantitative Modalities

- *Comment cards*—voluntary patient-enrollee ratings of service quality
- *Mail surveys*—questionnaires mailed to users for completion and return
- *Point-of-service interviews*—self-administered or interviewer-administered questionnaires completed usually following service delivery at the delivery site
- *Telephone interviews*—personal interviews with users over the telephone by trained interviewers

Critical considerations when comparing these optional measurement modalities involve expense, timeliness of feedback, required staff competencies to develop and administer the measurement instrument, desired depth of understanding, and complexity of the data capture effort. Work teams and quality circles have become a well-established part of CQI efforts, providing useful and timely consumer satisfaction information that is non-episodic. However, this particular method does not offer information that is necessarily generalizable or comprehensive. Comment cards are the least expensive and complex service evaluation technique; however, the results are often biased with respect to the type of consumers who are inclined to respond and the type of information typically provided. A qualitative approach is particularly useful for exploring patients' views in areas that have not been previously studied (Wensing and Elwyn, 2003). In general, any modality offers only a snapshot of the service experience and must be replicated over time in order to provide feedback useful to the CQI process.

A clear understanding of organizational capabilities and commitment together with the intended purpose of satisfaction measures is necessary to select the modality to be used. Selection of the appropriate data capture modality involves learning more about information-gathering techniques and choosing the right technique for the target group and desired depth of information sought. Trade-offs between budgetary constraints and methodological rigor are often central selection criteria.

Timing

Little attention has been paid to the appropriate timing of patient-enrollee survey administration and/or interviewing in the data collection process. Most marketing efforts have done collecting either with a point-of-service survey and/or with a short-term non–service-specific follow-up after discharge/encounter via mail or telephone. As we begin to use such data as part of the CQI process, more consideration should be given to the appropriate timing of such data collection. For instance, it may make sense to query emergency room visits at the point of service; however, follow-up of services with extended recovery periods may be more meaningful if they are conducted at clinically reasonable points in the recovery process (e.g., 6 weeks following care for hip replacements). However, considerations of the recovery process must be balanced with the ability for the patient to provide accurate recall. Survey vendors provide a data collection protocol as part of their service; the HCAHPS methodology also specifies data collection protocols and timing of survey implementation.

Validity and Psychometric Properties

Patient satisfaction survey instruments should be validated to ensure that the questions measure what they are intended to measure. The science has much improved since 1994 when a review of 195 studies of patient satisfaction showed that only 46% reported some validity or reliability data and only 6% reported evidence of measuring the intended domain (Sitzia, 1999). Cognitive testing of the survey items with the intended audience should be reviewed as part of an evaluation of a survey instrument under consideration. Survey instruments should also have adequate psychometric features (Streiner and Norman, 1989). For example, a high response rate to an item usually indicates that the question is relevant and understandable, while a low item response rate may suggest confusion with the item or response categories (Wensing and Elwyn, 2003). Questionnaires that are designed to measure different aspects of quality should demonstrate variation across patients (ability to discriminate) as well as variation between measurements at different points in time (e.g., responsiveness to change and interventions). Once valid and reliable consumer satisfaction measures have been produced, they become a valuable component of the feedback loop in the CQI process. Only through dissemination can this information actually be used for performance improvement.

SATISFACTION AND THE BALANCED SCORECARD

Kaplan and Norton developed the premise for the Balanced Scorecard (BSC) approach through a series of articles that were published in the *Harvard Business Review* in the early 1990s and later compiled this work with a more in-depth discussion of examples from the field in a book (1996). In addition to strict financial outcomes, health care financial managers need to consider and monitor intangible assets that have an impact on the organization's bottom line. These include clinical processes, staff skills, and patient satisfaction and loyalty. The BSC is an integrative approach to performance evaluation that examines performance related to finance, human resources, internal processes, and customers (Oliveira, 2001). The BSC is more than a measurement tool; it is a management system used to achieve long-term strategic goals by linking performance to outcomes and can be used to (1) guide current performance through feedback and (2) target future performance improvement. The instrumentation of a BSC focuses on a single strategy where multiple, relevant measures are linked together in a cause–effect network. Measures transcend the traditional financial accounting framework used to assess organizational performance, seeking to build internal assets and capabilities while forging the integration of strategic alliances. Leading (structure and process) and lagging (outcomes) measures are identified in four categories: financial performance, customer knowledge, internal business processes, and staff learning and growth. Customer satisfaction is typically included in the customer knowledge category. Indicators are selected by a designated group within an organization, and periodic reports are disseminated for monitoring and evaluative purposes.

Application of this innovative tool is occurring with greater frequency in health care (Hall et al., 2003; Pineno, 2002; Pink et al., 2001). Several major integrated delivery and hospital systems are currently implementing BSCs. Macdonald (1998) reported on the application of the BSC in aligning strategy and performance in long-term care at the Sisters of Charity of Ottawa Health Service. The section of their developed BSC addressing customer satisfaction is shown in **Table 6–2**.

TABLE 6–2 A Balanced Scorecard Example

Strategic Objective	Lag Indicators	Lead Indicators
Meet clients' needs, priorities, and expectations in a manner that exemplilfies the Sisters of Charity of Ottawa Health Service values of respect, compassion, social justice, and community spirit.	• Overall satisfaction—clients and families (all programs) • Satisfaction with physical, social, emotional, and spiritual care (all programs) • Percentage of patients satisfied with service in the language of their choice (all programs) • Percentage of patients who feel they are treated with respect; participate in decisions about their own care (all programs)	• Volunteer hours per patient day (percentage variance) (Human Resources) • Direct care hours worked per patient day (percentage variance) (Finance) • Staff stability ratio (Human Resources) • Number and nature of projects that focus on increasing patient, resident, or client quality of life (all programs and departments)

Source: Excerpted from Macdonald, 1998.

CASE-MIX ADJUSTMENT: ADDRESSING A SPECIAL ISSUE IN MEASURING CONSUMER SATISFACTION

Using performance measures to suggest improvement opportunities as part of CQI often results in internal staff criticism such as "my patients are sicker" or "my patients are different." Case-mix adjustment methodologies have been used to control for explainable differences in subpopulations of patients-enrollees so that valid comparisons may be made with adjusted performance measures. Case-mix and risk adjustment techniques are a common feature of the computer macros that estimate HCAHPS measures and are used to adjust consumer ratings and composites to allow for cross-plan comparisons (Landon et al., 2004). The HCAHPS comparison's case mix adjusts for consumer characteristics such as age, gender, education, self-reported health status, and proxy respondent.

Hargraves and colleagues (2001) examined patient characteristics thought to be associated with reports and ratings of hospital care and considered these as adjusters to hospital ratings and reports. Demographic and health status variables were evaluated by exploring how adjusting reports and ratings for hospital differences in such variables affects comparison of performance among hospitals. Their findings suggest that the demographic variables with the strongest and most consistent associations with patient-reported problems were age and reported health status. Patient gender and education sometimes predicted reports and ratings but not as consistently as the other two variables. However, overall, the impact of adjusting for patient characteristics on hospital rankings was small. Nevertheless, the authors recommend adjusting for the most important predictors, such as age and health status, to help alleviate concerns about bias. As with the earlier study, the authors also recommend that data be stratified by groups of patients (i.e., medical, surgical, obstetrics) to facilitate interpretation and target quality improvement efforts.

CONCLUSIONS

Patient satisfaction surveys are used increasingly to gauge consumer experience with health care. However, efforts to adequately measure consumer satisfaction are complex. As with any evaluative (whether formative or summative) effort, consideration must be given to the ultimate end use of the generated satisfaction measures. In doing so, key measures should be selected given the context of the particular health care service and/or procedure. Relevant consumers should next be identified and their input solicited. Assessment should be made of alternative modalities for gathering data from consumers. It is important that this choice be aligned with the intended use of this information in light of organizational constraints on resources, time, and internal capabilities. Then the collected satisfaction measures should be applied as part of the CQI process, and always with the goal of taking action to improve quality and safety.

REFERENCES

Balestracci, D. 2009. *Data Sanity: A Quantum Leap to Unprecedented Results.* Englewood, CO: Medical Group Management Association.

Blizzard, R. 2005. Healthcare panel: How do people choose hospitals? Retrieved April 21, 2011, from http://www.gallup.com/poll/19402/Healthcare-Panel-How-People-Choose-Hospitals.aspx

Cleary, P. D. 2003. A hospitalization from hell: A patient's perspective on quality. *Ann Intern Med*, 138(1): 33–39.

Davies, A. R., and Ware, J. E. 1988. Involving consumers in quality of care assessment. *Health Affairs*, 7(1): 33–48.

Donabedian, A. 1982. *The Criteria and Standards of Quality.* Ann Arbor, MI: Health Administration Press.

Fletcher, R. H., O'Malley, M. S., Earp, J. A., et al. 1983. Patients' priorities for medical care. *Med Care*, XXI: 234–242.

Ford, R. C., Bach, S. A., and Fottler, M. D. 1997. Methods of measuring patient satisfaction. *Health Care Manage Rev*, 22(2): 74–89.

Hall, L. M. et al. 2003. A balanced scorecard approach for nursing report card development. *Outcomes Management*, 7(1): 17–22.

Hargraves, J. L., Wilson, I. B., Zaslavsky, A., et al. 2001. Adjusting for patient characteristics when analyzing reports from patients about hospital care. *Med Care*, 39: 635–641.

Hunt, H. K. 1977. CS/D: Overview and future research directions. In Hunt, H. K. (Ed.), *Conceptualization and Measurement of Consumer Satisfaction and Dissatisfaction.* Cambridge, MA: Marketing Science Institute.

Kaplan, R. S., and Norton, D. P. 1996. *The Balanced Scorecard, Translating Strategy into Action.* Boston, MA: Harvard Business School Press.

Kaya, S., Cankul, H. I., Yigit, C., et al. 2003. Comparing patients' and physicians' opinions on quality outpatient care. *Mil Med*, 168: 1029–1033.

Kotler, P., and Armstrong, G. 1997. Consumer markets and consumer buying behavior. In *Marketing, An Introduction* (4th ed., Chap. 5). Englewood Cliffs, NJ: Prentice Hall.

LaBarbara, P. A., and Mazursky, D. 1983. A longitudinal assessment of consumer satisfaction/dissatisfaction: The dynamic aspect of the cognitive process, *J Market Res*, 20: 393–404.

Landon, B. E., Zaslavsky, A. M., Bernard, S. L., et al. 2004. Comparison of performance of traditional Medicare versus Medicare Managed Care. *JAMA*, 291: 1744–1752.

Liang, M. H., Lew, R. A., Stucki, G., et al. 2002. Measuring clinically important changes with patient-oriented questionnaires. *Med Care*, 40(4): II45–II51.

Macdonald, M. 1998. Using the balanced scorecard to align strategy and performance in long term care. *Healthcare Manage Forum*, 11(3): 33–38.

McGlynn, E. A. 1997. Six challenges for measuring the quality of health care. *Health Affairs*, 16(3): 7–21.

National Committee for Quality Assessment. 2003. *The State of Health Care Quality: Industry Trends and Analysis.* Washington, DC: NCQA.

Oliveira, J. 2001. The balanced scorecard: An integrative approach to performance evaluation. *Healthcare Financial Manage*, 55: 42–46.

Pascoe, G. C. 1983. Patient satisfaction in primary health care: A literature review and analysis. *Eval Program Plan*, 6: 185–210.

Pineno, C. J. 2002. The balanced scorecard: An incremental approach model to health care management. *J Health Care Finance*, 28(4): 69–80.

Pink, G. H et al. 2001. Creating a balanced scorecard for a hospital system. *J Health Care Finance*, 24(1): 55–58.

Savitz, L. A. 1994. *The Influence of Maternal Employment on Obstetrical Health Care Seeking Behavior.* Ann Arbor, MI: UMI Press.

Scalise, D. 2003. The patient experience. *Hosp Health Network*, 77(12): 41–48.

Schmittdiel, J., Selby, J. V., Grumbach, K., et al. 1997. Choice of a personal physician and patient satisfaction in a health maintenance organization. *JAMA*, 278: 1596–1599.

Schweikhart, S. B., Strasser, S., and Kennedy, M. R. 1993. Service Recovery in health service organizations. *Hosp Health Serv Admin*, 38(1): 3–23.

Sitzia, J. 1999. How valid and reliable are patient satisfaction data? An analysis of 195 studies. *Int Soc Qual Health Care*, 11(4): 319–328.

Streiner, D. L., and Norman, G. R. 1989. *Health Measurement Scales. A Practical Guide to Their Development and Use.* Oxford, UK: Oxford University Press.

Wensing, M., and Elwyn, G. 2002. Research on patients' views in the evaluation and improvement of quality of care. *Qual Saf Health Care*, 11: 153–157.

Wensing, M., and Elwyn, G. 2003. Improving the quality of health care: Methods for incorporating patients' views in health care. *BMJ*, 326: 877–879.

Woodbury, D., Tracy, D., and McKnight, E. 1997. Does considering severity of illness improve interpretation of patient satisfaction data? *J Healthcare Qual*, 20(4): 33–40.

Zifko-Baliga, G. M., and Krampf, R. F. 1997. Managing perceptions of hospital quality. *Market Health Serv*, 17(11): 28–35.

The Role of the Patient in Continuous Quality Improvement

Joanne F. Travaglia and Hamish Robertson

"It is much more important to know what sort of a patient has a disease than what sort of a disease a patient has."

—William Osler (Canadian physician, 1849–1919)

Health systems and services around the world have one primary function: to care for the health and well-being of individuals and populations in the most effective and efficient way possible. This is true whether the individuals involved are working in a laboratory, managing a hospital, triaging at an accident or disaster site, performing cardiac surgery, delivering meals, or counseling a patient with schizophrenia. Whatever the setting or the service, the measures of quality for the professional, staff member, team, ward, and/or service are generally clear. These measures are established by a range of mechanisms, including legislation, professional registration, peer and management review, government and organizational policies and guidelines, research and evidence-based practice, and reflective practice, to name a few.

Much less well defined is the role of the patient (and the patient's family and caregivers) in maintaining and improving the quality of health care (Peat et al., 2010; Schwappach, 2010). This lack of clarity arises from three sources. First, at least in part, it is a result of the variety of historical, philosophical, political, community, organizational, and managerial agendas that converge on this issue. Second, there exists a wide variety of policies (including no policy at all) governing patient involvement in health care services, and there is a similar range of mechanisms, methods, and tools by which services can increase patient involvement. Third, it remains difficult to link patient perceptions of quality and satisfaction, patient involvement in health care services, and the quality of outcomes either for patients as individuals or for patients in general.

Yet while this lack of clarity can make the involvement of consumers difficult, it does not negate the importance of their involvement in continuous quality improvement (CQI). One of the markers of CQI, compared to other quality systems, is that CQI acknowledges customer input as a vital source of evidence at every step of the improvement process. In health care, this input has traditionally taken a number of forms. At an institutional level, services have sought information from customers through surveys, market research, advertising, and outreach efforts. From the customer perspective, feedback has been provided via the same customer satisfaction surveys, but it is also measured via word of mouth referrals, complaints, service reputation, service demand, and litigation. (See Chapter 6.)

The value of these sources of information is unquestionable. Patient or consumer "involvement" in health care, however, is about more than the collection of patient satisfaction surveys. There is an increasing recognition that efforts to increase the safety and improve the quality of care have, to date, largely focused on technical, managerial, or professional levels. In some cases, this may leave the patient behind, or, at the very least, outside the improvement processes. A meta-analysis of eight public inquiries into large-scale breaches of patient safety around the world showed that there were common features in the breakdown of care. The inquiries included those of two hospitals in the United Kingdom (Bristol Royal Infirmary and the Bristol Royal Hospital for Sick Children, and the Victoria Infirmary, Glasgow), three from Australia (Campbelltown and Camden Hospitals, King Edward Memorial Hospital, and Royal Melbourne Hospital), and one each from Slovenia (Celje Hospital), New Zealand (Southland Mental Health Service), and Canada (Winnipeg Health Services Centre). The focus of the inquiries was equally varied and included reviews of pediatric cardiac surgery, the quality of general medical care, the provision of pathology services, hospital-acquired infections, the quality of maternity care, the conduct of nursing staff, and the provision of mental health services. Despite the diversity of country of origin, health care system, type of error(s), and clinicians involved, several key themes were identified across the inquiries. These themes included a lack of patient and family involvement, poor communication and teamwork, and inadequate quality monitoring processes (Hindle et al., 2006). This confluence of factors points clearly to the importance of the integral involvement of patients in the CQI process. The question remains, however, how do we best gain and maximize the benefit from the active involvement of patients in the quality improvement process?

In this chapter, we will begin by reviewing the rationale, models, mechanisms, and current evidence base for patient involvement in quality improvement. We will then present a model of patients' involvement in health care that defines three dimensions (active to passive involvement, proactive to reactive responses, and micro to macro levels). We will then consider the barriers to involvement in CQI by patients, and in particular vulnerable patients, and the ways in which health care services can address this issue.

PATIENT INVOLVEMENT IN HEALTH CARE IMPROVEMENT: A BRIEF OVERVIEW

The call for active patient involvement in CQI activities is in line with changes to the "traditional" patient–clinician relationship that have occurred over several decades. Rather than passive, unquestioning recipients of medical care, patients have demanded, and have even been encouraged (by some providers at least), to become active partners in both their health and their health care.

This space for engagement opened as a result of broader social changes. We will briefly consider five such changes, which impacted the way in which not only patients but health care as a whole was perceived. These changes included shifts in social structures, which in turn had an effect on the patient–clinician relationship.

From the late 1960s onward, individuals and groups became more critical of institutions of power, including medicine and health care (Illich, 1974). A greater questioning of the relationship between medical practitioners and their patients and other clinicians has led to a decline (albeit a slow one) in medical and provider dominance (Dent, 2006; Wade and Halligan, 2004). The increasing diversity of the health professions has meant that the disciplinary scope of the health sciences has expanded, with a consequent expansion in what are conceived of as legitimate forms of practice, thereby increasing patient choice (Borthwick et al., 2010).

Several unforseen global developments contributed to this shift in expertise. The emergence of HIV/AIDS in the 1980s produced profound social and clinical changes. Because of the rate of this condition's progression, the patients themselves knew more about the illness than the clinicians and researchers, introducing the concept of the lay (or patient) expert (Epstein, 1995). The slow response to the scale and severity of AIDS saw some significant shifts in political policy generally and health policy in particular. Not only did communities become directly engaged in providing education about and treatment of the disease, but attitudes and responses of health services and governments to patient involvement also changed as powerful community lobby groups emerged (Shilts, 2007). Similar trends developed in the United States in the 1990s relative to information services that became available to cancer patients and other seriously ill patients; these services continue to be rich sources of patient information, leading to greater patient empowerment. For example, the U.S. National Cancer Institute sponsors a "Cancer Information Service" that allows patients direct access to the latest information by cancer site and type, providing access to both physician- and patient-level information, including information on treatment options, treatment centers, and the latest news about clinical trials. These services can be accessed utilizing multiple modes—via the Internet (http://www.cancer.gov/cancertopics/factsheet/Information/CIS), via telephone (1-800-4-Cancer), and most recently using social media, such as Twitter and Facebook. This service provides patients with knowledge to help choose and even direct the level of care they are receiving, ensuring the highest level of quality and thereby playing a direct role in quality improvement. (See Chapter 1.)

The politicization of various groups and their own efforts to reestablish and legitimize their medical traditions as part of their disenfranchised cultures and epistemologies have contributed to the growth in the number of calls for patient involvement in health care. These calls have combined with a growing recognition of the impact of the social determinants of health (Bambra et al., 2010) and differences in access and quality of care (Betancourt and King, 2003). The concept of cultural safety in health care was developed by the late Irihapeti Ramsden in New Zealand and has now spread internationally as a way of conceptualizing the importance of indigenous perspectives, ideas, and values in health care systems. Ramsden's argument was that health care systems were already political and that for disenfranchised peoples to have their perspectives acknowledged by these systems was, in actuality, a political act of both self-definition and resistance (Ramsden, 1993; Ramsden, 2000a; Ramsden, 2000b).

The growth in "alternative" or complementary medicine since the 1980s has been associated with both globalization and the dissatisfaction felt by many people with mainstream medical care. It has, in effect, produced a secondary health care system, one directly controlled by the consumer (Mak and Faux, 2010; Senel, 2010). The emergence of invigorated cultural traditions means that mainstream systems need to address demands for the recognition and inclusion of, for example, traditional healers, medicines, and conceptual schemata (Gottlieb et al., 2008). Where medical systems have resisted these shifts, they have often been forced by political pressure and policy shifts to make some accommodations of these more patient-centered and patient-driven approaches.

Finally, the arrival of the Internet has changed patients' access to information in profound ways. Patients now have readily accessible information about their conditions (Bylund et al., 2010). They can also gain more information about the treatments, services, or clinicians available locally, nationally, and internationally. The media, both public and private, now produces or hosts regular programs, Web sites, and columns addressing health care and services. In addition to breaking news stories, there is now a constant stream of health-related programs ranging from documentaries to "reality" television programs on hospitals and clinicians, all the way to the cult of the celebrity clinician. Medicine has gone from the rarefied and private to the common and public.

It is not only the patients and the media who make use of this technology. Health departments and services use Web sites and social networking sites to distribute information. Prominent clinicians also use the technology; for example, Atul Gawande, a leading patient safety researcher, has a regular column in the *New Yorker*. Other researchers and practitioners use iTunes to disseminate their messages to clinicians and patients alike. The Institute for Healthcare Improvement (IHI) offers an online interprofessional educational community for clinicians

and students wanting to learn more about quality and safety (http://www
.ihi.org/IHI/Programs/IHIOpenSchool/).

For patients, the Internet has produced another profound effect. It has
become a platform whereby support and discussion groups have developed.
Even individuals with the rarest of conditions (given access to computers
and the World Wide Web) now have access to forums where they can
describe and discuss both the progressions and the symptoms of their illness; moreover, they can compare the type and quality of their treatments.

RATIONALE FOR PATIENT INVOLVEMENT IN CQI

As social and clinical relationships were changing, there was also increasing
public awareness and disquiet about the incidence of medical errors. Most
quality and safety practitioners and academics associate the birth of the current
patient safety movement with the Institute of Medicine's *To Err Is Human*
report (IOM, 2000). Although it was presenting data about error rates from
a much earlier study by Brennan et al. (1991), the IOM report galvanized
health care systems around the world into action; the report's metaphor of
hospital errors being the equivalent of a "jumbo jet full of patients crashing
every three days" drew widespread media and public attention.

Around the same time, a series of high-profile cases of negligence,
incompetence, and/or medical homicide began to appear in the press. The
Bristol Royal Infirmary inquiry (pediatric cardiac surgery) and Shipman
inquiry (general practice) in the United Kingdom (Department of Health,
2001; Smith, 2005), the King Edward Memorial inquiry (women and
infants) and Bundaberg Hospital inquiry (surgery) in Australia (Douglas
et al., 2001; Morris, 2005), the Cartwright inquiry (cervical screening)
in New Zealand (Cervical Cancer Inquiry, 1988), and the Manitoba
Coroner's inquest (pediatric cardiac surgery) in Canada (Sinclair, 1994)
were just some of the cases that increased public anxiety about the quality
and safety of care internationally. Added to these two factors were rising
levels of complaints and litigation faced by health services, both public and
private. The scene was set for new approaches to safeguarding patients.

Early on in the development of the patient safety movement, Vincent
and Coulter (2002) asked the question "Patient safety: what about the
patient?" Their argument was that "plans for improving safety in medical
care often ignore the patient's perspective" (p. 76) and that the active

role of patients in the safety of their care was something that health care services and clinicians needed to acknowledge and encourage.

Patient involvement in CQI and other quality and safety strategies therefore reflects a profound change in the health services approach to the provision of care. Health systems and clinicians now recognize that patients and their families can no longer be treated as passive recipients of care. In addition to the ethics involved, this perspective has a strong practical element. Patient involvement is about ensuring the accountability and transparency of services (Emanuel and Emanuel, 1997; Forrest, 2004). It is about the provision of patient-centered, as opposed to service-centered, care (Andrews et al., 2004; Berntsen, 2006; Robb et al., 2006). But it is equally about joining with patients as partners in the constant vigilance and heedfulness required to protect against errors. Simply stated, health practitioners, services, and managers needed patients to be involved in their care.

METHODS FOR INVOLVING PATIENTS IN CQI

What does patient involvement look like? The answer depends largely on the level and type of system under consideration. One way of assessing patient involvement in CQI is to focus on three levels: micro (direct clinician–patient interactions), meso (health service or system level), and macro (national or international) (modified from Bronfenbrenner, 1979).

Micro-Level Patient Involvement

At a micro level, patients can be directly involved in the decision making and management plans associated with their individual treatment and in ensuring that the intended treatment is given as planned and according to established protocols (that is, in the monitoring of the quality and safety of their care) (Longtin et al., 2010; Peat et al., 2010). Here terms such as the *engaged, active, vigilant,* or *empowered* patient are applied, as health services seek to educate and inform their patients to take on a self-management role, particularly in the case of chronic illness (Anderson, 2007; Coulter and Elwyn, 2002; Entwistle and Quick, 2006). Recently a new level of patient self-management, *personalization,* has been introduced that is associated with the CQI concept of mass customization (McLaughlin and Kaluzny, 2006). Personalization is a term that has been used in various industries, especially the computer industry. The association between personalization and mass customization is discussed in detail by Tseng and Piller (2003), who describe personalization as going beyond the traditional definition of customization by involving customers (patients) in intense communication and high levels of interaction (between customer and suppliers), including negotiating the selection of services with the customer. This terminology has begun to be adopted in medical care, especially with the advent of genomics as a way to develop personalized medicines and, by extension, personalized care (Hamburg and Collins, 2010). This concept is also evolving rapidly from medical genomics to patient care by expanding the concept of evidence-based medicine to include patient preferences in a greater way, using the terms *individualization of care* and *shared decision making* (Barratt, 2008; Robinson et al., 2008). See Chapters 1 and 10 for a detailed discussion of these concepts.

Patients are involved in helping clinicians reach accurate diagnoses, deciding on appropriate treatment and/or management strategies, choosing a suitably experienced and safe provider, and ensuring the appropriate administration of, monitoring of, and adherence to treatments or directions (DiGiovanni et al., 2003; Ubbink et al., 2009). At this level, patient involvement can contribute to reducing the inappropriate use of health care resources (such as the overuse of medications), which in turn can potentially reduce health care errors (Smith, 2009).

Patients are also increasingly called on to identify and notify unsafe acts on the part of clinicians, including, for example, a lack of hand hygiene (Bittle and LaMarche, 2009; "Care recipients," 2002). As with self-management of chronic conditions, patients are encouraged to participate in quality improvement programs through a combination of awareness raising, information, and educational programs (Anthony et al., 2003).

Meso-Level Patient Involvement

At the meso level, patient involvement in CQI is about the appropriate, effective, and safe provision of services. As consumers or customers, patients involved at this level are engaged in the planning, management, and evaluation of entire health systems or individual services. Such participation can take a variety of forms.

Individuals can be involved as members of the public, as patients, as caregivers or family members of individuals receiving care, as representatives of consumer organizations (such as advocacy and self-help groups), and as members and representatives of population groups or communities (Anderson et al., 2006; Conway et al., 1997; Draper, 1997). The perceived effectiveness of this last type of participation has been attributed (by patients) to their own participatory behavior and the availability of institutional participatory spaces—that is, the "opening up" of CQI mechanisms to patient involvement (Delgado-Gallego and Vazquez, 2009). It is important to note that there are criticisms of the "representativeness" of consumers, in particular that the patients involved tend to be either "professional" consumers or individuals who tend to mirror the socioeconomic and educational profiles of health care professionals (Coulter, 2002).

The mechanisms by which they are involved also vary. Participation can be a "one-off" involvement in a forum or workshop or attendance at a conference. It can involve participation in time-limited activities, such as membership of committees or groups, including, for example, sitting on public or service-level (e.g., root cause analysis) inquiries into breaches of patient safety or acting as members of patient safety committees in hospitals or services (Brennan and Safran, 2004; Connor et al., 2002; Hindle et al., 2006). Participation can also be anonymous and more passive or reactive. Feedback via patient satisfaction surveys (see Chapter 6), exit interviews, or questionnaires can contribute to quality efforts, as can involvement in focus groups or complaints and compliments letters (Ableson et al., 2001; Ciesla et al., 1992; Delbanco et al., 1995; Ervin, 2006; Mease et al., 2007; Rowe and Frewer, 2000; Saturno Hernandez, 1995). Patients are increasingly involved in more active CQI strategies, including the monitoring of service quality (Donabedian, 1983).

Macro-Level Patient Involvement

Macro-level involvement in CQI sees the patient involved in patient safety activities at a national or international level. Various examples exist and will be discussed in the following sections. The World Health Organization's (WHO) Patients for Patient Safety movement is one example of an international strategy aimed at ensuring that the patient's perspective is integrated in mechanisms to improve the quality and safety of care. The WHO's London Declaration is a pledge of partnership and a core document for its World Alliance for Patient Safety (Patients for Patient Safety, 2006). The document is available at http://www.who.int/patientsafety/patients_for_patient/London_Declaration_EN.pdf.

For both publicly funded and privately funded health care around the world, public reporting on the quality of care remains a contested issue (Duckett et al., 2008). The argument for the publication of such data is that it will make patients (often, in this context, referred to as consumers) more active participants in their choice of providers (Utzon and Kaergaard, 2009). Effective public reporting is said to (1) engage and involve health care systems and services from the initiation of the reporting program, (2) ensure the data reported are of the highest quality, (3) provide information in a way that is accessible and appropriate to consumers, and (4) to provide clinicians with detailed information on their individual performance (Tu and Lauer, 2009). Finally, in addition to input into direct service and health system delivery issues, some countries are grappling with the involvement of consumers and the public in "upstream" areas of patient safety such as health-related research (Andejeski et al., 2002).

FACTORS AFFECTING PATIENT INVOLVEMENT

What evidence is available to support the involvement of patients in the quality and safety of care? Rigorous evaluations of both educational campaigns (Schwappach, 2010) and patient involvement (Peat et al., 2010) were found to be lacking. Available evidence indicates that although patients tend to have a positive attitude toward the idea of being involved in their safety, their actual involvement varies (Schwappach, 2010).

From the patients' perspective, a number of factors contribute to their willingness to participate in patient safety and quality strategies. These include their sense of self-efficacy; their acceptance of a new, more active role as patients; the perceived preventability of incidents; and the perceived effectiveness of their actions (Peat et al., 2010; Schwappach, 2010). Health literacy is a significant factor in determining patient involvement at every level of care (Kripalani et al., 2010; Pappas et al., 2007; Peota, 2004; Rothman et al., 2009a; Rothman et al., 2009b). Factors inhibiting patient involvement range from the complexity of the patient's condition (e.g., the presence of comorbidities) to a perceived lack of confidence or skills to broader socioeconomic issues (such as social status and ethnicity) (Johnstone and Kanitsaki, 2009; Longtin et al., 2010). The health care setting (e.g., whether it is primary, secondary, or tertiary care, or whether the patient perceives it to be intimidating) and the actual task involved (e.g., whether "involvement" includes confronting clinicians) have been found to contribute to patients' willingness and ability to participate in CQI-related strategies (Burroughs et al., 2005; Davis et al., 2007).

Perceived power differentials between individuals from vulnerable communities and health services can cause anxiety, including fear of retribution. So too can the burden of having to represent the needs and concerns of an entire community, without adequate skills, support, or preparation (Abelson et al., 2004; Arnstein, 1969; Delgado-Gallego and Vazquez, 2009; Murie and Douglas-Scott, 2004).

Type of illness and socioeconomic factors contribute to health workers' support of patient involvement. Clinicians' attitudes toward patient involvement are influenced by organizational issues (e.g., lack of time or training) and personal beliefs; for example, they may fear losing control or specialization or may perceive the "stakes" as being too high (Longtin et al., 2010).

MEASURING PATIENT INVOLVEMENT IN CQI

In keeping with the London Declaration, patient satisfaction surveys have been implemented in many countries in an effort to quantify some of the many nonclinical outcomes of the patient experience and in an effort to increase the transparency of the consequences of health and medical treatments. There is an ongoing debate about whether "satisfaction" is an adequate conceptual schemata for what is at stake, and other terms such as *patient experiences* have been proposed (Hekkert et al., 2009). The use of "satisfaction" measures also indicates the influence of established models in the corporate world for gaining feedback from those paying for and/ or receiving the service in question. The type of data collected lends itself to the statistical analysis of key institutional issues against patients' demographic variables, with a prevailing assumption that objective, quantifiable data provide the necessary understanding. An important constraint is that most satisfaction surveys tend to produce relatively positive results, and institutional providers may themselves be dependent on positive indicators for funding, board approvals, and other systemic "rewards."

Thus, measuring CQI from the patient perspective is complicated. It is clear that patient experiences, satisfaction included, can be highly individual, contextual, and fundamentally phenomenological in character—falling in the problematic "subjective" domain. Even patient responses to adverse events, up to and including disability or death, can be seen to vary enormously depending on how the health providers respond to those errors. Consequently, the science of patient involvement generally—and patient "satisfaction" as a particular dimension of that experience—relies on a much broader understanding of what knowledge we are seeking, why we are seeking it, and how we go about acquiring the information to construct that knowledge. To use only, or even mainly, standard quantitative measures in the highly contextualized settings that health care involves (think appendectomy vs. chemotherapy, for example) does require a richer and more sophisticated information base than that generally produced from typically close-ended survey instruments. In the broader context, and given the information presented in this text, health care experiences do not reside on the same level as consumer-durable purchases and possess a richer set of conceptual and psychometric properties. As a result, we need to acknowledge that our science of measurement in patient involvement and satisfaction needs to address that multilayered complexity more directly and informatively. In essence there are multiple opportunities for more direct patient and caregiver involvement.

THE M-APR MODEL OF PATIENT INVOLVEMENT

Drawing on the evidence base, we developed a model of patient involvement that spans all levels and types of health care. The M-APR model of patient involvement looks at this issue at three levels—the "M"—micro, meso, macro; and across two dimensions—the "APR"—active/proactive and passive/reactive involvement. These dimensions indicate that patient, family, and public involvement and/or feedback into CQI can be achieved through a variety of mechanisms.

Active participation assumes the direct and ongoing involvement of patients and their families and caregivers in CQI activities, be it direct input and decision making about patients' individual care or the determination of ethical standards for professions or services. Passive involvement sees services and systems drawing on more removed, yet still useful, sources of patient feedback. Many services are most familiar, and most comfortable, with these sources, which include patient satisfaction surveys, exit interviews, patient focus groups, and more removed information provision via service report cards.

In proactive involvement, the patient is involved in attempting to prevent errors and addressing safety issues. These initiatives range from direct education and involvement in confronting potential sources of errors (e.g., addressing clinicians' hand hygiene or ensuring that the surgeon marks the appropriate limb or side of the body to be operated on), to involvement in CQI strategies and programs at service levels, to decision making about research directions at state, national, or international levels. In reactive approaches, the patient is involved in identifying the causes of errors that have already occurred, from the use of simple complaint letters to the analysis of incident reports; from involvement in root cause analysis programs to involvement in patient safety inquiries.

M-APR is intended to be a diagnostic rather than a prescriptive model. **Table 7–1** shows a summary of the model, along with some select examples. Examples, by necessity, reflect differences in the publicly vs. privately funded health systems.

Examples of Patient Involvement in CQI

In this section, we provide an overview of four very different strategies for patient involvement in CQI. These examples illustrate the different levels of the M-APR model and provide insights into mechanisms by which patients can contribute to ensuring the quality of health care for themselves and for the broader community.

Example 1: Partners in Health

For almost a decade, Kaiser Permanente in the United States has been promoting its Patients as Partners program. Led by Dr. David Sobel, this program focuses on the direct involvement of patients with long-term health conditions in their self-management and health literacy development. The concept is to reposition patients from being "consumers" of health services to being active partners in their own health treatment and management. The key concept is that patients with chronic conditions are already essentially responsible for 80% of their own diagnostic and treatment behaviors and that supporting this pattern can potentially improve care and save time, money, and resources.

This program grew out of work in the 1990s by Kate Lorig at the Stanford University Center for Research in Patient Education on a chronic disease self-management program and patient outcomes. The program at

TABLE 7-1 Dimension of Patient Involvement in Quality Improvement: The M-APR Model

Dimension	Micro	Meso	Macro	Dimension	Micro	Meso	Macro
Active	Patients are involved in every aspect of decision making for their own care. Patients and their families and caregivers are directly and continuously consulted in the provision of care and are considered part of the health care team.	Patients are full members of hospital or service boards.	Patients are full members of health system or professional ethics committees and review boards.	Passive	Service utilizes existing data sources such as patient satisfaction surveys or exit interviews.	Services utilize a patient-centered approach to all planning and quality improvement mechanisms.	Data on use of services by different population groups are compared. Performance data on clinicians and services are publicly available.
Proactive	Patients and their families and caregivers are educated and encouraged to confront clinicians or services that breach patient safety standards.	Patients and their families and caregivers are involved in service-level planning, in identifying areas for improvement in the quality or safety of services, and in establishing new approaches to and design of services.	Patients are involved in patient safety campaigns and organizations at a state, national, or international level. Patients are represented on boards of system-level quality improvement and monitoring agencies, including professional registration boards and accreditation bodies.	Reactive	Service utilizes existing or custom-made sources of information such as complaint letters.	Services analyze incident data to identify patient characteristics and population patterns in types and distribution of errors. Patients are involved in CQI strategies developed after occurrence of errors, including root cause analysis and incident reporting.	Patients are represented on public reports and reviews of the quality of care. Patients are full members of public patient safety inquiries.

Kaiser includes the Healthwise Handbook, initially available online, and a range of other print, Internet, and direct face-to-face supports. The concept of making low- and high-intensity interventions available was developed to cover a wide range of potential supports that could be adjusted to meet both patient and situational needs (e.g., clinician training, patient mailings, telephone calls, and face-to-face support groups).

Kaiser Permanente produced evidence to show that the strategy is highly effective and has lasting effects for patients as well as health service providers, including more appropriate utilization of services, improved accessibility, and measurable declines in selected types of service utilization. Satisfaction and behavioral indicators were positive, and return-on-investment measures ranged from 5:1 to 10:1 across the range of strategies. A randomized, controlled trial compared program subjects with wait-list controls. For participating patients with conditions including lung disease, heart disease, diabetes, and arthritis, the results showed improvements over 6 months in their exercise levels, their communication with physicians, self-reported health, and other measures. In addition, the program saw reductions in the number of hospital, outpatient, and emergency room admissions (Lorig et al., 1999). Although Kaiser is obviously a very large and influential health care provider, by its own estimate, up to 80% of the changes it implemented could also be implemented by smaller, less well-resourced providers where economics of scale and integration factors might not be as readily available (Sobel, 2003; Sofaer et al., 2009).

Example 2: National Patient Safety Goals in the United States

A second example of a patient involvement strategy is based on the accreditation requirements of health services and programs in the United States. The Joint Commission (TJC) has a specific National Patient Safety Goal (NPSG 13) that addresses this issue. It states that services should "encourage patients' active involvement in their own care as a patient safety strategy," with a more specific subclause (NPSG.13.01.01) that they should "define and communicate the means for patients and their families to report concerns about safety and encourage them to do so." In 2010, this goal became part of TJC's standards for accreditation of health care services. TJC published its *Patients as Partners: Toolkit for Implementing the National Patient Safety Goal* in 2007. This work grew out of the establishment of NPSG 13, which specifically addresses the idea of patients and their families and caregivers as having an important and tangible role in the identification of potential errors in patient treatment and care.

Patients as Partners has been supported by a range of related publications aimed at improving the capacity of patients and caregivers to identify patient safety issues as they see them developing. The program also involves training packages and accreditation for health service providers, including strategies for implementing, monitoring, and evaluating their performance. As with other patient safety systems around the world, being able to capture data and quantify the results of interventions is a crucial aspect of systemic change and program validation.

One of the key issues identified by TJC has been the diversity of patients, families, and caregivers in terms of their cultures and the variety of languages spoken and read. The focus on both English-language materials and materials for other important groups, such as Spanish speakers, has been integrated into the focus of this work. Central to this work is not simply the shifting demography of the United States (and other immigrant-receiving countries) but also the centrality of effective communication in patient safety improvements. If patients are to be actively engaged as partners, then key communication issues such as language have to be incorporated from the beginning.

While TJC is not the only accreditation organization in the United States, it is an important organization, both nationally and internationally, in promoting patient safety and supporting the role of patients, families, and caregivers in the processes associated with patient safety's systemic development. The establishment of tangible measures of patient involvement, in addition to other indicators, means that patient involvement is more likely to occur and produce systemic change (The Joint Commission, 2010).

Example 3: Patients as Partners Program

Impact British Columbia, a not-for-profit health service provider organization specifically established to work across British Columbia's health system to support service improvement, has recently implemented a Patients as Partners program based on the British Columbia Primary Health Care Charter. The charter is predicated on the understanding that only 15% of the population has *no* engagement with the primary health care system in any given year. One of the program's goals is therefore to raise the level of patient involvement and self-management through such means as outreach programs that people can access from close to home. The training programs include patients, caregivers, and health care providers. In addition, while acute care is a major focus of the health system generally, chronic conditions contribute to a large proportion of the costs of health care and high average costs per patient, especially when patients with multiple conditions are more effectively taken into account.

The specified principles at Impact are as follows:

- People are treated with respect and dignity.
- Health care providers communicate and share complete and unbiased information with patients and families in ways that are affirmative and useful.
- Individuals and families build on their strengths through participation in experiences that enhance control and independence.
- Collaboration among patients, families, and providers occurs in policy and program development and professional education, as well as in the delivery of care.

The scope of the program aims to meet tangible goals for improving patient access to self-treatment programs, including training programs for both patients and staff on self-management programs, patient satisfaction measures, and patient and staff confidence measures in utilizing the programs. The focus is on British Columbians who are English speakers, once again acknowledging the key part that communication, generally, and language, in particular, play in these processes of patient engagement, empowerment, and quality improvement.

Beyond the individual level, communities are engaged in allowing providers to define their local community and its constituents. Broad targets are identified for outreach activities to community organizations and related bodies (health and nonhealth) and for the need to train health professionals in developing skills for community engagement (Impact British Columbia, 2007).

Example 4: From Partners to Owners

Historically, health services for native peoples in the United States were provided by the U.S. Indian Health Service. This did not produce successful outcomes for many groups, including the Alaskan native communities, regardless of how well-intentioned providers were. The South Central Foundation (SCF) and the Alaska Native Tribal Health Consortium signed an agreement in 1999 taking over the management of *all* Indian Health Service programs on the Alaska Native Health Campus (ANHC). These included the Alaska Native Medical Center (ANMC), the Native Primary Care Center, and the South Central Foundation's main administration building, as well as other facilities based in Anchorage. The realization of the goal of health service *ownership* by a not-for-profit organization has since seen a significant philosophical and pragmatic shift in the design and delivery of health care services to Alaskan native peoples seeking treatment at the SCF/ANHC services.

The reorientation has focused on the owners/patients as the central component in the health system's design and delivery of services. Native people were asked how they would like care to be provided, and the results have been substantial. Outcome measures were included from the outset of the change program, and key measures such as satisfaction (of patients and staff), access, quality, and utilization are all very high. The change model has also produced significant reductions in features such as patient backlogs, HIV-positive patient admissions, and emergency department admissions.

The shift from a "patient-centered" to a "patient-driven" system has produced significant and meaningful changes across the spectrum of Alaskan native health care and established a model of innovation and change management that is attracting national and international attention. The direct and practical involvement of patients has improved measures across all domains of care for both patients and providers (Eby, 2007; Gottlieb, 2007; Gottlieb et al., 2008; The SouthCentral Foundation, 2010).

CONCLUSIONS

As we have shown, the involvement of patients in CQI and other forms of quality improvement is no longer in question. What is also without dispute is that, despite a decade of sustained effort by governments, services, and clinicians, error rates have not significantly been reduced (Wachter, 2010) across the board, and disparities in the quality and accessibility of care continue. Determining the best way to involve consumers in reducing those errors, improving the quality of care they receive, and maximizing the benefits of that involvement, remain problematic. Each health care system and service, across the world, will rightly need to take into account its unique funding and governance structures, planning strategies, and quality improvement mechanisms in deciding which patient involvement strategy is most suitable to its needs. Whatever the particulars involved, whatever method or mechanism the service chooses, it is clear that patients will have a greater level of involvement in their care and in ensuring higher quality. The years of token and "one-size-fits-all" involvement are over.

Cross-Reference to the Companion Casebook

(McLaughlin, C. P., Johnson, J. K., and Sollecito, W. A. [Eds.]. 2012. *Implementing Continuous Quality Improvement in Health Care: A Global Casebook.* Sudbury, MA: Jones & Bartlett Learning.)

Case Study Number	Case Study Title	Case Study Authors
16	The Lewis Blackman Hospital Patient Safety Act: It's Hard to Kill a Healthy 15-Year-Old	*Julie K. Johnson, Helen Haskell, and Paul Barach*

REFERENCES

Abelson, J., Forest, P. G., Casebeer, A., et al. 2004. Will it make a difference if I show up and share? A citizen's perspective on improving public involvement processes for health system decision-making. *J Health Serv Res Policy*, 9: 205–212.

Ableson, J., Forest, P. G., Smith, P., et al. 2001. *A Review of Public Participation and Consultation Methods Working Paper 01-04.* Hamilton, Ontario, Canada: McMaster University Centre for Health Economics and Policy Analysis.

Andejeski, Y., Breslau, E. S., Hart, E., et al. 2002. Benefits and drawbacks of including consumer reviewers in the scientific merit review of breast cancer research. *J Womens Health Gender-Based Med*, 11: 119–136.

Anderson, B. 2007. Collaborative care and motivational interviewing: Improving depression outcomes through patient empowerment interventions. *Am J Managed Care*, 13: S103–S106.

Anderson, E., Shepherd, M., and Salisbury, C. 2006. "Taking off the suit": Engaging the community in primary health care decision-making. *Health Expectat*, 9: 70–80.

Andrews, J., Manthorpe, J., and Watson, R. 2004. Involving older people in intermediate care. *J Advanced Nurs*, 46: 303–310.

Anthony, R., Miranda, F., Mawji, Z., et al. 2003. John M. Eisenberg Patient Safety Awards. The LVHHN patient safety video: Patients as partners in safe care delivery. *Joint Commission J Qual Safety*, 29: 640–645.

Arnstein, S. 1969. A ladder of citizen participation in the USA. *J Am Instit Planners*, 57: 176–182.

Bambra, C., Gibson, M., Sowden, A., et al. 2010. Tackling the wider social determinants of health and health inequalities: Evidence from systematic reviews. *J Epidemiol Community Health*, 64: 284–291.

Barratt, A. 2008. Evidence-based medicine and shared decision making: The challenge of getting both the evidence and preferences into health care. *Patient Educ Counseling*, 73: 407–412.

Berntsen, K. J. 2006. Implementation of patient centeredness to enhance patient safety. *J Nurs Care Quality*, 21: 15–19.

Betancourt, J. R., and King, R. K. 2003. Unequal treatment: The Institute of Medicine report and its public health implications. *Public Health Rep*, 118: 287–292.

Bittle, M. J., and LaMarche, S. 2009. Engaging the patient as observer to promote hand hygiene compliance in ambulatory care. *Joint Commission J Qual Patient Safety*, 35: 519–525.

Borthwick, A. M., Short, A. J., Nancarrow, S. A., et al. 2010. Non-medical prescribing in Australasia and the UK: The case of podiatry. *J Foot Ankle Res*, 3: 1.

Brennan, P. F., and Safran, C. 2004. Patient safety. Remember who it's really for. *Int J Med Informatics*, 73: 547–550.

Brennan, T. A., Leape, L. L., Laird, N. M., et al. 1991. Incidence of adverse events and negligence in hospitalized patients. Results of the Harvard Medical Practice Study I. *N Engl J Med*, 324(6): 370–376.

Bronfenbrenner, U. 1979. *The Ecology of Human Development: Experiments by Nature and Design.* Cambridge, MA: Harvard University Press.

Burroughs, T. E., Waterman, A. D., Gallagher, T. H., et al. 2005. Patient concerns about medical errors in emergency departments. *Acad Emerg Med*, 12: 57–64.

Bylund, C. L., Gueguen, J. A., D'Agostino, T. A., et al. 2010. Doctor-patient communication about cancer-related Internet information. *J Psychosoc Oncol*, 28: 127–142.

Care recipients urged to "speak up" for safer health care. 2002. *Joint Commission Perspectives*, 22: 3.

Cervical Cancer Inquiry, Cartwright Inquiry. 1988. *The Report of the Committee of Inquiry into Allegations Concerning the Treatment of Cervical Cancer at the National Women's Hospital and into Other Related Matters. Report of the Cervical Cancer Inquiry, CCR.* Auckland, New Zealand: Government Printing Office.

Ciesla, J. R., Samuels, M. E., and Stoskopf, C. H. 1992. The role of the Medical Care Advisory Committee in the administration of state Medicaid programs. *Eval Health Profess*, 15: 282–298.

Connor, M., Ponte, P. R., and Conway, J. 2002. Multidisciplinary approaches to reducing error and risk in a patient care setting. *Crit Care Nurs Clin North Am*, 14: 359–367.

Conway, T., Hu, T. C., and Harrington, T. 1997. Setting health priorities: Community boards accurately reflect the preferences of the community's residents. *J Community Health*, 22: 57–68.

Coulter, A. 2002. Involving patients: Representation or representativeness? *Health Expectations*, 5: 1.

Coulter, A., and Elwyn, G. 2002. What do patients want from high-quality general practice and how do we involve them in improvement? *Br J Gen Pract*, 52: S22–S26.

Davis, R. E., Jacklin, R., Sevdalis, N., et al. 2007. Patient involvement in patient safety: What factors influence patient participation and engagement? *Health Expectations*, 10: 259–267.

Delbanco, T. L., Stokes, D. M., Cleary, P. D., et al. 1995. Medical patients' assessments of their care during hospitalization: Insights for internists. *J Gen Intern Med*, 10: 679–685.

Delgado-Gallego, M. E., and Vazquez, M. L. 2009. Users' and community leaders' perceptions of their capacity to influence the quality of health care: Case studies of Colombia and Brazil. *Cadernos de Saude Publica*, 25: 169–178.

Dent, M. 2006. Disciplining the medical profession? Implications of patient choice for medical dominance. *Health Sociol Rev*, 15: 458–468.

Department of Health. 2001. *Learning from Bristol: The Report of the Public Enquiry into Children's Heart Surgery at the Bristol Royal Infirmary, 1984–1995.* London: The Stationery Office.

DiGiovanni, C. W., Kang, L., and Manuel, J. 2003. Patient compliance in avoiding wrong-site surgery. *J Bone Joint Surg Am Vol,* 85-A: 815–819.

Donabedian, A. 1983. Quality assessment and monitoring. Retrospect and prospect. *Eval Health Profess,* 6: 363–375.

Douglas, N., Robinson, J., and Fahy, K. 2001. *Inquiry into Obstetric and Gynaecological Services at King Edward Memorial Hospital 1990–2000.* Perth, Australia: Health Department of Western Australia.

Draper, M. 1997. *Involving Consumers in Improving Hospital Care: Lessons from Australian Hospitals.* Canberra, Australia: Commonwealth Department of Health and Aged Care.

Duckett, S. J., Collins, J., Kamp, M., et al. 2008. An improvement focus in public reporting: The Queensland approach. *Med J Aust,* 189: 616–617.

Eby, D. K. 2007. Primary care at the Alaska Native Medical Center: a fully deployed "new model" of primary care. *Int J Circumpolar Health,* 66: 4–13.

Emanuel, E. J., and Emanuel, L. L. 1997. Preserving community in health care. *J Health Policy Law,* 22: 147–184.

Entwistle, V. A., and Quick, O. 2006. Trust in the context of patient safety problems. *J Health Organ Manage,* 20: 397–416.

Epstein, S. 1995. The construction of lay expertise: AIDS activism and the forging of credibility in the reform of clinical trials. *Sci Technol Hum Values,* 20: 408–437.

Ervin, N. E. 2006. Does patient satisfaction contribute to nursing care quality? *J Nurs Admin,* 36: 126–130.

Forrest, E. 2004. Patient-public involvement. *Health Serv J,* 114: 26–27.

Gottlieb, K. 2007. The family wellness warriors initiative. *Alaska Med,* 49: 49–54.

Gottlieb, K., Sylvester, I., and Eby, D. 2008. Transforming your practice: What matters most. *Fam Pract Manage,* 15: 32–38.

Hamburg, M. A., and Collins, F. S. 2010. The path to personalized medicine. *N Engl J Med,* 363(4): 301–304.

Hekkert, K. D., Cihangir, S., Kleefstra, S. M., et al. 2009. Patient satisfaction revisited: A multilevel approach. *Soc Sci Med,* 69: 68–75.

Hindle, D., Braithwaite, J., Iedema, R., et al. 2006. *Patient Safety: A Comparative Analysis of Eight Inquiries in Six Countries.* Sydney: Centre for Clinical Governance Research in Health, University of NSW and Clinical Excellence Commission.

Illich, I. 1974. Medical nemesis. *Lancet,* 1: 918–921.

Impact British Columbia. 2007. *Primary Health Care Charter: A Collaborative Approach.* Vancouver, British Columbia: Ministry of Health.

Institute of Medicine. 2000. *To Err Is Human: Building a Safer Health System.* Washington, DC: National Academies Press.

The Joint Commission. 2010. *The Joint Commission—National Patient Safety Goals.* Oakbrook Terrace, IL: Author.

Johnstone, M.-J., and Kanitsaki, O. 2009. Engaging patients as safety partners: Some considerations for ensuring a culturally and linguistically appropriate approach. *Health Policy,* 90: 1–7.

Kripalani, S., Jacobson, T. A., Mugalla, I. C., et al. 2010. Health literacy and the quality of physician-patient communication during hospitalization. *J Hosp Med,* 5: 269–275.

Longtin, Y., Sax, H., Leape, L. L., et al. 2010. Patient participation: Current knowledge and applicability to patient safety. *Mayo Clinic Proceedings,* 85: 53–62.

Lorig, K. R., Sobel, D. S., Stewart, A. L., et al. 1999. Evidence suggesting that a chronic disease self-management program can improve health status while reducing hospitalization: A randomized trial. *Med Care,* 37(1): 5–14.

Mak, J. C., and Faux, S. 2010. Use of complementary and alternative medicine by patients with osteoporosis in Australia. *Med J Aust,* 192: 54–55.

McLaughlin, C., and Kaluzny, A. (Eds.). 2006. *Continuous Quality Improvement in Health Care: Theory, Implementations, and Applications.* Sudbury: Jones & Bartlett Publishers.

Mease, P., Arnold, L. M., Bennett, R., et al. 2007. Fibromyalgia syndrome. *J Rheumatol,* 34: 1415–1425.

Morris, A. 2005. *Bundaberg Base Hospital Commission of Inquiry.* Brisbane, Australia: Bundaberg Base Hospital Commission of Inquiry.

Murie, J., and Douglas-Scott, G. 2004. Developing an evidence base for patient and public involvement. *Clin Governance Int J,* 9: 147–154.

Pappas, G., Siozopoulou, V., Saplaoura, K., et al. 2007. Health literacy in the field of infectious diseases: The paradigm of brucellosis. *J Infect*, 54: 40–45.

Patients for Patient Safety, World Health Organization World Alliance for Patient Safety. 2006. London Declaration. Geneva: World Health Organization World Alliance for Patient Safety.

Peat, M., Entwistle, V., Hall, J., et al. 2010. Scoping review and approach to appraisal of interventions intended to involve patients in patient safety. *J Health Serv Res Policy*, 15(1): 17–25.

Peota, C. 2004. Health literacy and patient safety. *Minnesota Med*, 87: 32–34.

Ramsden, I. 1993. Cultural safety in nursing education in Aotearoa New Zealand. *Nurs Praxis N Z*, 8: 4–10.

Ramsden, I. 2000a. Cultural safety/Kawa Whakaruruhau ten years on: A personal overview. *Nurs Praxis N Z*, 15: 4–12.

Ramsden, I. 2000b. Defining cultural safety and transcultural nursing. *Nurs N Z*, 6: 4–5; author reply 5.

Robb, G., Seddon, M., and Effective Practice Informatics and Quality. 2006. Quality improvement in New Zealand healthcare. Part 6: keeping the patient front and centre to improve healthcare quality. *N Z Med J*, 119: U2174.

Robinson, J. H., Callister, L. C., Berry, J. A., et al. 2008. Patient-centered care and adherence: Definitions and applications to improve outcomes. *J Am Acad Nurse Pract*, 20: 600–607.

Rothman, R. L., Yin, H. S., Mulvaney, S., et al. 2009a. Health literacy and quality: Focus on chronic illness care and patient safety. *Pediatrics*, 124(3): S315–S326.

Rothman, R. L., Yin, H. S., Mulvaney, S., et al. 2009b. Health literacy and quality: Focus on chronic illness care and patient safety. *Pediatrics*, 124(3), S315–S326.

Rowe, G., and Frewer, L. J. 2000. Public participation methods: A framework for evaluation. *Sci Tech Hum Values*, 25: 3–29.

Saturno Hernandez, P. J. 1995. Methods of user participation in the evaluation and improvement of the quality of health services. *Revista Espanola de Salud Publica*, 69: 163–175.

Schwappach, D. L. B. 2010. Review: Engaging patients as vigilant partners in safety: A systematic review. *Med Care Res Rev*, 67: 119–148.

Senel, H. G. 2010. Parents' views and experiences about complementary and alternative medicine treatments for their children with autistic spectrum disorder. *J Autism Develop Disord*, 40: 494–503.

Shilts, R. 2007. *And the Band Played On: Politics, People, and the AIDS Epidemic, 20th-Anniversary Edition.* New York: St. Martin's Griffin.

Sinclair, C. M. 1994. *Report of the Manitoba Pediatric Cardiac Surgery Inquest.* Winnipeg, Canada: Manitoba Provincial Court.

Smith, J. 2005. *Shipman: The Final Report.* London: HMSO.

Smith, L. H. 2009. National patient safety goal #13: Patients' active involvement in their own care: Preventing chemotherapy extravasation. *Clin J Oncol Nurs*, 13: 233–234.

Sobel, D. 2003. *Learning from Kaiser Permanente—How Can the NHS Make Better Use of Its Resources and Improve Patient Care?* London: National Primary and Care Trust Development Programme.

Sofaer, S., Shaller, D., Ojeda, G., et al. 2009. *From Patients to Partners: A Consensus Framework for Engaging Californians in Their Health and Health Care.* Berkeley: California Program on Access to Care CPAC at the University of California Berkeley.

The SouthCentral Foundation. 2010. *The SouthCentral Foundation—About Us.* Anchorage, AK: Author.

Tseng, M., and Piller, F. 2003. *The Customer Centric Enterprise: Advances in Mass Customization and Personalization.* New York: Springer.

Tu, H. T., and Lauer, J. R. 2009. Designing effective health care quality transparency initiatives. *Issue Brief/Center Study Health Syst Change*, July: 1–6.

Ubbink, D. T., Knops, A. M., Legemate, D. A., et al. 2009. Choosing between different treatment options: How should I inform my patients? *Nederlands Tijdschrift voor Geneeskunde*, 153: B344.

Utzon, J., and Kaergaard, J. 2009. Publication of healthcare quality data to citizens—Status and perspectives. *Ugeskrift for Laeger*, 171: 1670–1674.

Vincent, C. A., and Coulter, A. 2002. Patient safety: What about the patient? *Qual Saf Health Care*, 11(1): 76–80.

Wachter, R. M. 2010. Patient safety at ten: Unmistakable progress, troubling gaps. *Health Aff (Millwood)*, 29(1): 165–173.

Wade, D. T., and Halligan, P. W. 2004. Do biomedical models of illness make for good healthcare systems? *BMJ*, 329: 1398–1401.

CHAPTER 8

A Social Marketing Approach to Continuous Quality Improvement Initiatives

Carol E. Breland and Mike Newton-Ward

"The aim of marketing is to know and understand the customer so well that the product or service fits him or her and sells itself."

—Peter Drucker

BACKGROUND AND DEFINITIONS

Imagine a typical scenario in which hospital management has recently implemented a continuous quality improvement (CQI) initiative to decrease the incidence of hospital-acquired infections. Their data suggest that poor hand-washing techniques by staff and bacteria on portable equipment are to blame. The CQI plan is to provide hand-washing training, implement mandatory hand-washing for doctors when entering and leaving a patient room, and ensure more thorough cleaning of portable X-ray machines that come into the patient rooms.

However, the census at the hospital has increased recently due to a closure of a nearby hospital. The housekeeping staff is struggling to keep up with the demand, so staff members have responded by shortening the time they spend cleaning rooms between patients. They do not have time to measure the disinfectant product they mix with water and do not want to run out, so they just guess at the amount, resulting in a less effective cleaning product. They defer the floor mopping, reasoning that the patient is not on the floor so it will not matter anyway. However, every time someone drops something on the floor, there is a risk of contamination. In addition, the cleaning staff has never been instructed to clean the remote control device, and thus infection-causing agents are being transferred from patient to patient.

Without a better understanding of these "background issues," the CQI team will be disappointed in the latest data showing that infection rates have not decreased. A meeting might be held to determine how to improve the process for hand-washing and how to check for bacteria more often on equipment. Formal brainstorming, perhaps using a traditional CQI tool such as a fishbone diagram, prior to the implementation phase might have led to improved outcomes. Alternatively, or as an adjunct to brainstorming, social marketing behavior theories and techniques could also have been used as a way to ensure greater success by including formative research and data gathered on multiple target audiences. Using this process, the team might have discovered that the housekeeping staff was unknowingly undermining their efforts. Through better understanding of the behavior of the housekeeping staff, a plan could be developed to remove some of the barriers to proper cleaning, such as having the disinfectant premeasured and stored nearby and having a separate designated mop team to ensure that rooms are mopped thoroughly.

The primary goal of this chapter is to introduce social marketing as a novel approach that can be used in conjunction with other more traditional techniques to implement and help to ensure the broadest acceptance and adoption of CQI initiatives.

Because it is a unique application in CQI, we will first define social marketing concepts and processes. Social marketing is a behavioral change methodology firmly planted in the theory and processes of commercial marketing. When sown in the abundant fields of psychology, public health, sociology, economics, and communications, social marketers have access to a rich harvest of many broad and diverse methods for influencing behaviors that improve outcomes that benefit society. An excellent definition of social marketing is found in Philip Kotler and Nancy R. Lee's book *Social Marketing: Influencing Behaviors for Good*: "Social marketing is a process that applies marketing principles and techniques to create, communicate, and deliver value in order to influence target audience behaviors that benefit society (public health, safety, the environment, and communities) as well as the target audience" (2008, p. 7).

The terminology and application of social marketing has evolved since the 1970s, when the term *social marketing* was first introduced by Philip Kotler and Gerald Zaltman in the *Journal of Marketing* (Kotler and Zaltman, 1971). Over the past 40 years, the field has undergone constant growth and refinement. This evolution includes the extension of business concepts of commercial marketing, which was the traditional form of marketing prior to the 1970s, to nontraditional settings such as nongovernmental organizations (NGOs) and nontraditional fields of marketing application such as public health. It has also included internal growth through lessons learned from ever-broadening applications within these nontraditional settings. For example, during the 1980s, some major health-related organizations, such as the Centers for Disease Control and Prevention (CDC) and the World Health Organization (WHO), began to consider implementing social marketing concepts. The ideas spread further in the 1990s when universities such as the University of South Florida in Tampa, Florida, and the University of Strathclyde in Glasgow, Scotland, began to create academic programs in social marketing (Kotler and Lee, 2008). The journal *Social Marketing Quarterly* was founded, and a pivotal text by Alan Andreasen, *Marketing Social Change: Changing Behavior to Promote Health, Social Development, and the Environment* (Andreasen, 1995) was introduced.

Social marketing has produced some well-known health behavior change campaigns, such as the antitobacco "Truth" campaign (Evans et al., 2002), the "VERB: It's What You Do" adolescent physical activity campaign (Wong et al., 2004), the "Save the Crabs, Then Eat 'Em" campaign for protecting the Chesapeake Bay area (Landers et al., 2006), the "Back to Sleep" campaign for sudden infant death syndrome prevention (Cotroneo et al., 2001), and the "Click It or Ticket" campaign for seat belt use to save lives (Williams et al., 2002). Social marketing is sometimes confused with *social media marketing*, a new term that describes the use of social media networking sites such as Facebook or Twitter, in marketing campaigns (Uhrig et al., 2010). Social marketing also should not be confused with communication-only campaigns that rely on advertisements, public service announcements, or printed materials, but that do not address the barriers and facilitators for behaviors. It is important to note that all types of marketing efforts in this area (e.g., public health, education, health services) are using the same fundamental concepts and principles (Siegel and Doner, 1998), as all are rooted in the science of commercial marketing.

To further understand how social marketing has evolved, some discussion of traditional commercial marketing is helpful. The most important distinction between traditional commercial marketing and social marketing is the product or service being sold. Social marketers hope to promote (sell) a good behavior, with no real goal of financial gain, while commercial marketers are focused on selling a good or service, irrespective of its benefit to society, for financial gain. The competitor of the commercial marketer is usually another similar product or company, whereas in social marketing, it is usually a competing behavior. For example, the social marketer working on an antismoking campaign, perhaps in a public health school or agency, is interested in decreasing smoking behavior and replacing it with a healthy behavior. In contrast, marketers who work for tobacco companies have a completely different goal, such as increasing use of the particular brand of cigarettes that will lead to the greatest profitability for the tobacco company, which is the ultimate goal of most commercial marketing campaigns. Commercial marketing, using the four Ps (Product, Place, Price, Promotion), employs a range of proven techniques that are all essential in creating an effective marketing campaign to increase the use of a product and increase the financial gain of a company. These techniques include marketing mix, branding, exchange, audience targeting and segmentation, and consumer research, survey, evaluation, and monitoring. Social marketing uses the same concepts but with the goal of gaining an outcome that improves society—for example, better health in a community.

When considering the application of social marketing methods to health initiatives, it is not just individual health behaviors that can be improved by understanding and addressing the factors that produce the behavior. Improvement can also be addressed at the organization level. For example, a common goal in all health care clinics is to emphasize proper hand-washing behavior to control the spread of infection (Dauer, 2007). To encourage this behavior, health care providers are regularly trained on the importance of hand-washing, and reminder messages are usually posted near sinks. Thus, health care is similar to other noncommercial settings that can be described as having standards that are based on behaviors that can be influenced (for the good) by social marketing techniques (Mah et al., 2006). As stated by Kotler and Lee:

> We also join the voices of many who are advocating for an expanded role for social marketing and social marketers, challenging professionals to take this technology "upstream" and influence other factors that affect positive social change, including laws, enforcement, public policy, built environments, business practices, and the media. (2008, p. 3)

For example, if refraining from smoking in the workplace can become the standard of behavior through social marketing and public policy, then it follows that health care practices can be improved, resulting in better patient outcomes, through the same methods.

HALLMARKS OF SOCIAL MARKETING

Understanding the application of elements of social marketing to changes in both individual health behavior and health care practices takes some realignment of traditional attitudes toward promoting such changes. Behavior change requires more than the conviction of the agency, committee, or organization that change is needed. Social marketers seek to understand the needs of the individuals they are interested in and to get agreement from those individuals that change is both needed and achievable. Therefore, social marketing strategies are fundamentally consumer-focused, voluntary, use-proven, consumer-driven commercial marketing techniques that take into consideration the individual's ability and desire to change and that are designed to change behavior over time instead of all at once. Parallels to CQI begin to become apparent from this definition; its focus is on consumers/customers and the ultimate goal of making gradual behavior changes (i.e., continuous improvements in health or social behaviors).

Social marketing borrows the best practices from the commercial marketing field. Commercial marketers are experts at looking through the eyes of the individual and seeing what drives that person's desire for a product. For example, often in commercials there is an emphasis on being accepted by the group, by the opposite sex, or by one's self. Images are

Know your AUDIENCE (really!), and put them at the center of every decision you make.

It's about ACTION.

There must be an EXCHANGE.

COMPETITION always exists.

Keep the four Ps of marketing (PRODUCT, PRICE, PLACE, PROMOTION) and policy in mind.

FIGURE 8–1 Basic Marketing Principles

Source: Social Marketing National Excellence Collaborative, 2002.

presented of being included in a family gathering, getting a promotion at work, or getting a date, with the message that gaining these experiences hinges on wearing the right cologne or using the best toothpaste. While these products are certainly no guarantee that the desires of the individual will be met—and, of course, usually fail—still the commercial marketers know, based on their audience research, that the individual will keep trying to meet some very basic human needs for acceptance and success and will still want to buy their product.

Social marketers can use these same techniques to meet some of the same desires but by promoting voluntary behavior changes that encourage health, better health outcomes, true well-being, and a better society. The approach is summarized in "The Basics of Social Marketing" (Social Marketing National Excellence Collaborative, 2002), in which the authors introduce several important principles (see **Figure 8–1**).

Although the details of the campaign may vary, the goal of using social marketing to achieve behavior change is "to figure out how to make behavior change EASY, FUN, and POPULAR" (Social Marketing National Excellence Collaborative, 2002).

SOCIAL MARKETING APPLICATIONS TO CQI IN HEALTH CARE

Why use social marketing, a discipline designed for influencing health behaviors, in CQI initiatives? As we have noted, there are several parallels between CQI and the approaches and methods of social marketing, but these are just a starting point for where social marketing can be applied to CQI in health care. Social marketing may actually hold the keys to improving some processes that have been resistant to improvement initiatives and improving health outcomes as well. Social marketing is a methodology that draws from human behavior theory; as humans are involved in endeavors to improve quality not only in industrial processes but in the provision of health services, it stands to reason that social marketing techniques can be applied to CQI initiatives that require behavior change. Change and improvement are the fundamental basis of all CQI initiatives. As stated in Chapter 1:

> CQI is simultaneously two things: a management philosophy and a management method. It is distinguished by the recognition that the customer requirements are the key to customer quality and that ultimately customer requirements will change over time because of changes in education, economics, technology, and culture. Such changes, in turn, require continuous improvements in the administrative and clinical methods that affect the quality of patient care. . . . Change is fundamental of the health care environment, and the organization's systems must have both a will and the way to master such change effectively. (pp. 8–9)

Traditionally, CQI approaches emphasize managerial and professional processes to build a structural framework to implement changes. Individuals are needed to provide input into what changes need to be made and the best methods for changing them. In his plenary address to the First Annual European Forum on Quality Improvement in Health Care in 1996, Dr. Donald M. Berwick, then-President of the Institute for Healthcare Improvement, outlined some fundamental concepts needed for change (Berwick, 1996, p. 619). The following quotes from his address are particularly relevant to this discussion:

- "Real improvement comes from changing systems, not changing within systems."
- "To make improvement, we must be clear about what we are trying to accomplish, how we will know that a change has led to improvement, and what change we can make that will result in an improvement."
- "You win the Tour de France not by planning for years for the perfect first bicycle ride but by constantly making small improvements."

Other efforts of CQI are to deemphasize individual blame, recognize individual contributions, decentralize responsibility, and rely on hard data such as surveys, patient data, and equipment costs in making decisions.

Similarly, social marketing emphasizes first building a foundation for the change framework using behavior change models such as the social norms theory, the health belief model, the theory of planned behavior, and the social cognitive theory to explore the benefits, barriers, and competition of the behavior change (Kotler and Lee, 2008, pp. 167–171). These models seek to understand the readiness of their audience to change, what perceptions they have of the desired behavior change, what the seriousness of the change is (what will happen if the change does not occur), and how they will be perceived by their peer group if they change. By considering some of these change models in implementing CQI initiatives, there is a much stronger understanding of the motivations of those who are involved in designing and implementing CQI.

A key question that must be asked in all CQI initiatives is "How do we know if a change is an improvement?" (Langley et al., 2009). A logical consequence of that question is that behavior change will not always happen as quickly or as widely as it should, especially if there is disagreement about whether the change being proposed is an improvement. For example, Atul Gawande (2009) describes this concept in detail in regard to the introduction of surgical checklists. The concept is also the subject of Case 9 in the companion casebook (McLaughlin et al., 2012); in that case, it is illustrated how a social marketing approach can explain behaviors related to the use of surgical checklists and motivate their greater use.

Social marketing, like CQI, also relies heavily on data when formulating the design and goals of the program. Formative research may consist of reviews of published research, Internet and in-person surveys, focus groups, social media networking data, and social, economic, consumer, and population studies, enabling researchers to learn about their audience before planning the behavior change campaign. CQI initiatives could use these additional types of data to better understand how the patients and employees may act as barriers to or may benefit from their planned program. In a hypothetical example, a hospital management team might hope to improve utilization of current intensive care unit medication pumps and defer buying new equipment. The benefits that health care management would plan to obtain through CQI might be improved customer satisfaction, both external (patients and their families) and internal (employees); more efficient use of resources, including time and equipment; and greater compliance with the CQI program. By adding some social marketing methods, such as conducting formative research on the target audience, compliance with CQI implementation can be increased. For example, using a focus group of the nurses who use the medication pumps to assess how equipment is used and why some types of pumps seem to be in high demand when other equipment remains in the closet, an improvement team may better understand its target audience and obtain better outcomes from its CQI program.

For health care service provider managers, other scenarios where social marketing theories and techniques could be used are numerous—for example, decreasing the rate of hospital readmissions for patients discharged with incisions, decreasing the rate of medication noncompliance or multi-drug interactions after hospital discharge, and improving surgical safety outcomes by implementing a simple safety checklist.

The evolutionary process from commercial marketing to social marketing, and in turn from traditional social marketing to CQI, is gaining momentum in the same way that other CQI processes have evolved exponentially in health care in the past several years. Nationally, social marketing has already benefited the quality improvement process. Between 2005 and 2007, the Social Marketing National Excellence Collaborative trained staff from a majority of Quality Improvement Organizations (QIOs) to apply the social marketing process to the items in their scope of work, developed by the Centers for Medicare and Medicaid Services (CMS). The collaborative conducted a series of trainings around the country. QIO staff created social marketing plans for issues such as the implementation of electronic medical records by private physician practices, reduction of pressure ulcers among nursing home patients, improved management of oral medication in home health clients, improved care of hospital patients with pneumonia, and improved validity rate of chart abstracts submitted to CMS. (For a further discussion of QIOs, see Chapter 15.) When applying social marketing methods to CQI initiatives, the same formal processes should be followed as in any social marketing campaign. The first step is developing a strategic marketing plan. One good starting place is the Web site of the Academy for Educational Development (http://www.aed.org/Publications/loader.cfm?url=/commonspot/security/getfile.cfm&pageid=33595), where the "Twelve Strategic Questions" are found (Smith and Strand, 2008, p. 16):

1. What is the social problem I want to address?

2. Who/what is to blame?

3. What action do I believe will best address that problem?

4. Who is being asked to take that action? (audience)

5. What does the audience want in exchange for adopting this new behavior? (key benefit)

6. Why will the audience believe that anything we offer is real and true? (support)

7. What is the competition offering? Are we offering something the audience wants more? (competition)

8. What marketing mix will increase benefits the audience wants and reduce behaviors they care about?

9. What is the best time and place to reach members of our audience so that they are most disposed to receiving the intervention? (aperture)

10. How often, and from whom, does the intervention need to be received if it is to work? (exposure)

11. How can I integrate a variety of interventions to act over time in a coordinated manner to influence the behavior? (integration)

12. Do I have the resources to carry out this strategy, and if not, where can I find useful partners?

Note that answers to these questions need to be determined through audience research, not by the best guesses or the impressions of the planning team.

Once the basic questions have been considered, a more substantial detailed plan is required (Kotler and Lee, 2008, p. 36):

1. Describe the plan background, purpose, and focus.

2. Conduct a situational analysis.

3. Select target markets.

4. Set objectives and goals.

5. Identify the competition and target market barriers and motivators.

6. Craft a desired positioning.

7. Develop a strategic marketing mix (the four Ps).

8. Outline a plan for monitoring and evaluation.

9. Establish budgets and find funding sources.

10. Complete an implementation plan.

There are two basic types of research objectives that are critical in a social marketing campaign. The first type develops the target audience and proper audience segmentation. This is often called formative research, which was introduced earlier in this chapter. Formative research in social marketing aligns with the Plan, Do, Study, Act (PDSA) approach that is used in CQI and, in particular, the improvement model described by Langley et al. (2009). Formative research can utilize primary data (data collected just for the initiative at hand) or secondary data (data collected in a different but similar research study). It is prudent to use both types of data. As noted by Berwick (1996), the primary purpose of collecting and analyzing these data is learning about improvement and using the data to implement further improvements in a PDSA cycle—a direct parallel to the purpose and use of formative research in social marketing.

The second type of research focuses on the collection and evaluation of data during the pretesting part of the campaign; it is used for continuous monitoring and improvement during and after the campaign and most often utilizes primary data. Once again, this process is directly parallel to the use of primary data collection in CQI to measure the baseline and track the impact of improvements over time—such as in a health care process—using control charts or other quantitative CQI tools, as described in Chapter 3. In social marketing settings, data for this research may be gathered from focus groups, online and in-person surveys, personal interviews, Web site hits and feeds, and blogs.

Applying Social Marketing to a Health Care CQI Initiative

Armed with the strategies just discussed, a CQI initiative using a social marketing approach can begin to take shape. One initiative where social marketing would be a good adjunct to CQI would be an intervention to reduce medical errors in hospitals across the country and the world. The recently published study of a successful intervention for the reduction in surgical errors using a simple checklist, a standard CQI tool (see Chapter 3), provides an excellent opportunity for introduction of social marketing concepts and demonstrates how social marketing methods can be adapted to health care procedures related to health promotion interventions involving the redesign of human engineering methods (Haynes et al., 2009).

Creating a social marketing campaign for achieving a reduction in surgical errors is simple to organize into basic, logical steps of planning, action, and evaluation. Following the model noted previously from Kotler and Lee's social marketing primer, the process is broken down into an executive summary and 10 basic steps.

Although social marketing has had numerous health applications such as those described earlier to address automobile safety, smoking cessation, and other vital issues, it is still relatively new in its application to CQI in health care. To illustrate how it might be applied to a significant lifesaving issue, the following scenario is presented (see also Case 9 in the companion casebook; McLaughlin et al., 2012). The U.S.-based scenario utilizes a current, real-world, health care CQI initiative that has received much attention in medical care publications as well as popular media. This CQI initiative is designed to improve patient outcomes and customer satisfaction in hospitals where surgical procedures take place using a surgical safety checklist designed and tested by the WHO (Haynes et al., 2009). As Atul Gawande (2007) noted in the popular press, if a new drug was found to be as effective in saving lives as checklists are, there would be a nationwide marketing campaign urging doctors to use it. In this scenario, we do just that. A social marketing strategy will be employed to determine the appropriate target audiences; important marketing objectives; the most effective marketing mix; the most efficient methods of data collection, monitoring, and evaluation; an adequate budget and timelines; and a comprehensive implementation plan.

Social Marketing Strategy Steps

Step 1: Describe the Plan Background, Purpose, and Focus

Every year, 44,000–98,000 deaths attributable to medical errors occur in hospitals in the United States (Agency for Healthcare Research and Quality, 2000). This issue, which is also addressed elsewhere in this text, is an important target of CQI initiatives in health care. Surgical errors that involve operating on the incorrect patient or on the incorrect limb or organ are completely avoidable. Other errors, such as administration of incorrect medications, lack of adequate blood supplies, incorrect surgical instrument counts, and use of nonsterile instruments, contribute to additional injuries and expenses due to complications.

The implementation of a simple surgical checklist, created and published by the WHO, has been shown to reduce surgery-related errors by improving medical team communication through confirmation of specific safety checks during surgical procedures. An example of the checklist is found on the WHO Web site (http://www.who.int/patientsafety/safesurgery/en/index.html). Between October 2007 and September 2008, eight hospitals around the world implemented the 19-item WHO safe-surgery checklist. Over the course of just 1 year, the average death rate at these hospitals declined from 1.5% to 0.8%, and the average complication rate declined from 11% to 7%.

In our hypothetical scenario, our hospital has determined that there is a need for a social marketing effort to encourage surgical service providers to adopt this checklist—or at least a modified version of the checklist that meets their needs. The surgical team is composed of multiple specialties that work fairly well together but still need improved communication to achieve better outcomes for patients and create a safer environment in the operating room. Social marketing can address the need to position the issue, identify the exchange being asked of affected staff, identify beliefs that promote or hinder acceptance of the checklist, identify cost-effective strategies, and set up specific, measureable goals to evaluate the outcome of the initiative.

Step 2: Conduct a Situation Analysis

Performing a SWOT analysis (Strengths, Weaknesses, Opportunities, and Threats) will identify any internal or external environmental influences on the initiative. Here is a list of possible issues:

- *Strength*: Everyone on the surgical team is interested in patient safety.
- *Weakness*: The team is composed of different disciplines—surgeons, nurses, technologists, and anesthesiologists or nurse anesthetists.
- *Opportunities*: The health care reform bills passed in 2010 in the United States have provisions to provide incentives and penalties for preventable medical errors.
- *Threats*: Other hospitals may not require the use of a checklist. The surgeon may decide to take his or her business to these other hospitals.

Step 3: Select Target Markets

Several target audiences are involved in this initiative, and they may be in various states of readiness to change:

- *Surgeon* (a physician and the most senior-level person on the team): Does not see a need for change
- *Anesthetist* (either a physician or an advanced practitioner nurse): Is not comfortable with change
- *Cardiac perfusionist* (a surgical specialist): Is indifferent to change
- *Circulating nurse* (the surgical procedure manager): Is ready for change, as surgical errors impact her outcomes
- *Surgical medical equipment technician* (the person responsible for equipment): Is ready for change but has feelings of powerlessness
- *Scrub nurse* (the person responsible for assisting the surgeon): Thinks about change but does not want to disrupt the status quo

Based on these characterizations of the potential target audiences, the most suitable person to initiate change on this team is the circulating nurse.

Step 4: Set Objectives and Goals

The objective of the social marketing strategy is to improve the use of the surgical safety checklist, thus increasing effective implementation of the checklist and ultimately decreasing the number of medical surgical errors and improving patient outcomes and customer satisfaction. After conducting some formative research (personal communications: Edward Dauer, MD, April 18, 2009; Robert S. Smith, MD, and Dori Smith, CRNA, November 27, 2008), with clinicians who are familiar with the role of, or are themselves, surgical team members, the choice of the primary target audience is confirmed to be the circulating nurse. In deciding upon basic goals to be achieved, it is critical that goals be SMART: Specific, Measureable, Attainable, Relevant, and Time-sensitive. This requires the choice of several short-term, intermediate, and long-term goals. In the following examples, the goals set will be incorporated into the monitoring and evaluation plan that will create data from the campaign, providing vital real-time sampling of the initiative, in the same way CQI methods elicit feedback. The chosen goals are as follows:

- *Short term*: (1) All team members will be trained on the checklist within 1 month by the quality assurance manager at the regular weekly staff meeting. (2) Each surgical team will complete a checklist for one surgery per day for the 10 working days during the month, beginning on the first of the month, for a total of 10 different types of surgeries, each month for 3 months. (3) The circulating nurse will receive additional training on team leadership. (4) The circulating nurse will record the surgery information and report to the nurse manager and CQI team on the success or difficulties encountered at each instance, weekly.

- *Intermediate*: (1) At the end of 6 months, each surgical team will complete a checklist on 50% of the surgeries performed during the month. (2) The circulating nurse will record the surgery information and report on the success or difficulties encountered at each instance, twice a month.
- *Long term*: (1) At the end of 12 months, each surgical team will complete the checklist on each of the surgeries they perform. (2) The circulating nurse will lead a discussion of the pros and cons of the surgical safety checklist. (3) The average mortality rate will decline by 40%. (4) The average complication rate will decline by 30%.

Step 5: Identify the Competition and Target Market Barriers and Motivators

Understanding the reasons for current behaviors is one of the key concepts that a social marketing approach can bring to CQI. Often, the challenge is simply that changing procedures causes a disruption in the comfortable established workflow, as in this example, where the target audience is the circulating nurse. Barriers to the desired behavior change may involve a circulating nurse with a personality characteristic that makes him or her less disposed to change of any type. Teams may have worked out their group dynamics already, and the circulating nurse may be reluctant to introduce change in the group because it may cause discord or change the agreed-upon decision-making chain within the group. Surgical teams work together in close proximity in a closed environment, and change may be viewed as causing unnecessary disruption or delay in a carefully timed and orderly environment. It is important to uncover motivators for your target audience, such as pride in overseeing surgeries that avoid the embarrassment and stress of errors, and to then give tools that empower the nurse with methods for improvement that are easy to perform.

Step 6: Craft a Desired Position

After determining how your target audience perceives the CQI initiative, you may need to reposition the behavior you want to obtain. Positioning refers to how a behavior is viewed (e.g., "cool," evidence-based, desirable) compared to competing behaviors. As previously stated, the surgical safety checklist may be viewed as an unnecessary intrusion into the already tightly packed surgical procedure schedule. The circulating nurse is aware of the many times that errors have been caught at the last minute and avoided, but his or her stress and anxiety in dealing with such instances may be less intense than the stress of interrupting the established workflow during each surgery. The checklist needs to be repositioned from a burdensome bureaucratic task to a method of enhanced communication that all team members can benefit from and that will contribute to increased patient safety, which enhances everyone's job satisfaction and decreases stress from possible situations where errors have to be caught and averted.

Step 7: Develop a Strategic Marketing Mix

This is where the advantages of adding a combination of the commercial marketing techniques of the four Ps, Product, Place, Price, and Promotion (supplemented by a fifth P, advocacy for Policy change), enhance customization of your CQI initiative. Your Product (what you are trying to "sell") is the acceptance and use of the surgical safety checklist. Tangible activities that support adoption of the behavior might include training in the use of the checklist and blog postings from other clinicians about how they successfully incorporated use of the list. The Place, or location where you will perform the campaign, should be where the behavior is to be performed—in this case, the work environment (i.e., the surgical suite). You have already identified some of the "costs," the Price, for performing the behavior, such as change in the established workflow. Any monetary incentives that might be available for adherence to the checklist, such as extra time off or a cash bonus, should also be considered here, as well as nonmonetary incentives, such as employee recognition. Other approaches that address the identified cost might include having the team discuss how they can best use the checklist to minimize disruptions or hearing from successful users of the checklist. The Promotion consists of the messages and methods for communicating to support doing the desired behavior. It may be as simple as a large laminated checklist posted in the surgical break room, daily email reminders sent to the circulating nurse's computer, or brightly colored reminder stickers or stars posted at the top of the surgical schedule clipboard.

Step 8: Outline a Plan for Monitoring and Evaluation

By identifying our goals, we have already begun the process for creating a plan for monitoring and evaluation. A simple flowchart of inputs, outputs, and outcomes will help identify other goals and establish a system of continuous monitoring of the CQI initiative. The social media networking field has exploded, and there are numerous opportunities to use these platforms (e.g., a Facebook page) and devices (e.g., a Web-enabled mobile phone) to gain information about attitudes and beliefs about the surgical safety checklist. A link could be set up on the hospital Web site leading employees to information about other hospitals' implementation of the checklist. The circulating nurse could create a blog that might be shared with other nurses on a nursing social networking Web site. Another link could be created on the Web site leading to a survey that records patient satisfaction data during the implementation of the checklist period. A sample evaluation plan is shown in **Table 8–1**. Note that this plan includes and tracks the goals defined in Step 4.

Step 9: Establish Budgets and Find Funding Sources

Monetary considerations are often a barrier when a social marketing approach is proposed, as budgets are so often tight and marketing a quality improvement initiative may seem unnecessary and expensive. The costliest parts of the process are often the marketing research, developing tangible products, producing communication materials (and purchasing time, if mass media is used), and evaluation. However, much marketing research on your target audience may already be available commercially. Using secondary resources is often a cost-effective method for researching your target audience. Internal and external partners can often assist in developing materials or conducting evaluations. In addition, this type of campaign is very limited in scope and is generally quite inexpensive. It is important to remember that social marketing is as much a mindset and a way to think about problems and solutions as it is a series of tasks or tangible offerings that cost money.

TABLE 8–1 Sample Evaluation Plan

Goal	Measurement Item	Method	Who Will Take Measurements
Short-Term Goals			
1. Team member training	a. Number of members trained b. Knowledge and attitude pretest c. Knowledge and attitude posttest	a. Observation (qualitative) b. Web-based survey on computers in training room c. Web-based survey on computers in staff meeting room	a. QA manager b. Self-administered c. Self-administered
2. Completion of checklist for 10 surgeries each month for first 3 months	a. Number completed b. Whether completed correctly c. 10 different types of surgery included d. Quality of team interaction while using checklist	a. Review of checklists by hand b. Review of checklists by hand and observation during surgery; review of data entered into Web-enabled mobile phone or hand-held device such as iPod or Zune by surgical team c. Review of checklists by hand d. Observation	a–d. QA manager
3. Circulating nurse to receive additional leadership training	a. Whether attended training b. Knowledge pretest and posttest	a. Observation b. Role-play and Web-based survey	a. QA manager b. Course trainer
4. Circulating nurse records and reports information for first 3 months	a. If recording completed b. Accuracy of record c. If report occurred weekly	a–c. Observation–data entered in mobile phone or hand-held device	a–c. QA manager

(continues)

Intermediate Goals

Goal	Measures	Data Source	Responsible
1. At the end of 6 months, team to complete a checklist on 50% of all surgeries.	a. Number completed b. If completed correctly c. Different types of surgery included and if 50% used checklist d. Quality of team interaction while using checklist	a. Review of checklists by hand b. Review of checklists by hand and observation during surgery; review of data entered into Web-enabled mobile phone or hand-held device such as iPod or Zune by surgical team c. Review of checklists by hand d. Observation	a–d. QA manager
2. The circulating nurse reviews information for second 3 months and reports twice a month.	a. If recording completed b. Accuracy of record c. If report occurred biweekly	a–c. Observation—data entered in mobile phone or hand-held device	a–c. QA manager

Long-Term Goals

Goal	Measures	Data Source	Responsible
1. At the end of 12 months, checklist will be completed on all surgeries.	a. Number completed b. If completed correctly c. Different types of surgery included and if 100% used checklist d. Quality of team interaction while using checklist	a. Review of checklists by hand b. Review of checklists by hand and observation during surgery; review of data entered into Web-enabled mobile phone or hand-held device such as iPod or Zune by surgical team c. Review of checklists by hand d. Observation	a–d. QA manager
2. The circulating nurse will lead a discussion of the pros and cons of the surgical safety checklist.	a. Team members attending b. List of pros/cons	a. Observation b. Review of data from discussion on pros/cons	a–b. QA manager
3. The average mortality rate will decrease by 40% by the end of 12 months.	Death rate due to surgical errors	Review of patient records	QA manager
4. The average complication rate will decrease by 30% by the end of 12 months.	Rate of medical complications due to surgical errors	Review of patient records	QA manager

Step 10: Complete an Implementation Plan

This final step in the plan is the actual blueprint for the campaign. Here is where formative research, objectives and goals, target audience decisions, and methods for data monitoring and evaluation come together. The implementation plan identifies who will do which activities during what time frame. It also considers how to sustain your efforts. A unified social marketing strategy would be focused on a local target audience, the circulating nurse in your surgical department. In exchange for disrupting the comfortable established workflow, the circulating nurse gains the responsibility for leading the team in an important patient safety initiative and provides simple, effective tools for improving surgical safety. The strategy will be implemented in three distinct phases: (1) a training phase where the circulating nurse is named as the safety leader and other team members acknowledge his or her role; (2) a pilot run where the surgical checklist is only implemented in a portion of all surgeries and where the circulating nurse will record information for data analysis by the CQI team; and (3) a phase where the entire team comes together with the circulating nurse as the team leader to give feedback on the initiative to the CQI team.

CONCLUSIONS

As with other innovations in health care, the use of social marketing as a CQI technique evolved over time as a result of cross-disciplinary thinking/learning. Similar to the way that measuring patient feedback grew out of traditional commercial market research, social marketing applications have been adapted to address health and other social issues. Just as commercial marketing first evolved to social marketing, and later from health care applications in general to specific use in CQI, there is every reason to believe that social marketing will continue to grow as a new technique and set of tools for helping to further the adoption of improvements in health care.

In this brief overview of the social marketing approach as applied to CQI, it is difficult to examine all the possibilities and uncover all nuances that the fusion of these two powerful strategies make possible. Using a scenario based on the use of the surgical safety checklist, a simple CQI method is given strength and accountability through proven social marketing methods to change behavior for the betterment of the common good—a safer surgical environment not only for patients but also for the team members performing the surgery. The use of social marketing in conjunction with CQI represents an important step in the further evolution of both fields. It is the hope that this introduction to social marketing may spark many new ideas and methods of improvement in medical environments that may be encountered by various medical specialties and situations. The use of social marketing applications not only may improve outcomes of specific CQI initiatives, but in the longer term may help to foster greater diffusion of the CQI philosophy and processes throughout the health care community.

Cross-References to the Companion Casebook

(McLaughlin, C. P., Johnson, J. K., and Sollecito, W. A. [Eds.]. 2012. *Implementing Continuous Quality Improvement in Health Care: A Global Casebook.* Sudbury, MA: Jones & Bartlett Learning.)

Case Study Number	Case Study Title	Case Study Authors
3	Clemson's Nursing Home: Working with the State Quality Improvement Organization's Restraint Reduction Initiative	*Franziska Rokoske, Jill A. McArdle, and Anna P. Schenck*
9	Forthright Medical Center: Social Marketing and the Surgical Checklist	*Carol E. Breland*

REFERENCES

Agency for Healthcare Research and Quality. 2000. 20 tips to help prevent medical errors. Patient fact sheet. Retrieved March 25, 2011, from http://www.ahrq.gov/consumer/20tips.htm

Andreasen, A. 1995. *Marketing Social Change: Changing Behavior to Promote Health, Social Development, and the Environment.* San Francisco: Jossey-Bass.

Berwick, D. 1996. A primer on leading the improvement of systems. *BMJ*, 312(7031): 619–622.

Cotroneo, S., Hazel, J., and Chapman, S. 2001. Partnering for social change: Back to Sleep—Reducing the risk of sudden infant death syndrome (SIDS). *Soc Market Q*, 73: 119–121.

Dauer, E. 2007. Medical errors in hospitals: Cause and prevention. Program on Health Outcomes presentation at UNC School of Public Health, Chapel Hill, North Carolina, October 5, 2007. Retrieved March 26, 2011, from http://www.sph.unc.edu/pho/edward_a._dauer_fall_2007_10477.html

Evans, W., Wasserman, J., Bertolotti, E., et al. 2002. Branding behavior: The strategy behind the Truth^SM Campaign. *Soc Market Q*, 83: 17–29.

Gawande, A. 2007. The checklist. *New Yorker*, December 10, 2007.

Gawande, A. 2009. *The Checklist Manifesto*. New York: Metropolitan Books.

Haynes, A. B., Weiser, T. G., Berry, W. R., et al. 2009. A surgical safety checklist to reduce morbidity and mortality in a global population. *N Engl J Med*, 360: 491–499.

Kotler, P., and Lee, N. R. 2008. *Social Marketing: Influencing Behaviors for Good* (3rd ed.). Thousand Oaks, CA: Sage.

Kotler, P., and Zaltman, J. 1971. Social marketing: An approach to planned social change. *J Market*, 35: 3–12.

Landers, J., Mitchell, P., Smith, B., et al. 2006. "Save the crabs, then eat 'em": A culinary approach to saving the Chesapeake Bay. *Soc Market Q*, 123: 15–18.

Langley, G. L., Nolan, K. M., Nolan, T. W., et al. 2009. *The Improvement Guide: A Practical Approach to Enhancing Organizational Performance* (2nd ed.). San Francisco: Jossey-Bass.

Mah, W. M., Deshpande, S., and Rothschild, M. L. 2006. Social marketing: A behavior change technology for infection control. *Am J Infect Control*, 34: 452–457.

McLaughlin, C. P., Johnson, J. K., and Sollecito, W. A. (Eds.). 2012. *Implementing Continuous Quality Improvement in Health Care: A Global Casebook*. Sudbury, MA: Jones & Bartlett Learning.

Siegel, M., and Doner, L. 1998. *Marketing Public Health: Strategies to Promote Social Change*. Gaithersburg, MD: Aspen Publishers.

Smith, W. A., and Strand, J. 2008. Social marketing behavior: A practical resource for social marketing professionals [Electronic version]. Washington, DC: Academy for Educational Development. Retrieved March 25, 2011, from http://www.aed.org/Publications/loader.cfm?url=/commonspot/security/getfile.cfm&pageid=33595

Social Marketing National Excellence Collaborative. 2002. *The Basics of Social Marketing*. [Electronic version]. Seattle: University of

Washington. Retrieved March 6, 2011, from http://www.
turningpointprogram.org/toolkit/pdf/SM_Basics_web.pdf

Uhrig, J., Bann, C., Williams, P., et al. 2010. Social marketing web-
sites as a platform for disseminating social marketing. *Soc Market Q,*
16(1): 2–20.

Williams, A. F., Wells, J. K., and Reinfurt, D. W. 2002. Increasing seat
belt use in North Carolina. In Hornik, R. C. (Ed.), *Public Health
Communication: Evidence for Behavior Change* (pp. 85–96). Mahwah,
NJ: Lawrence Erlbaum Associates.

Wong, F., Huhman, M., Asbury, L., et al. 2004. VERB™—A social
marketing campaign to increase physical activity among youth
[Electronic version]. *Prevent Chron Dis*, 13: A10.

Assessing Risk and Harm in the Clinical Microsystem

Paul Barach and Julie K. Johnson

"Medicine used to be simple, ineffective, and relatively safe. Now it is complex, effective, and dangerous."

—Sir Cyril Chantler

Modern medical care is complex, expensive, and at times dangerous. Across the world, hospital patients are harmed 9.2% of the time, with death occurring in 7.4% of these events. Furthermore, it is estimated that 43.5% of these harm events are preventable (de Vries et al., 2008; Landrigan et al., 2010). The rates could be debated, as they depend on the methods used in the studies as well as unknown levels of underreporting; however, what is clear is that we need to change and improve our health care systems dramatically. Most significantly, the study of patient safety has identified the need to design better systems to prevent errors from causing patient harm. From all perspectives (patients' and providers' as well as the health care system's), the current level of avoidable harm is unacceptable and financially ruinous.

The goal of this chapter is to discuss how to develop resilience in health care providers while embedding a vision of zero avoidable harm into the culture of the health care system. Achieving this vision requires a risk management strategy that includes (1) identifying risk—finding out what is going wrong; (2) analyzing risk—collecting data and using appropriate methods to understand what it means; and (3) controlling risk—devising and implementing strategies to better detect, manage, and prevent the problems from occurring (Dickson, 1995).

This chapter begins with the background and definitions of risk management. We discuss the universal ingredients of individual accidents, organizational accidents, and human error. We then discuss models of risk management, focusing on how to create a culture of safety and engagement and present strategies for applying concepts to clinical microsystem settings. The chapter concludes with a discussion of the role of disclosure of adverse events as part of a risk management strategy.

RISK MANAGEMENT—BACKGROUND AND DEFINITIONS

Traditionally, risk has been seen as exposure to events that may threaten or damage the organization (Walshe, 2001). Essentially, risk is the chance of something happening that will have an impact on key elements. It can be measured in terms of consequences and likelihood. The task of risk management, therefore, becomes balancing the costs and consequences of risks against the costs of risk reduction. The goal in clinical risk management should be to improve care and protect patients from harm; however, a perverse incentive for the organization as well as for those who work within the organization is that risk management may become a financially driven exercise (Vincent, 1997). Clinical risk management is the culture, process, and structures that are directed toward the effective management of potential opportunities and adverse events. We measure risk in terms of the likelihood and consequences of something going wrong, which is in contrast to how we measure quality (i.e., the extent to which a service or product achieves a desired result or outcome). Quality is commonly measured by whether a product or service is safe, timely, effective, efficient, equitable, and patient centered (Institute of Medicine, 2001).

There is substantial evidence that the majority of harm caused by health care is avoidable and the result of systemic problems rather than poor performance or negligence by individual providers. The past several years have seen an increase in proposed or operative legislation, including a near-miss reporting system, changes in mandated reporting systems, and the creation of state agencies dedicated to the coordination of patient safety research and implementation of change. There is clear policy guidance and a compelling ethical basis for the disclosure of adverse events to patients and their families. Mechanisms have been developed to involve all stakeholders—the government, health care professionals, administrators and planners, providers, and consumers—in ongoing, effective consultation, communication, and cultural change. These cultural and regulatory devices have helped engender more trust, which is an essential element in developing and sustaining a culture of safety.

Accidents

Research in managing risk has focused on the culture and structure of the organization. Perrow advanced the Normal Accidents Theory, which describes accidents as inevitable in complex, tightly coupled systems such as chemical plants and nuclear power plants (Perrow, 1984). These accidents occur irrespective of the skill and intentions of the designers and operators; hence, they are normal and difficult to prevent. Perrow further argues that as the system gets more complex, it becomes opaque to its users so that people are less likely to recognize and be afraid of potential adverse occurrences. There are three universal ingredients of accidents:

1. *All human beings, regardless of their skills, abilities, and specialist training, make fallible decisions and commit unsafe acts.* This human propensity for committing errors and violating safety procedures can be moderated by selection, training, well-designed equipment, and good management, but it can never be entirely eliminated.

2. *All man-made systems possess latent failures to some degree.* This is true no matter how well designed, constructed, operated, and maintained a system may be. These unseen failures are analogous to resident pathogens in the human body that combine with local triggering factors (e.g., life stress, toxic chemicals)

to overcome the immune system and produce disease. Adverse events such as cancers and heart attacks in well-defended systems do not arise from single causes but from multifactorial reasons. The adverse conjunction of such factors, each necessary but insufficient alone to breach the defenses, are behind the majority of adverse events.

3. *All human endeavors involve some measure of risk.* In many cases, the local hazards are well understood and can be guarded against by a variety of technical or procedural countermeasures. No one, however, can foresee all the possible adverse scenarios, so there will always be defects in this protective armor.

These three ubiquitous accident ingredients reveal something important about the nature of making care safer (Bernstein, 1996). We can mitigate the risk of adverse events by process improvement, standardization, and an in-depth understanding of the safety degradations in systems, but we cannot prevent all risk. Embracing this uncertainty and training to cope with it, as opposed to focusing solely on minimizing it, is essential in high-risk, highly coupled industries.

Outside health care, the most obvious impetus of the renewed interest in human error and impact of the organizational dynamics has been the growing concern over the terrible cost of human error that led to disasters. Examples include the Tenerife runway collision in 1977 (540 fatalities), the Three Mile Island nuclear disaster in 1979, the Bhopal methyl isocyanate tragedy in 1984, the Challenger space shuttle accident in 1986 (Vaughn, 1996), and the Chernobyl nuclear disaster in 1986 (Reason, 1997). There is nothing new about tragic accidents caused by human error, but in the past, the injurious consequences were usually confined to the immediate vicinity of the disaster. Today the nature and scale of potentially hazardous technologies in society and hospitals means that human error can have adverse effects way beyond the confines of the individual provider and patient settings. For example, *Pseudomonas aeruginosa* contamination of a single damaged bronchoscope has the potential to infect dozens of patients (DiazGranados et al., 2009). In recent years, there has been a noticeable spirit of glasnost within the medical profession concerning the role played by human error in causing medical adverse events (Millenson, 1997).

The Organizational Accident

Certain systems have been designed and redesigned with a wide variety of technical and procedural safeguards (e.g., operating rooms), yet they are still subject to accidents and adverse events (e.g., fire in the operating room, wrong-patient procedure, drug errors). These types of accidents and adverse events have been termed *organizational accidents* (Perrow, 1984; Reason, 1997). Organizational accidents are mishaps that arise not from single errors or isolated component breakdowns, but from the insidious culture change due to an accumulation of failures lying mainly within the managerial and organizational spheres. Such latent failures may subsequently combine with active failures and local triggering factors to penetrate or bypass the system defenses. Bosk (1979), in his classic study of surgical teams, *Forgive and Remember*, demonstrates how the underlying culture acts to acculturate newcomers and suppress external views for change while enabling substandard practices to go unchecked.

The etiology of an organizational accident can be divided into five phases (Perrow, 1984):

1. Organizational processes giving rise to latent failures

2. Conditions that produce errors and violations within workplaces (e.g., operating room, pharmacy, intensive care unit)

3. The commission of errors and violations by "sharp end" individuals (The "sharp end" refers to the personnel or parts of the health care system in direct contact with patients. In contrast, the "blunt end" refers to the many layers of the health care system that affect the individuals at the sharp end. These colloquial terms are more formally known as "active errors," which occur at the point of contact between a human and some aspect of a larger system, and "latent errors," which are the less apparent failures of the organization.)

4. The breaching of defenses or safeguards

5. Outcomes that vary from a "free lesson" to a catastrophe

Viewed from this perspective, the unsafe acts of those in direct contact with the patient are the end result of a long chain of events that originate higher up in the organization. One of the basic principles of error management is that the transitory mental states associated with error production—momentary inattention, distraction, preoccupation, forgetting—are the least manageable links in the error chain because they are both unintended and largely unpredictable (Hollnagel et al., 2006). These errors have their cognitive origins in highly adaptive mental processes (Sagan, 1993). Such states can strike health care providers at any time, leading to slips, forgetfulness, and inattention. The system must be designed to mitigate the impact of these momentary lapses in awareness and to maintain the integrity of patient care.

Human Error and Performance Limitations

Although there was virtually no research in the field of safety in medicine and health care delivery until the mid-1980s, in other fields, such as aviation, road and rail travel, nuclear power, and chemical processing, safety science and human factor principles have been applied to understand, prevent, and mitigate the associated adverse events (e.g., crashes, spills, and contaminations). The study of human error and of the organizational culture and climate, as well as intensive crash investigations, have been well developed for several decades in these arenas (Rasmussen, 1990; Sagan, 1993). The presumption of increasing risk in health care, associated with an apparent rise in the rate of litigation in the 1980s and attributable to the media's amplified attention to the subject, has brought medical adverse events to the attention of both clinicians and the general public (Kasperson et al., 1988).

In parallel with these developments, researchers from several disciplines have developed increasingly sophisticated methods for analyzing all incidents (Turner and Pidgeon, 1997). Theories of error and accident causation have evolved and are applicable across many human activities, including health care (Reason, 1997). These developments have led to a much broader understanding of accident causation, with less focus on the individual who commits an error at the "sharp end" of the incident and more on preexisting organizational and system factors that provide the context in which errors and patient harm can occur. An important consequence of this has been the realization that rigorous and innovative techniques of accident analysis may reveal deep-rooted, latent, and unsafe features of organizations. James Reason's "Swiss cheese" model captures these relationships very well (Reason, 1990). Understanding and predicting performance in complex settings requires a detailed understanding of the setting, the regulatory environment, and the human factors that influence that performance.

MODELS OF RISK MANAGEMENT

Risk management deals with the fact that adverse events, however rare, do occur. Furthermore, risk management as a concept means that we should never ignore the possibility or significance of rare, unpredictable events. Using a creative analogy, Nassim Nicholas Taleb (2010) argues that before Europeans discovered Australia, there was no reason to believe that swans could be any color but white. However, when they discovered Australia, they found black swans. Black swans remind us that things do occur that we cannot possibly predict. Taleb continues the analogy to say that his "black swan" is an event with three properties: (1) the probability is low based on past knowledge, (2) the impact of the occurrence is massive, and (3) it is subject to hindsight bias; that is, people do not see it coming, but after its occurrence, everyone knew it was likely to happen.

In general, risk management models take into consideration the probability of an event occurring, which is then multiplied by the potential impact of the event. **Figure 9–1** illustrates a simple risk management model that considers the probability of an event (low, medium, or high) and the impact of the consequences (limited/minor, moderate, or significant).

		Probability		
		Low	Medium	High
Impact	Significant	Considerable management required	Substantial management and monitoring of risks	Extensive management crucial
	Moderate	May accept risks but monitor them	Management effort worthwhile	Management effort required
	Limited/Minor	Accept risks	Accept but monitor risks	Manage and monitor risks

FIGURE 9–1 Risk Management Model

Assigning an event to one of the cells is not an exact science, but the matrix offers a guideline to an appropriate response to the risk. The individual unit or organization would need to determine how to translate each cell into action (e.g., what is required for "extensive management" of events with a significant negative impact and high likelihood of occurring).

ENGINEERING A CULTURE OF SAFETY

How do we create an organizational climate in health care that fosters safety? What are the ingredients of a safety culture? While national cultures arise largely out of shared norms and values, an organizational culture is shaped mainly by shared practices. And practices can be shaped by the implementation and enforcement of rules. Culture can be defined as the collection of individual and group values, attitudes, and practices that guide the behavior of group members (Helmreich and Merritt, 2001). Acquiring a safety culture is a process of organizational learning that recognizes the inevitability of error and proactively seeks to identify latent threats. Characteristics of a strong safety culture include (Pronovost et al., 2003):

1. A commitment of the leadership to discuss and learn from errors

2. Communications founded on mutual trust and respect

3. Shared perceptions of the importance of safety

4. Encouragement and practice of teamwork

5. Incorporation of nonpunitive systems for reporting and analyzing adverse events

Striving for a safety culture is a process of collective learning. When the usual reaction to an adverse incident is to write another procedure and to provide more training, the system will not become more resistant to future organizational accidents. In fact, these actions may deflect the blame from the organization as a whole. There is a long tradition in medicine of examining past practices to understand how things might have been done differently. However, morbidity and mortality conferences, grand rounds, and peer reviews share many of the same shortcomings, such as a lack of human factors and systems thinking, a narrow focus on individual performance that excludes analysis of the contributory team factors and larger social issues, retrospective bias (a tendency to search for errors as opposed to the myriad system causes of error induction), and a lack of multidisciplinary integration into the organization-wide culture (Small and Barach, 2002).

If clinicians at the sharp end are not empowered by managerial leadership to be honest and reflective on their practice, rules and regulations will have a limited impact on enabling safer outcomes. Health care administrators need to understand the fundamental dynamics that lead to adverse events. Employing tools such as root cause analysis and failure mode and effects analysis can help clinicians and others better understand how adverse events occur (Dekker, 2004).

Collecting and learning from near misses is essential. Definitions vary somewhat, but we define a near miss as any error that had the potential to cause an adverse outcome but did not result in patient harm (Barach and Small, 2000). It is indistinguishable from a fully fledged adverse event in all but outcome (March et al., 1991). Near misses offer powerful reminders of system hazards and retard the process of forgetting to be afraid of adverse events. A comprehensive effort to record and analyze near-miss data in health care has, however, lagged behind other industries (e.g., aviation, nuclear power industry) (Small and Barach, 2002). Vital but underappreciated studies suggest that near misses are quite common. In a classic study, Heinreich (1941) estimated there are approximately 100 near misses for every adverse event resulting in patient harm.

A focus on learning from near misses offers several advantages (Barach and Small, 2000):

1. Near misses occur 3–300 times more often than adverse events, enabling quantitative analysis.

2. There are fewer barriers to data collection, allowing analysis of interrelations of small failures.

3. Recovery strategies can be studied to enhance proactive interventions and to deemphasize the culture of blame.

4. Hindsight bias is more effectively reduced.

If near misses and adverse events are inevitable, how do we learn from them once they occur? The next section discusses an approach for learning from events using a microsystem framework.

APPLYING RISK MANAGEMENT CONCEPTS TO IMPROVING QUALITY AND SAFETY WITHIN THE CLINICAL MICROSYSTEM

The clinical microsystem—as a unit of research, analysis, and practice—is an important level at which to focus patient safety interventions. Chapter 13 in this text provides a detailed definition of the clinical microsystem, the small team of providers and staff providing care for a defined population of patients. Most patients and caregivers meet at this system level, and it is here that real changes in patient care can (and must) be made. Errors and failure occur within the microsystem, and ultimately it is the well-functioning microsystem that can prevent or mitigate errors and failure to avoid causing patient harm. Safety is a property of the clinical microsystem that can be achieved only through a systematic application of a broad array of process, equipment, organization, supervision, training, simulation, and teamwork changes. The scenario included in **Exhibit 9–1** illustrates a patient safety event in an academic clinical microsystem and how the resulting analysis can allow a microsystem to learn from the event. Throughout the story, as told from the perspective of a senior resident physician in pediatrics, there are many system failures.

Many methods are available to explore the causal system at work (Dekker, 2002; Reason, 1995; Vincent, 2003; Vincent et al., 1998), and they all suggest the importance of holding the entire causal system in our analytic frame, not just seeking a "root" cause. One method that we have found to be useful for systematically looking at patient safety events builds on William Haddon's overarching framework (1972) on injury epidemiology (Mohr et al., 2003).

Haddon, as the first Director of the National Highway Safety Bureau (1966 to 1969), was interested in the broad issue of injury that results from the transfer of energy in such ways that inanimate or animate objects are damaged. The clinical microsystem offers a setting in which this injury can be studied. According to Haddon, there are a number of strategies for reducing losses:

- Prevent the marshaling of the energy.
- Reduce the amount of energy marshaled.
- Prevent the release of the energy.

EXHIBIT 9-1 Patient Safety Scenario—Interview with a Third-Year Pediatrics Resident

---

Resident: I had a patient who was very ill. We thought that an abdominal CT would be helpful and it needed to be infused. He was 12 years old and was completely healthy up until 3 months ago and since then has been in our hospital and two other hospitals, pretty much the entire time. He has been in respiratory failure, he's had mechanical ventilation (including oscillation), he's been in renal failure, he's had a number of ministrokes, and when I came on service he was having diarrhea—3 to 5 liters/day—and we still didn't know what was going on with him.

He was a very anxious child. Understandably, it's hard for the nurses, and for me, and for his mother to deal with. He thought of it as pain, but it was anxiety and it responded well to anxiolytics.

When I came in that morning, it hadn't been passed along to nursing that he was supposed to go to CT that morning. I heard the charge nurse getting the report from the night nurse. I said, "You know that he is supposed to go for a CT today." She was already upset because they were very short staffed. She heard me and then said that she was not only the charge nurse, but also taking care of two patients, and one had to go to CT. She went off to the main unit to talk to someone. Then she paged me and said, "If you want this child to have a scan, you have to go with him." I said, "OK." Nurses are the ones who usually go. But it didn't seem to be beyond my abilities . . . at the time.

So, I took the child for his CT and his mom came with us. We gave him extra Ativan on the way there, because whenever he had a procedure he was extra anxious. When we got there, they weren't ready. We had lost our spot from the morning. My patient got more and more anxious and was actually yelling at the techs, "Hurry up!" We went into the room. He was about 5 or 6 hours late for his study and we had given him contrast enterally. The techs were concerned that he didn't have enough anymore and wanted to give him more through his G-tube. I said, "That sounds fine." And they mixed it up and gave it to me to give through his G-tube. I went to his side and—not registering that it was his central line—I unhooked his central line, not only taking off the cap but unhooking something, and I pushed 70 cc of the gastrografin in. As soon as I had finished the second syringe I realized I was using the wrong tube. I said, "Oh no!" Mom was right there and said, "What?" I said, "I put the stuff in the wrong tube. He looks OK. I'll be right back, I have to call somebody."

I clamped him off and I called my attending and the radiologist. My attending said that he was on his way down. The radiologist was over by the time I had hung up the phone. My patient was stable the whole time. We figured out what was in the gastrografin that could potentially cause harm. We decided to cancel the study. . . . I sent the gastrografin—the extra stuff in the tubes—for a culture just in case he grew some kind of infection and then we would be able to treat it and match it with what I had pushed into the line. I filled out an incident report. I called my chiefs and told them. . . . They said, "It's OK. He's fine, right?" I said, "Yes." They came up later in the evening just to be supportive. They said, "It's OK. It's OK to make a mistake."

Interviewer: What was your attending's response?

Resident: The attending that I had called when I made the mistake said, "I'm sorry that you were in that situation. You shouldn't have been put in that situation." Another attending the next day was telling people, "Well, you know what happened yesterday," as if it were the only thing going on for this patient.

(continues)

EXHIBIT 9-1 Patient Safety Scenario—Interview with a Third-Year Pediatrics Resident *(continued)*

I thought it was embarrassing that he was just passing on this little tidbit of information as if it would explain everything that was going on. As opposed to saying, "Yes, an error was made, it is something that we are taking into account." And he told me to pay more attention to the patient. Yes, I made the mistake, but hands-down I still and always did know that patient better than he did. I just thought that was mean and not fair. And the only other thing I thought was not good was the next morning when I was prerounding some of the nurses were whispering and I just assumed that was what they were whispering about. I walked up to them and said, "I'm the one who did it. I made a mistake. How is he doing?" I tried to answer any questions they had and move on.

Interviewer: How did the nurses respond when you said that you made a mistake?

Resident: The nurse that had sent me down with him told me, "It's OK, don't worry about it." The others just listened politely and didn't say anything.

Interviewer: How did the mother respond to you the next day?

Resident: The next day, I felt really bad. I felt very incompetent. I was feeling very awkward being the leader of this child's care—because I am still at a loss for his diagnosis. And after the event, when the grandma found out—she was very angry. I apologized to the mom and I thought it would be overdoing it to keep saying, "I am so sorry." So, the next day I went into the room and said to the mom, "You need to have confidence in the person taking care of your son. If my mistake undermines that at all, you don't have to have me as your son's doctor and I can arrange it so that you can have whoever you want." She said, "No. No, it's fine. We want you as his doctor." Then we just moved on with the care plan. That felt good. And that felt appropriate. I couldn't just walk into the room and act like nothing had happened. I needed her to give me the power to be their doctor. So, I just went and asked for it.

- Modify the rate or spatial distribution of release of the energy.
- Separate in time and space the energy being released and the susceptible structure.
- Use a physical barrier to separate the energy and the susceptible structure.
- Modify the contact surface or structure with which people can come in contact.
- Strengthen the structure that might be damaged by the energy transfer.
- When injury does occur, rapidly detect it and counter its continuation and extension.
- When injury does occur, take all necessary reparative and rehabilitative steps.

All these strategies have a logical sequence that is related to the three essential phases of injury control relating to preinjury, injury, and postinjury.

Haddon developed a three-by-three matrix with factors related to an auto injury (human, vehicle, and environment) heading the columns and phases of the event (preinjury, injury, and postinjury) heading the rows. **Figure 9–2** shows how the Haddon Matrix can be used to analyze an auto accident (Haddon, 1972). The use of the matrix focuses the analysis on the interrelationship between the factors and phases. A mix of countermeasures derived from Haddon's strategies is necessary to minimize loss. Furthermore, the countermeasures can be designed for each phase—preevent, event, and postevent. This approach confirms what we know about adverse events in complex environments—it takes a variety of strategies to prevent and/or mitigate harm. Understanding injury in its larger context helps us recognize the basic nature of "unsafe" systems and the important work of humans to mitigate the inherent hazards (Dekker, 2002).

We can also use the Haddon Matrix to guide the analysis of patient safety adverse events. Translating this tool from injury epidemiology

		FACTORS		
		Human	Vehicle	Environment
PHASES	Preinjury	Alcohol intoxication	Braking capacity of motor vehicles	Visibility of hazards
	Injury	Resistance to energy insults	Sharp or pointed edges and surfaces	Flammable building materials
	Postinjury	Hemorrhage	Rapidity of energy reduction	Emergency medical response

FIGURE 9–2 Haddon Matrix Used to Analyze Auto Accident

Source: Haddon, W. A. 1972. Logical framework for categorizing highway safety phenomena and activity. *J Trauma*, 12(2): 197.

to patient safety, we have revised the matrix to include phases labeled *preevent*, *event*, and *postevent* instead of *preinjury*, *injury*, and *postinjury*. The revised factors, *patient–family*, *health care professional*, *system*, and *environment*, replace *human*, *vehicle*, and *environment*. Note that we have added a fourth factor, system, to refer to the processes and systems that are in place for the microsystem. This addition recognizes the significant contribution that systems make toward harm and error in the microsystem. "Environment" refers to the context (enablers and barriers) that the microsystem exists within. **Figure 9–3** shows a completed matrix using the pediatric case. The next step in learning from errors and adverse events is to develop and execute countermeasures to address the issues in

		FACTORS			
		Patient/Family	Health Care Professional	System	Environment
PHASES	Preevent	• Consent (process, timing) • Anxiety • Patient lines • Mother's presence	• Not familiar with procedure • Lack of MD–RN communication • Focus on anxiety and not on procedure • Assumed roles, made assumptions • Arrogance/respect	• Several lines in patient • Silos	• Nurse shortage • Scheduling delays • Manufacturing (performance shaping factors, human factors) • Lack of process for risk analysis
	Event	• Anxiety (patient's and parent's) • No shared expectations • No active participation	• Fatigue • Aware of limitations • Training	• Work hours • Protocols • Standardization • Double-checking	• Work hours for residents • Rushed • No other clinician
	Postevent	• Lack of explanation • Disclosure • Who should talk to family?	• Guilt • Lack of confidence • Loss of face	• Lack of understanding of errors/ systems • Lack of supportive environment for resident • Incidence report morbidity and mortality • Analysis of event	• Regulatory

FIGURE 9–3 Completed Patient Safety Matrix

		FACTORS		
		Patient/Family	Health Care Professional	Systems/Environment
PHASES	Preevent	• Orientation to the process (process mapping)	• Probablistic risk assessment • Scenario building • Hazard analysis • Checklists	• Failure modes effects analysis • Human factors engineering
	Event	• Interview	• Crew resource management • Checklists	• Root cause analysis
	Postevent	• Interview • Focus group interviews	• Microsystem analysis • Morbidity and mortality conference	• Root cause analysis • Artifact analysis

FIGURE 9-4 Patient Safety Matrix with Tools for Assessing Risk and Analyzing Events

each cell of the matrix. **Figure 9-4** provides a list of tools that would be appropriate to assess each "cell" of the matrix as part of a microsystems risk assessment framework.

Microsystems and Macrosystems

Health care organizations are composed of multiple, differentiated, variably autonomous microsystems. These interdependent small systems exhibit loose and tight coupling (Weick and Sutcliffe, 2001). Several assumptions are made about the relationship between these microsystems and the macrosystem (Nelson et al., 2002):

1. Bigger systems (macrosystems) are made of smaller systems.

2. These smaller systems (microsystems) produce quality, safety, and cost outcomes at the front line of care.

3. Ultimately, the outcomes from macrosystems can be no better than the microsystems of which they are formed.

These assumptions suggest that it is necessary to intervene within each microsystem in the organization if the organization as a whole wants to improve. A microsystem cannot function independently from the other microsystems it regularly works with or its macrosystem.

From the macrosystem perspective, senior leaders can enable an overall patient safety focus with clear, visible values, expectations, and recognition of "deeds well done." They can set direction by clearly expecting that each microsystem will align its mission, vision, and strategies with the organization's mission, vision, and strategies. Senior leadership can offer each microsystem the flexibility needed to achieve its mission and ensure the creation of strategies, systems, and methods for achieving excellence in health care, thereby stimulating innovation and building knowledge and capabilities. Finally, senior leaders can pay careful attention to the questions they ask as they nurture meaningful work and hold the microsystem's leadership accountable to achieve the strategic mission of providing safer care.

Table 9–1 builds on the research of high-performing microsystems (Mohr, 2000; Mohr and Batalden, 2002; Mohr et al., 2004) and provides specific actions that can be further explored to apply patient safety concepts to understanding the impact and performance of clinical microsystems. It also provides linkages to the macrosystem's ongoing organization-centered and issue-centered quality efforts, which can either support or conflict with this approach, as discussed in greater detail in Chapter 13. **Table 9–2** provides a set of accountability questions that senior leaders might ask as they work to improve the safety and quality of the organization.

Promoting System Resilience Across and Between the Microsystems

Microsystems usually coexist with multiple other microsystems within the organization. Patients are aware of the gaps and handoffs between microsystems as they navigate the health care system, such as when they transfer from inpatient care back into the community. Patients are aware of the challenges of "synthesizing" knowledge across the various microsystems they encounter. Models developed by Zimmerman and Hayday (1999) for understanding and supporting work on the relationships across microsystems offer insight into the generative work of interdependence. Understanding the dynamics of effective organizational relationships can be helpful in thinking about how to foster relationships between microsystems within the same organization and across differing organizations. These cross-microsystem relationships

TABLE 9-1 Linkage of Microsystem Characteristics to Patient Safety

Microsystem Characteristics	What This Means for Patient Safety
1. Leadership	• Define the safety vision of the organization
	• Identify the existing constraints within the organization
	• Allocate resources for plan development, implementation, and ongoing monitoring and evaluation
	• Build in microsystems participation and input to plan development
	• Align organizational quality and safety goals
	• Engage the board of trustees in ongoing conversations about the organizational progress toward achieving safety goals
	• Recognition for prompt truth-telling about errors or hazards
	• Certification of helpful changes to improve safety
2. Organizational support	• Work with clinical microsystems to identify patient safety issues and make relevant local changes
	• Put the necessary resources and tools in the hands of individuals
3. Staff focus	• Assess current safety culture
	• Identify the gap between current culture and safety vision
	• Plan cultural interventions
	• Conduct periodic assessments of culture
	• Celebrate examples of desired behavior, for example, acknowledgment of an error
4. Education and training	• Develop patient safety curriculum
	• Provide training and education of key clinical and management leadership
	• Develop a core of people with patient safety skills who can work across microsystems as a resource
5. Interdependence of the care team	• Build PDSA* cycles into debriefings
	• Use daily huddles to debrief and to celebrate identifying errors
6. Patient focus	• Establish patient and family partnerships
	• Support disclosure and truth around medical error
7. Community and market focus	• Analyze safety issues in community, and partner with external groups to reduce risk to population

(continues)

TABLE 9–1 Linkage of Microsystem Characteristics to Patient Safety *(continued)*

Microsystem Characteristics	What This Means for Patient Safety
8. Performance results	• Develop key safety measures
	• Create feedback mechanisms to share results with microsystems
9. Process improvement	• Identify patient safety priorities based on assessment of key safety measures
	• Address the work that will be required at the microsystem level
10. Information and information technology	• Enhance error-reporting systems • Build safety concepts into information flow (e.g., checklists, reminder systems)

*PDSA: Plan Do Study Act

are fundamentally related to improving handoffs, but this inquiry can also provide opportunities for learning about systemic problems within the institution and interventions to improve quality and safety.

An effective collaborative relationship is based on the underlying assumption that collaboration is a more effective approach to achieve a goal than multiple individual efforts. Weick suggests that leaders today need to develop groups that are also respectful of the interactions that hold the group together (Weick, 1993, 1995). Resilient groups

TABLE 9–2 Questions Senior Leaders Could Ask About Patient Safety

What information do we have about errors and patient harm?

What is the patient safety plan?

How will the plan be implemented at the organizational level and at the microsystem level?

What type of infrastructure is needed to support implementation?

What is the best way to communicate the plan to the individual microsystems?

How can we foster reporting—telling the truth—about errors?

How will we empower microsystem staff to make suggestions for improving safety?

What training will staff need?

Who are the key stakeholders?

How can we build linkages to the key stakeholders?

What stories can we tell that relate the importance of patient safety?

How will we recognize and celebrate progress?

have respectful interactions that are founded on three major elements (Weick, 1996):

1. *Trust*—a willingness to base beliefs and actions on the reports of others

2. *Honesty*—reporting so that others may use one's observations in developing and enhancing their own beliefs

3. *Self-respect*—integrating one's perceptions and beliefs with the reports of others without depreciating them or oneself

Four aspects of the relationship can help generate creative responses to the diagnosed challenges facing entities needing to work better together (Zimmerman and Hayday, 1999):

1. The separateness or differences of the two microsystems

2. The talking–listening–tuning opportunities that the two microsystems have

3. The action opportunities that the two entities have

4. The reasons they have to work together

Balanced attention to each of these aspects enables creative work.

The conditions also must be present for relationships to develop across organizations (Kaluzny, 1985). For voluntary interactions—which may be quite different than those mandated by an external power—several conditions must be met. There must be an internal need for resources, a commitment to an external problem, and the opportunity to change. In addition, there must be a consensus regarding both the external problem(s) facing the organizations and the specific goals and services for developing a joint effort. The 2000 Institute of Medicine report *To Err Is Human* brought patient safety to the forefront of the agenda and set the stage for discussing specific goals and strategies for achieving those goals.

Mitchell and Shortell (2000) provide a synthesis of the literature on the success of community health partnerships that suggests several factors that influence the success of interorganizational relationships. These factors are:

- Context
- Strategic intent

- Resource base
- Membership heterogeneity
- Coordination of skills
- Response to accountability

Context refers to the environment in which the partnership exists—the internal and external stakeholders, their historical relationships and influence, the presence or absence of human and financial resources, the political environment, public sentiments, and the current challenges facing the community. Strategic intent—a similar concept to a consensus on the external problem(s) facing the organizations—refers to the reasons the interorganizational relationship is formed. A diversified resource base helps ensure that the collaborative is able to pursue the strategic intent without getting sidetracked by pursuing the goals of a single funding agency. Membership heterogeneity refers to the balance of the participating members in regard to the number and types of participants. Informal as well as formal communication mechanisms ensure that the collaborators meet their own goals and are held accountable to demonstrate their progress internally and externally.

ROLE OF RISK MANAGEMENT AND PATIENT DISCLOSURE

When patients seek medical care, they entrust their health to us. Health care providers have a responsibility or "fiduciary duty" to act in the best interests of the patient (Kraman and Hamm, 1999). Properly assessing the type of procedure planned (e.g., invasive vs. noninvasive), patient risk factors, type of drug to use (e.g., hypnotic vs. analgesic), and type of team and level of support are all critical. When assessing the level of risk of the procedure, we should ask, What are the desired clinical effects? How quickly are effects desired? What is the desired duration of effects? And are there any adverse "other" clinical effects?

Injured patients and their families want to know the cause of their bad outcomes, especially if the adverse event was caused by an error (Studdert et al., 2004). The most important factor in the decision to file lawsuits is not negligence but ineffective communication between patients and providers (Wu et al., 1997). Malpractice suits often result when an unexpected adverse outcome is met with no effort to apologize, with a lack of empathy from physicians and a perceived or actual withholding of essential information (Barach, 2005; Wu et al., 1997).

Studies consistently show that health care providers are understandably reticent about discussing errors, believing they have no appropriate assurance of legal protection (LeBlang and King, 1984). This reticence, in turn, impedes systemic and programmatic efforts to prevent medical errors. A growing initiative in health care has been to encourage open and frank discussion with patients and their families after an adverse event; this initiative has met with salutary effects. The lack of evidence that disclosure adversely impacts claims, case resolution, and patient and family perceptions is changing organizational practices.

Evidence from the University of Michigan supports an aggressive disclosure policy (Clinton and Obama, 2006). In 2002, the University of Michigan Health System launched a program with three components: (1) acknowledge cases in which a patient was hurt because of medical error and compensate these patients quickly and fairly, (2) aggressively defend cases that the hospital considers to be without merit, and (3) study all adverse events to determine how procedures and systems can be improved.

Disclosing an adverse event should occur when the adverse event (1) has a perceptible effect on the patient that was not discussed in advance as a known risk, (2) necessitates a change in the patient's care, (3) potentially poses an important risk to the patient's future health, even if that risk is extremely small, and (4) involves providing a treatment or procedure without the patient's consent (Cantor et al., 2005). From an ethical perspective, the disclosure process should begin at the time of discussing the consent form and interventions with the patients (Barach and Cantor, 2007).

CONCLUSIONS

The health care system has begun to approach patient safety in a more systematic way, but we continue to tolerate an extraordinary level of risk and preventable harm. There is a clear need to improve the safety of care, as patients still suffer harm from medical care at alarmingly high rates. Strong leadership is needed to change organizational cultures to achieve a vision of zero tolerance of preventable harm. The application of safety science principles, methods, and analytical tools in the health sector promises the development of a coherent bundle of interrelated strategies for change.

Much work is needed to change the mental model of clinicians and providers toward a system-based metaphor. The traditional approach within medicine and health care was to stress the individual's responsibility for errors and to encourage the belief that the way to eliminate adverse events was for individual clinicians to perfect their practices. This simplistic approach fails to address the important and complex systematic flaws that contribute to the genesis of adverse events, and also perpetuates a myth of infallibility that is a disservice to both clinicians and their patients. The focus on the actions of individuals as the sole cause of adverse events inevitably results in continued system failures, resulting in the injury and death of patients and the tendency for clinicians to blame themselves for this harm. The efforts of the innumerable government bodies around the world to align external financial, regulatory, and educational incentives are beginning to have an impact on clinicians' and providers' interest in embracing the safety themes described in this chapter.

Cultural and process changes require profound alterations in management thinking, staff empowerment, and communications skills within and across disciplines. Attributing errors to system failures does not absolve clinicians of their duty of care or their fiduciary duty to act in the best interests of their patients. In fact, acknowledging system failures adds to that duty a responsibility to admit errors, investigate them collaboratively, and participate in redesign for a safer system. One way to achieve this is to deconstruct errors and failures at the front lines of health care as a way to assess risk and develop further strategies for managing risk. Such understanding and corrective efforts can be made to embed quality and safety into the microsystem.

Cross-Reference to the Companion Casebook

(McLaughlin, C. P., Johnson, J. K., and Sollecito, W. A. [Eds.]. 2012. *Implementing Continuous Quality Improvement in Health Care: A Global Casebook.* Sudbury, MA: Jones & Bartlett Learning.)

Case Study Number	Case Study Title	Case Study Authors
16	The Lewis Blackman Hospital Patient Safety Act: It's Hard To Kill A Healthy 15-Year-Old	*Julie K. Johnson, Helen Haskell, and Paul Barach*

REFERENCES

Barach, P. 2005. The Unintended Consequences of Florida Medical Liability Legislation. *Perspectives on Patient Safety.* Retrieved March 6, 2010, from http://www.webmm.ahrq.gov/perspective .aspx?perspectiveID=14

Barach, P., and Cantor, M. 2007. Adverse event disclosure: Benefits and drawbacks for patients and clinicians. In Clarke, S., and Oakley, J. (Eds.), *Informed Consent and Clinician Accountability: The Ethics of Report Cards on Surgeon Performance.* Cambridge, UK: Cambridge University Press.

Barach, P., and Small, S. 2000. Reporting and preventing medical mishaps: Lessons from non-medical near miss reporting systems. *BMJ,* 320: 759–763.

Bernstein, P. 1996. *Against the Gods. The Remarkable Story of Risk.* New York: Wiley.

Bosk, C. 1979. *Forgive and Remember: Managing Medical Failure.* Chicago: University of Chicago Press.

Cantor, M. D., Barach, P., Derse, A., et al. 2005. Disclosing adverse events to patients. *Jt Comm J Qual Patient Saf,* 31(1): 5–12.

Clinton, H. R., and Obama, B. 2006. Making patient safety the centerpiece of medical liability reform. *N Engl J Med,* 354(21): 2205–2208.

Dekker, S. 2002. *The Field Guide to Human Error Investigations.* Aldershot, UK: Ashgate Publishing Limited.

Dekker, S. 2004. *Ten Questions About Human Error: A New View of Human Factors and System Safety.* Mahwah, NJ: Erlbaum.

de Vries, E., Ramrattan, M., Smorenburg, S. M., et al. 2008. The incidence and nature of in-hospital adverse events: A systematic review. *Qual Saf Health Care,* 17: 216–223.

DiazGranados, C. A., Jones, M. Y., Kongphet-Tran, T., et al. 2009. Outbreak of *Pseudomonas aeruginosa* infection associated with contamination of a flexible bronchoscope. *Infect Control Hosp Epidemiol,* 30(6): 550–555.

Dickson, G. 1995. Principles of risk management. *Qual Healthcare,* 4: 75–79.

Haddon, W. J. 1972. A logical framework for categorizing highway safety phenomena and activity. *J Trauma,* 12(2): 193–207.

Heinreich, H. 1941. *Industrial Accident Prevention.* New York: McGraw-Hill.

Helmreich, R., and Merritt, A. 2001. *Culture at Work in Aviation and Medicine.* Burlington, VT: Ashgate.

Hollnagel, E., Woods, D. D., Leveson, N. (Eds.). 2006. *Resilience Engineering: Concepts and Precepts.* Aldershot, UK: Ashgate.

Institute of Medicine. 2000. *To Err Is Human: Building a Safer Health System.* Washington, DC: National Academies Press.

Institute of Medicine. 2001. *Crossing the Quality Chasm: A New Health System for the 21st Century.* Washington, DC: National Academies Press.

Kaluzny, A. 1985. Design and management of disciplinary and interdisciplinary groups in health services: Review and critique. *Med Care Rev,* 42(1): 77–112.

Kasperson, R., Renn, O., Slovic, P., et al. 1988. Social amplification of risk: A conceptual framework. *Risk Anal,* 8: 177–187.

Kraman, S. S., and Hamm, G. 1999. Risk management: Extreme honesty may be the best policy. *Ann Intern Med,* 131(12): 963–937.

Landrigan, C. P., Parry, G. J., Bones, C. B., et al. 2010. Temporal trends in rates of patient harm resulting from medical care. *N Engl J Med,* 363(22): 2124–2134.

LeBlang, T., and King, J. L. 1984. Tort liability for nondisclosure: The physician's legal obligations to disclose patient illness and injury. *Dickinson Law Rev,* 89: 1–18.

March, J., Sproull, L., and Tamuz, M. 1991. Learning from samples of one or fewer. *Organ Sci,* 2: 1–3.

Millenson, M. 1997. *Demanding Medical Excellence: Doctors and Accountability in the Information Age.* Chicago: The University of Chicago Press.

Mitchell, S. M., and Shortell, S. M. 2000. The governance and management of effective community health partnerships. *Milbank Q,* 78(2): 241–289.

Mohr, J. 2000. *Forming, Operating, and Improving Microsystems of Care.* Hanover, NH: Center for the Evaluative Clinical Sciences, Dartmouth College.

Mohr, J., Barach, P., Cravero, J. P., et al. 2003. Microsystems in health care: Part 6. Designing patient safety into the microsystem. *Joint Commiss J Qual Safety,* 29(8): 401–408.

Mohr, J., and Batalden, P. 2002. Improving safety at the front lines: The role clinical microsystems. *Qual Safety Health Care,* 11(1): 45–50.

Mohr, J., Batalden, P., and Barach, P. 2004. Integrating patient safety into the clinical microsystem. *Quality Safety Health Care*, 13(2): ii34–ii38.

Nelson, E., Batalden, P., Huber, T. P., et al. 2002. Microsystems in health care: Part 1. Learning from high-performing front-line clinical units. *Joint Commiss J Qual Improv*, 28(9): 472–493.

Perrow, C. 1984. *Normal Accidents, Living with High-Risk Technologies.* New York: Basic Books.

Pronovost, P., Weast, B., Holzmueller, C. G., et al. 2003. Evaluation of the culture of safety: Survey of clinicians and managers in an academic medical center. *Qual Safety Health Care*, 12: 405–410.

Rasmussen, J. 1990. The role of error in organising behaviour. *Ergonomics*, 33: 1185–1199.

Reason, J. 1990. *Human Errors.* New York: Cambridge University Press.

Reason, J. 1995. Understanding adverse events: Human factors. In Vincent, C. (Ed.), *Clinical Risk Management* (pp. 31–54). London: BMJ Publications.

Reason, J. 1997. *Managing the Risks of Organizational Accidents.* Aldershot, UK: Ashgate.

Sagan, S. D. 1993. *The Limits of Safety.* Princeton, NJ: Princeton University Press.

Small, D., and Barach, P. 2002. Patient safety and health policy: A history and review. *Hematol Oncol Clin North Am*, 16: 1463–1482.

Studdert, D. M., Mello, M. M., and Brenna, T. A. 2004. Medical malpractice. *N Engl J Med*, 350(3): 283–292.

Taleb, N. N. 2010. *The Black Swan: The Impact of the Highly Improbable.* New York: Random House.

Turner, B., and Pidgeon, N. 1997. *Man-Made Disasters.* London: Butterworth and Heinemann.

Vaughn, D. 1996. *The Challenger Launch Decision: Risky Technology, Culture, and Deviance at NASA.* Chicago: University of Chicago Press.

Vincent, C. 1997. Risk, safety, and the dark side of quality. *BMJ*, 314: 1775–1776.

Vincent, C. 2003. Understanding and responding to adverse events [see comment]. *N Engl J Med*, 348(11): 1051–1056.

Vincent, C., Taylor-Adams, S., Stanhope, N., et al. 1998. Framework for analysing risk and safety in clinical medicine. *BMJ*, 316(7138): 1154–1157.

Walshe, K. 2001. The development of clinical risk management. In Reason, C. (Ed.), *Clinical Risk Management: Enhancing Patient Safety*. London: BMJ Books.

Weick, K., and Sutcliffe, K. 2001. *Managing the Unexpected: Assuring High Performance in an Age of Complexity*. Ann Arbor: University of Michigan Business School.

Weick, K. E. 1993. The collapse of sensemaking in organizations: The Mann Gulch disaster. *Adm Sci Q*, 38: 628–652.

Weick, K. E. 1995. *Sensemaking in Organizations*. Thousand Oaks, CA: Sage.

Weick, K. E. 1996. Prepare your organization to fight fires. *Harvard Business Rev*, May–June.

Wu, A. W., Cavanaugh, T. A., McPhee, S. J., et al. 1997. To tell the truth: Ethical and practical issues in disclosing medical mistakes to patients. *J Gen Intern Med*, 12(12): 770–775.

Zimmerman, B., and Hayday, B. 1999. A board's journey into complexity science. *Group Decis Making Negotiat*, 8: 281–303.

Implementation

CQI, Transformation, and the "Learning" Organization

Vaughn M. Upshaw, David P. Steffen, and Curtis P. McLaughlin

"The entire global business community is learning to learn together, becoming a learning community."

—Peter Senge (The Fifth Discipline, 1990)

While the advent of continuous quality improvement (CQI) in health care organizations was once viewed as a panacea for many health care quality problems, realities have challenged many of these initial high expectations. Health care organizations and providers can no longer view CQI and performance improvements as optional or sufficient (Fawcett et al., 2009). Consider a few of these realities (The Advisory Board Company, 1997; Batalden, 1996).

- "Quality" has been superseded by "value" as the key criterion by which to judge organizational performance, and cost reduction must be accomplished while achieving essential outcomes.
- Organizations are characterized by "right sizing," "downsizing," layoffs, and mergers in health services, with resultant declines in employee satisfaction and loyalty, particularly among physicians.
- Health care organizations are increasingly viewed as complex, "wicked" systems demanding application of advanced, "adaptive"

techniques to generate large-scale systems change in addition to incremental process improvements.

- Outcomes are demanded of the health care system as a whole; therefore, individual organization improvements must be paired with boundary-spanning improvement initiatives.
- Health information systems that are robust and interoperable are a requirement for improvement processes and reporting to payers, policy makers, and patients.
- Unprecedented leadership is needed by organizational management and physicians to engage all staff in the effort to institutionalize quality improvement and improve systems.
- Improvement initiatives are often short-lived and may avoid dealing with the substantive challenges facing the organization.
- "Integration" has not fulfilled expectations, and there is increasing interest and experimentation in the "unbundling of provider risk." Yet, at the same time, management experts are arguing that cost controls call for bundled payments that require an organization's management to take responsibility for process efficiency and effectiveness (Bohmer, 2009; Christensen et al., 2009; Porter and Teisberg, 2004; Shih et al., 2008).
- Informed patients are increasingly demanding personalization of their care and practicing assertive self-care, which challenges the traditional hierarchy and perception of health care professionals' and patients' roles.

Each institution delivering health care needs a comprehensive approach to continuous improvement that goes beyond small changes that incrementally reduce variance to improve quality, but instead aggressively promotes quality of health services through a systematic process of organizational learning.

The objective of this chapter is to assess the underlying dimensions of the transformation in health care services, explore the changing roles for CQI, evaluate new approaches to transformation and organizational learning, and identify strategies for securing effective team engagement and clinical leadership in organizational learning and change.

Organizational learning has been defined as "a process of increasing knowledge and innovating work routines through the interplay of action and reflection that is more extensive than individually focused training and repetition" (Carroll and Edmondson, 2002, p. 55). Organizational learning encompasses CQI teams (see Chapters 2 and 4); improvement collaboratives (see Chapters 1 and 14), such as the Institute for Healthcare Improvement's Breakthrough Series; and many health care reengineering efforts. It may take on different names, but the process is generic. For example, in the United Kingdom, the health system has adopted the term *clinical governance*, a mandated multiprofessional approach to learning and improvement (Heard et al., 2001). The aim of clinical governance is to establish a culture of quality improvement through the "10 Cs," which are:

1. Clinical performance

2. Clinical audit

3. Clinical risk management

4. Complaints

5. Continuing health needs assessments

6. Changing practice through evidence

7. Continuing education

8. Clinical leadership

9. Culture of excellence

10. Clear accountability

The first seven of these points appear to relate to what Bohmer (2009) calls the "signal detection" component of organizational learning. In his model of organizational learning, the organization must first observe "process anomalies." When identified, these anomalies lead to the creation of new knowledge that must then be transferred to implementers, who then change their behaviors (p. 170).

TRANSFORMING HEALTH CARE

A fundamental change accompanying the transition of health care is that the locus of control for technological decision making in health services has moved from individual autonomy for physicians to organizational strategies such as evidence-based medicine, CQI, and transparency (Hurley, 1997; Nash and Quigley, 2008). Managers assume that greater control over costs and quality will be achieved by implementing evidence-based care, clinical protocols, and financial control mechanisms, such as pay-for-performance, capitation, or prior approvals. However, the dynamic nature of work processes within health care organizations may or may not be consistent with the implementation or use of these approaches. For example, the greater role of the patient in health care decision making and CQI (see Chapter 7) must be considered in implementing these approaches (Barratt, 2008). The challenge is to effectively and efficiently provide a continuum of clinical products, each with sufficient variability to adapt to the individual needs of patients and providers.

The practice and management of health care services will undergo continued refinements and further codification. However, these changes will be successful only if they are accompanied by organizational learning as a way to hasten the adoption of evidence-based practices while accommodating the personalization of care to meet the uncertainties of the care delivery process, which at times involves unique needs and situations. In other words, what is needed is an institutional commitment to expand the organization's capacity to maintain or improve performance, building from its own experience and reflection; recognizing the inherent skill, insights, and knowledge of individuals within the organization; and using these qualities to meet the challenges of new situations (Bohmer, 2009; Carroll and Edmondson, 2002; DiBella et al., 1996). Appropriately practiced in health services, CQI is one of the building blocks for institutional knowledge and learning, but it will not succeed without active participation from physicians and other professionals who bring intellectual capital and provide key leadership to facilitate learning and innovation. In addition, CQI strategies are unlikely to be successful if leaders apply the techniques without taking into account contextual factors, such as the financial condition of the health care organization, strategic challenges, and market conditions (Alexander et al., 2007).

Traditionally, managers merely consulted or hired a health care professional to determine whether managerial strategies would be in serious conflict with physicians' methods, norms, or values; organizational values; or the patient's interests. Health care managers were neither concerned with nor technically prepared to evaluate clinical performance. However, the growth of evidence-based care has allowed managers and payers to assume greater organizational responsibility and control over many clinical issues.

Why the change? The continuous and significant introduction of science and technology into the art of medicine over the last 50 years has made possible, perhaps inevitable, a shift from the craft or guild structure of medicine toward an industrial structure. As introduced in Chapter 1, most sectors are in some stage of the transition to mass customization or mass personalization (Boynton et al., 1993; Swensen et al., 2010). Manufacturing industries went through the first step, adopting mass production approaches, in the late 19th and 20th centuries.

Medicine and many other professional services have made this transition much later because of insufficient predictability of cause and effect, the natural variability inherent in their work processes, and the high degree of autonomy and highly decentralized local organizational structures (McLaughlin, 1996). The historical analogy—the craft guild—was especially applicable to physician practices that were often referred to as a cottage industry. As with most technological change, the transition did not take place until all the factors—technical, economic, and social—were aligned.

In the latter part of the 20th century, hospitals served as the industrializing institutions of health care. They amassed large amounts of capital and absorbed the emerging technologies quickly. Some even experimented with mass production; for example, the surgicenter focused on cataract removal (McLaughlin et al., 1995). However, they tended not to employ physicians but rather continued to operate as the physician's workplace. As the hospital became increasingly corporate, an uneasy truce developed between the craft orientation of the physicians and the hospital's industrial model. Health care went through a period of rapid technological change where the increased technical capacity also meant increasing costs. Employer concerns about rising health care costs and the obvious excesses of fee-for-service medicine created a demand for improving the evidence base for clinical care. This has been followed by performance-based reimbursement mechanisms that are designed to deliver "value," which is defined as producing high-quality health outcomes at a reasonable cost over time.

ACCEPTING CONTINUOUS IMPROVEMENT

Hospitals were once considered impersonal at best and, at worst, dangerous. In fact, some still are considered to be not nearly as safe as they should be, especially in the global arena. As noted in Chapter 2, the rate of diffusion of CQI is not what it should be or could be given the current state of knowledge about the impact of CQI in health care. For example, a study published in 2010 of more than 2,300 admissions in 10 North Carolina hospitals found that patient harms remained common with little evidence of improvement during the study period from 2002 to 2007 (Landrigan et al., 2010). This is evidence of a broad issue that is prevalent not only in these 10 hospitals but across a wide spectrum of health care. Organizations made little effort to promote institutional learning, and the institution had little or no control over the performance of professional personnel. Even today, hospitals find that variable needs of individual patients and providers are often poorly accommodated. Information flows and patient referrals are fragmented and unreliable, and glaring differences in costs and outcomes are evident to those paying claims. Because of the craft nature of medicine, best practices are not easily disseminated nor widely adopted. Each provider has considerable autonomy over his or her work, often maintaining practices that are questionable or simply obsolete (Davies and Harrison, 2003).

The adoption and institutionalization of continuous improvement has provided an opportunity to better manage professional personnel. The alternative is a "culture of entrapment" in which autonomy works against learning and where shallow but plausible justifications impede even obviously necessary improvements (Gawande, 2009; Weick and Sutcliffe, 2003). Continuous improvement assumes capabilities for process dynamism and institutional learning. Teams within the institution, usually multidisciplinary teams, work cooperatively on the improvement of the institution's processes. Establishing ownership of patient-level processes that integrate professionally dominated knowledge and skills is one of CQI's objectives. One might even go so far as to classify this as capturing a competitive edge in intellectual capital. This was not a problem when the intellectual capital was assumed to be that of the professionals and not the institution. Although there have been many examples of greater sharing and collaboration in 21st-century medical care, due to competitiveness there is not as much sharing as we would like, and there is a need for even greater collaboration (McLaughlin and Johnson, 1995).

Continuous Improvement and Clinical Care

Fully integrated systems may have multiple internal perspectives seeking to improve a single treatment process. For example, units concerned with epidemiological research, cost containment, cost analysis, and care delivery may all undertake CQI activities for a particular disease process. These four perspectives are likely to differ not only in the approaches they use but also with respect to evaluative standards, quality criteria, economic criteria, the relevant time horizon, and the relationship to the population served. Although difficulties can result when these perspectives are at odds with one another, the opportunity for organizational learning greatly improves once these groups communicate with each other and share their respective views.

Continuous improvement is well aligned with many elements of managing care, such as prospective reimbursement, bundling, capitation, pay for performance, and prior approvals. By continually seeking to reduce errors and improve processes, CQI offers an opportunity to facilitate the larger transformation of health care organizations. Under prospective reimbursement systems, institutions are paid a flat amount for a specific type of admission based on a measure of industry best practices, and it is assumed that institutions will exercise sufficient control over their processes to operate within that cost range. Under bundling, institutions receive a single payment for comprehensive services provided to a patient under a diagnostic category for a complete episode of care. This would typically include hospital costs, physician and other services, and the costs of any readmissions that occur within a set time period after discharge. Under capitation, providers receive a flat monthly fee for providing a specified set of services to enrolled individuals during that period. Providers are expected to profit on the basis of their ability to appropriately and efficiently manage the care for people enrolled. Other cost-containment procedures, such as prior approvals for admissions and surgical procedures, assume that employers or their representatives possess sufficient technical knowledge to accept or countermand the decisions of the clinician. Prior approvals assume institutional knowledge is superior to the professional training and knowledge of providers.

Fundamental to efficient care management and to CQI are the mutability and dynamic nature of clinical processes and the ability of both institutions and clinicians to improve their performance over time. Both CQI teams and health care managers consistently seek to identify and implement evidence-based best practices, using such tools as checklists, clinical guidelines, and clinical pathways and processes such as product and case management. Nevertheless, many clinicians perceive both CQI and health care management processes as a challenge to their personal and professional autonomy and financial security.

CQI allows all personnel, not just physicians, an opportunity to engage in shaping and transforming how the organization provides health services. It builds institutional skills needed to detect anomalies and analyze processes, and it provides a mechanism for providers to retain their sense of autonomy and maintain control over organizational activities that affect clinical outcomes. To be successful, CQI efforts must challenge institutional cultures where admitting mistakes is discouraged. In order to learn and improve, all participants (providers, administrators, researchers, and other staff) must be able to discuss errors openly and feel supported in disclosing problems to prevent future errors from occurring (Deming, 1986; Stroud et al., 2009).

FROM MASS CUSTOMIZATION TO MASS PERSONALIZATION AND BEYOND

Patients and providers are quite variable, and both expect care that adapts to a range of conditions including differences in anatomy, physiology, cognitive style, psychological status, family setting, and economic resources. Patients and providers will evaluate their health care experiences in terms of how those needs are met. One concern is that health care managers and clinical health providers will never agree on the role of variability in an efficient system. Management tends to follow industrial models that focus on the importance of reducing unnecessary variability rather than coping with inherent variability. Health care providers, on the other hand, adapt clinical approaches in order to appropriately address inherent interpatient variability, often ignoring issues of unnecessary variability. Because insurers have a tendency to manage in the industrial model, they generally ignore or penalize inherent variability, creating potential barriers to mass personalization, a concept introduced in Chapter 1.

Historically, health care's production processes and target markets have influenced the industry's perception of variability and variation. As discussed earlier, health care started in a guild, or cottage industry, phase in which wide variation in price, process, and outcomes was standard. For a limited number of highly specific medical procedures (e.g., cataracts in surgicenters), health care then dabbled in mass production, which strives for little or no variation in order to reduce costs. The widespread adoption of process enhancement techniques, such as CQI, facilitated the move to mass customization, with its multiple, planned, small variations from a standard module. Now, necessity dictates that health care must advance to mass personalization, which values individually determined variations from a standard, produced by consultation between provider and patient. In the same way that evidence-based medicine has changed the locus of control in medical care, personalization, and the associated concepts of individualization and shared decision making, will build on that change to put more control in the hands of care providers and their patients (Barratt, 2008; Pfaff et al., 2010).

While each of these production strategies values producing goods and/ or services at the lowest possible price, their markets differ. Mass production targets a mass market, customization a market of few, and mass personalization a market of one (Kumar, 2007). A market of one refers to a market of one person at a time, with meaningful exchange of information and co-configuration and cocreation of products.

The Impact of Personalization on Health Care Organizations

Personalization in health care, as described here, is a broad concept that encompasses the terms *individualization* and *personalized medicine*, which is commonly linked to genomic medicine (Hamburg and Collins, 2010; Moldrup, 2009; Pfaff et al., 2010). Personalization can be seen as the ultimate vision for the health care system, and mass customization is the key process for realizing personalization. In this vision, the health care organization becomes better able to meet the needs of clients and evolves to be more nimble. Mass customization has been defined as "developing, producing, marketing, and delivering affordable goods and services with enough variety and customization that nearly everyone finds exactly what they want" (Piller and Tseng, 2010, p. 1). A number of economic sectors have embraced the concept of mass customization, including computer hardware (Dell Computers), harvesting machinery (John Deere), commercial airplanes

(Boeing), electronics (Sony), and trucks (Peterbilt). These companies have made the paradigm shift that health care needs to make, seeing differences among demands of customers as new, valuable opportunities rather than as an irritating burden or a threat. In health care, mass customization has been described as "a conscious effort to introduce ever-increasing levels of personalization and variety of outcomes. Configuring and delivering modules of services in response to patient needs and preferences accomplish it" (Kaluzny and McLaughlin, 2003, p. 1).

Leaders in the health care industry that have been able to organize processes to maximize quality while limiting cost have been termed *accountable care organizations* (ACOs) or *accountable health systems* (Devers and Berenson, 2009; Shortell and Casalino, 2008). Examples include both large health plans such as Kaiser Permanente and the Mayo Health System as well as smaller hospital and physician groups. The key features of these organizations are that they can deliver and manage care across the continuum of care, budget prospectively, and be large enough to engage in excellent performance measurement and quality improvement. These characteristics form the foundation for personalization. Financial incentives are being utilized to encourage patients to select ACOs for their health care.

Despite the progress toward systems and accountable care, the majority of health care providers are in single or small-group practices that have not adopted this type of thinking or practice. In addition to necessary changes in mindset, there are a number of barriers to mass customization that must be overcome, including (Piller and Tseng, 2010):

- Increased cost secondary to decreased economies of scale
- Increased complexity of processes for workers
- Heightened customer need for increased speed
- Increased interest, assertiveness, and responsibility by patients
- Patients' lack of knowledge of medical options, inability to decide precisely what they want from among the options, or unrealistic views of risks vs. benefits
- Lack of provider knowledge of patients and their desires as well as systems to capture and characterize these factors
- Difficulty of provider "synchronization" of consumer choice (i.e., reconciling patient's desire for features, product attributes, and options with an appreciation of willingness to pay)

Consumers' lack of knowledge regarding what is available and what they truly want could well be the biggest limiting factor in personalization (Svensson and Jensen, 2003). "Elicitation" of customer desires and subsequent "co-configuration" of patient care will be a much more important and in-depth process in which health care providers must involve themselves. Providers will need to engage with the patient on a more egalitarian basis, really get to know the patient (including the patient's social situation), outline options that tailor standard care (evidence-based medicine) so that it fits the patient and the health care institution can provide it well, and answer questions and come to a care decision with the patient and the health care team. Given the increasing restraints on provider–patient in-person interactions, much of this process will use electronic information sources and systems to accomplish the preliminary stages, and what is learned will be captured and processed for future encounters.

Personalization is utilizing technology and other organizational resources to take into account differences among individual patients. If personalization is executed successfully by the health care institution, it is beneficial to both patients and the health care system, providing desired care for patients and better care outcomes and more information—with which to consistently improve patient outcomes—for the health care system and providers.

It would be difficult, if not impossible, to attain and maintain personalization as a focus at all times. However, achieving "a perfect state" of mass customization is not what is important (Piller and Tseng, 2010). Rather, it is about gaining and maintaining the mindset of "mass customization thinking" that uses CQI and other powerful quality enhancement strategies toward the ultimate goal of the health care system, creating value for patients, providers, and payers.

Factors Influencing Personalization of Health Care

A number of factors are making personalization more possible for the health care system. Included in this are better, more robust information systems, including the electronic medical record; advances in genetics and genomics; the ability to better match pharmaceutical products with individual patient needs and physiology (Hamburg and Collins, 2010); increased patient self-care interest and use of the Internet for health information; sharing of potential therapeutic medical interventions among support group members; and openness of providers and payers to alternative therapies (Barratt, 2008; Pfaff et al., 2010; Piller and Tseng, 2010).

Personalization is a logical extension of evidence-based medicine, beginning with a standard mode of treatment and then adjusting it based upon individual characteristics and desires. Evidence-based medicine has developed enough standardization in health care to establish a consistent foundation from which to personalize care (Kaluzny and McLaughlin, 2003). These standardized core processes or services are akin to the "modules" in manufacturing that can be counted on as well-established units that are easily modifiable to adapt care to an individual.

Mass customization and personalization can only be achieved in a learning organization with strong, visionary leadership and excellent management. Only these types of organizations possess the type of openness to change and the unified strategic vision that are needed to practice "customization thinking" and significantly modify and coordinate their processes and workforce efforts and time. This customization of care for patients needs to be a strategic priority for the health care system in order for it to achieve value.

The Future of Personalization in Health Care

It is informative to identify where industry is going in the future relative to personalization because health care will likely be following in the same manner, considering that CQI in health care evolved from industry applications (see Chapter 1). Kumar (2007) indicates that after 20 years of mass customization, there are "unmistakable signs" of movement into the mass personalization zone. He predicts that organizations not incorporating this strategy will "soon be struggling for survival" (Kumar, 2007, p. 546). Furthermore, once personalization is achieved by a high proportion of providers of goods and services, it will be considered an expected characteristic that only varies by price (i.e., a "commodity"). Any further differentiation of products and producers will then be based on different customers' values, likely in the emotional sphere.

At least part of health care may become concerned with "emotional economy," emphasizing the importance of the "narrative" of the experience of a particular service, as other more basic expectations around price, performance, and health outcome are considered a given. The health care organization that has established excellent elicitation and configuration relationships and processes with patients will be ahead of the curve as a learning organization that will know where patients' values will be leading their health care choices and the industry in the future.

This move toward personalization will be a significant change, the scope of which may well challenge the adequacy of CQI in many institutions. This is because the tendency of continuous improvement efforts is incrementalism—starting with the existing process and improving it, rather than radically changing the process altogether so that it better integrates new technologies, especially information technologies. As well described by Ellen Gaucher (1994):

> Within health care, some of our processes are so bad that we could spend the rest of our professional careers trying to continuously improve them. We need to throw them out and begin with a clean sheet of paper and make sure we understand what the elements of each of these processes are. We need to redesign them to be effective in the long run.

Business, health policy, and political figures have all taken up major change issues. Now with better data in hand about variability in health care and the human cost of medical error, and with improved methods and electronic modes of disseminating this information, the political and public policy pendulum has swung toward forcing some rationalization of the fragmented health care system. Along with these external calls for change at the national level, advocacy, regulatory, and quality monitoring organizations have increasingly recommended or mandated institutionalized learning processes for organizations and professions. From among the more than 40 such groups in the United States, the most notable public and private entities that exert significant influence on health care quality include the Quality Improvement Organizations (QIOs) of the Centers for Medicare and Medicaid Services, the Agency for Healthcare Research and Quality, the National Quality Forum, the Institute of Medicine's Roundtable on Value and Science-Driven Health Care, the Institute for Healthcare Improvement, the Leapfrog Group, and The Joint Commission. To provide a detailed example, Chapter 15 describes the significant role that QIOs are playing to improve quality on a regional and national level in the United States.

THE TASK AHEAD

Efforts focused on continuous improvement need to recognize the inherent transitional nature of health care delivery. As discussed in Chapter 3, understanding causes of variation is a critical component of CQI efforts. However, CQI must go beyond the basic understanding and control of variation to foster change and innovation, and we must be prepared for major paradigm shifts such as mass personalization. Continuous improvement efforts must shift their focus from simply avoiding unnecessary variation to ensuring organizational learning as a means of providing health services. Health care managers must recognize that their role is not just to minimize costs but to develop the institutional and professional knowledge that will result in the coordinated care delivery that can provide quality and efficient care to a defined population. Increasingly, care is being personalized so that it meets and adapts to specific needs without compromising overall standards for cost and quality. The challenge for hospitals, health care organizations, and other providers is to add value. They must demonstrate that services are efficient and that they are improving health outcomes for individuals, target populations, and, in some instances, the larger community. The value proposition reemerged as a key consideration in health care CQI in 2010 and is discussed in greater detail in Chapter 20.

All stakeholders, including hospitals, insurers, and professional groups, must see themselves in a transition process that customizes care for the individual while improving the health status of the population, given available resources. Simultaneously, purchasers, consumers, competitors, and regulators will require information with which to assess the cost, quality, utilization, and availability of health services.

Information systems must be flexible, interoperable, expandable, available, and user-friendly. Information technology must provide information that is accurate, timely, useful for decision makers at all levels, accessible, and able to accommodate the demands of providers, managers, and employees. Information systems are critical to monitoring and improving the long-term performance of an organization. They must provide feedback that can be integrated back into the system in a timely and functional manner. Further details on the role of information technology and CQI are presented in Chapter 12.

Concurrent with the increased need for information, health care organizations are realizing that they must reduce and reorganize staffing within the organization. Large numbers of categorically skilled employees who provide institutionally based services are no longer required, but employees are needed who can perform multiple functions, work in cross-disciplinary teams, and operate in smaller units. Reducing workforces, retraining and reassigning personnel, and requiring new working relationships all contribute to concerns about workplace quality of life. To make these changes successfully, clinicians and managers must foster quality work, reward loyal and high-level performance, secure commitment from employees, and build a spirit of learning and empowerment while undergoing continuous and fundamental transitions.

MANAGING TRANSFORMATION AND LEARNING

To succeed in a rapidly changing environment, health care organizations need to smoothly manage the transformation process and take on the challenge of becoming what Peter Senge (1990, p. 3) described as "learning organizations," places where "people continually expand their capacity to create the results they truly desire, where new and expansive patterns of thinking are nurtured, where collective aspiration is set free and where people are continually learning to learn together."

As presented in **Figure 10–1**, health services are in the process of transitioning from a professional model characterized by individual responsibility, professional autonomy, and accountability to a transformational model characterized by shared responsibility and collaborative decision making, continuous innovation, and learning. Traditional CQI provides important skills needed to make the transition, but transformational models provide organizations the opportunity to ensure that both incremental and radical learning occur in order to meet the challenges of an uncertain and complex environment. Through organizational learning, health care organizations can better face the reality of managing costs, providing high-quality services, and improving outcomes while accommodating individual needs through case management, patient education, and support of patient decision making.

Professional	CQI	Transformational
• Individual responsibility	• Collective responsibility	• Leaders and employees share overall responsibility, as well as take individual responsibility
• Professional leadership	• Managerial leadership	
• Autonomy	• Accountability	
• Administrative authority	• Participation	
• Professional authority	• Performance and process expectations	• People at multiple levels assume leadership
• Goal expectations		
• Rigid planning	• Flexible planning	• Outcome and value driven
• Responses to complaints	• Benchmarking	• Shared decision making
• Retrospective performance appraisal	• Concurrent performance appraisal	• Continuous planning
		• Future orientation
• Quality assurance	• Continous improvement	• Performance enhancement appraisals
		• Continuous innovation

FIGURE 10–1 Emergence of Transformational Models for Organizational Performance

Figure 10–1 presents the following distinguishing characteristics of the transformational model that are fundamental to CQI:

- *Shared responsibility by leaders and employees, as well as individual responsibility.* Operating under transformational models, health care managers and clinical leaders share responsibility for accomplishing the organizational mission with other personnel. Everyone understands that they are important to the success of the organization, and they know what role they play in that success. Individuals, teams, units, and departments are committed to carrying out their responsibilities.
- *Leadership by people at multiple levels.* Leadership roles for making decisions and guiding change must be afforded to people working in managerial or clinical roles, line staff, and field positions. Changes and decisions designed by people in offices apart from where the work is performed usually have limited effect. Their role should be limited to determining and communicating the broader environmental context in which local decision making takes place. For real innovation and improved performance, people working directly with problems and systems need to be involved in designing

and deciding how to improve processes and quality. These are the people on the sharp end of processes.

- *Outcome- and value-driven process.* People throughout transformative health care organizations demonstrate commitment to achieving outcomes, improving quality, and adding value. Employees, providers, and managers recognize that improving outcomes means that individual expectations for quality and clinical services, such as disease treatment and management, meet and exceed standards.

- *Shared decision making.* It is critically important that people understand the core business, values, and mission of the organization so that they can participate in the decisions that affect them. Straight talk about what is occurring in the environment, how the organization is positioned to respond, and what people need to do to make necessary changes must be modeled and supported by managers and leaders. People need to understand their roles in helping the organization succeed, but they also need to define their roles and how they will contribute.

- *Continuous planning.* People must be motivated to make change and able to participate meaningfully in the change process. In general, participation will be more effective when the issues and changes are not routine (Schwarz, 1989). Transformational change in organizations prepares people to participate in planning and anticipating next steps in an evolutionary change process. When the organization is undergoing regular and dynamic change, people from across the organization must be informed and involved in deciding what changes should be made, in what order, and by what methods. Through functional and cross-functional teams, providers and managers can involve others in mapping strategies and preparing for new challenges (Carroll and Edmondson, 2002).

- *Future orientation.* Unlike what has come before, health service organizations must be defining what the future will be and setting their sights on how they will make that happen. A potential danger for the transformative organization is that it might achieve its objectives for the immediate future and turn its attention to categorizing its accomplishments. Such a retrospective orientation will slow the organization and reduce people's motivation to stay ahead of the trends in the ever-changing health care sector. Transformational leadership continually brings forward the vision of the future organization and indicates how the organization can get from where it is in the present to where it wants to be in the future.

- *Performance enhancement appraisals.* In addition to rewarding and assessing performance improvements for individual employees and teams, transformational organizations need to commit real resources and support structures to recognizing creativity and innovation. We need to look beyond improving how we get things done, to question and explore new ways of doing what needs to be done. Employees need to know that they will be rewarded for going outside the traditional structures to redesign and recreate the organization. Such changes will improve more than employee performance; they will increase employee dedication and contributions to the organization's future success. Commitment is greater in organizations that are actively managing change, obviously uncomfortable with the status quo, and creating a new standard for performance (McNeese-Smith, 1996; Pascale et al., 1997).

  Some of that uneasiness could be mitigated by training staff to understand that health care has two types of processes side by side, ranging from evidence-based to discovery (Bohmer, 2009) and exhibiting a continuum of complexity and uncertainty (Green et al., 2001).

- *Continuous innovation.* To excel in the future, health service organizations will need to establish systems that reward people for good work to recognize efforts that surpass expectations. Transformative models provide support for people to demonstrate creativity and innovation that extend beyond standard performance. Clear systems for highlighting outstanding performance and contributions of providers, administrators, and employees can energize others and provide standards against which to assess poor performance (Pascale et al., 1997).

PHYSICIAN LEADERS AND TRANSFORMATION

There are multiple roles for physicians in leading and managing within transforming organizations. Physicians may be designers of change, developing incentives, exploring opportunities, and gathering resources to promote transitions. Physicians may also serve in stewardship roles to ensure that there is a broad commitment to organizational learning, or they may contribute by performing in teaching roles where they demonstrate vision and values related to the work of the organization (Barnsley et al., 1998).

To secure physician leadership, it is important to identify what will make it attractive for physicians to participate in planning and leading organizational change and then provide them opportunities to exercise leadership within the transformational organization. It will be important, for instance, for physicians to see that they have a central role in making and controlling key decisions that affect the provision of health services. It is also important for physicians to help identify where targeted cost savings can occur that will enhance efficiencies without compromising patient care. Both physicians and managers will want to see the organization enhance its performance, but physicians have a particularly important role in designating common measures for preventive care activities and setting targets for meeting clinical care goals. Other areas of interest to physician leaders include improving patient satisfaction, utilization rates, and resource consumption.

Physicians have central roles in helping to define what the overall goals should be with regard to health status and quality outcomes. To foster participation in the design, planning, and implementation of transformational strategies, physicians need to understand how their participation will contribute to the change process. They should have access to trained facilitators and coaches who can support their efforts and identify strategic opportunities to develop their leadership competencies.

Physician leaders are important in promoting both technical and adaptive changes in health care organizations. Technical changes are those that take advantage of existing management structures and systems to promote incremental changes within the organization; when the issue is clear, there are proven methods of addressing it. Adaptive changes are more radical, requiring people to collectively identify the root causes of an issue and then discard those things that are not working and take risks to determine new, untested courses of action (Heifetz et al., 2009). When physicians are engaged in identifying and structuring processes that lead to better clinical outcomes—such as using existing evidence-based practices or standardizing mechanisms for reporting—they are champions for *technical* changes that will improve individual health as they control costs.

Health care providers who persuade others to explore new, previously resisted, approaches to care—such as expanding the institutional boundaries by creating new community partnerships or blending nontraditional approaches with standard medical practices—are engaged in *adaptive* change.

Organizational strategies can complement physician roles to improve the value of clinical care if they are well designed. Ensuring that the organization's incentive structures and strategies are consistent and complementary can have a significant influence on physician performance. One organization, for example, treating both capitated and fee-for-service clients, was successful in controlling costs when the same incentives were provided to physicians regardless of the patient's source of reimbursement (Flood et al., 1998).

Beyond the physician's role in the provision of care, there are additional areas in which physicians have an interest. For example, providers are concerned with issues such as market growth, percentage of revenue allocated to medical costs, administrative costs, and financial returns. These factors directly influence organizational decision making and clinical activities. As a result, all participants need to know that their interests are being protected as the organization develops strategies for enhancing growth, value, and outcomes while reducing costs.

To secure a shared vision around which to align strategies for improving organizational performance, managers, providers, and employees must participate in developing a common view of the future, clarifying the values associated with the core business, and articulating shared beliefs and values about how to achieve high-quality health care outcomes at a reasonable cost. The successful health care organizations will be those able to transition from focusing exclusively on standardization of all processes to reducing instances of *poor* care for individuals (Carroll and Edmondson, 2002).

Strategies for Learning

To develop an organizational culture that promotes learning and teaching, managers and physicians need key strategies that support such activity. Because people generally act as if their beliefs are a "truth" that is obvious and based upon real data, organizational leaders need techniques that help people learn how to achieve desired results. **Figure 10–2** presents the ladder of inference (Argyris, 1990) and illustrates why most people do

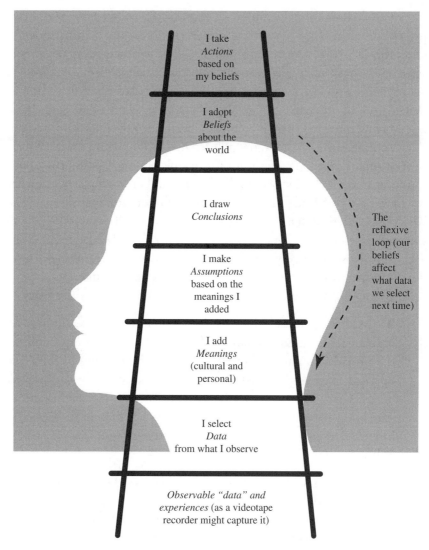

FIGURE 10–2 The Ladder of Inference

Source: From *The Fifth Discipline Fieldbook* by Peter M. Senge, Charlotte Roberts et al., copyright © 1994 by Peter M. Senge, Charlotte Roberts, Richard B. Ross, Bryan J. Smith, and Art Kleiner. Used by permission of Doubleday, a division of Random House, Inc.

not recognize that beliefs and truth are not the same thing. Furthermore, this model demonstrates why it is important to clarify perceptions, check perceptions against facts, and assess the influence of cultural beliefs and attitudes (Senge et al., 1994).

As you can see from Figure 10–2, the world of observable data is not perceived in the same way by all observers. Individuals independently select the data perceived to be important, add their own cultural and personal meanings, make assumptions and draw independent conclusions, adopt their own beliefs, and, finally, take action based upon these beliefs. When working in teams, all members may have access to the same data, but every member may act differently in response to the same information. When people move up the ladder of inference without being aware of their own or others' thinking, it can lead to people stating a position without clarifying their interests behind the position. For example, a provider might declare that evidence-based practices do not work with her clients. This position sets up tension between the provider and others who believe evidence-based practice can be applied in all settings. The ladder of inference can be useful in helping the provider explain the reasoning behind her position and in helping others better understand her interests.

The ladder of inference can improve communication in three ways:

1. By becoming aware of one's own thinking and reasoning, an individual learns to be more *reflective*. In the preceding example, the provider might ask herself what data she is using to form her opinion. Having identified the data she has selected, she can also ask herself what these data mean and what assumptions she has made based on these interpretations. In working her way up the ladder of inference, the provider is better able to understand how she arrived at her position.

2. Once a person has reflected upon his or her own thoughts and reasoning, that individual can better *advocate* for his or her position to others. If the provider in our example understands how she arrived at her position, she is better able to articulate what led her to her conclusion. Having a number of geriatric patients with comorbidities, for instance, may lead our provider to conclude that evidence-based practices are too narrowly focused to accommodate the needs of her patients.

3. As individuals better understand how to reflect upon and advocate for their own positions, they are also better able to *inquire* into the thinking and reasoning of other members of the team. Others working with a provider who is reluctant to follow evidence-based practices can use the ladder of inference to better understand how that provider came to his or her conclusions.

In combination, the skills of reflection, advocacy, and inquiry are important communication skills that facilitate team and organizational learning. To improve learning within the organization, managers and physician leaders can stimulate communication in a number of ways.

- *Test assumptions by gathering facts.* Once people have described their beliefs, others can ask them to provide evidence for their conclusions. Often people have come to conclusions based in part on evidence and in part on assumptions. Only by having open discussions where people can explain what facts they used and how they reached their conclusions is it possible to learn what data they selected, what data they ignored, and what data are missing.

- *Engage people in a discussion of what they assume to be true.* Physicians and other clinicians need to listen to others' views of reality. All people witnessing the same event do not necessarily have the same understanding of what has occurred. Differences emerge based upon our own experiences, biases, and beliefs. Therefore, the physician and other clinicians must invite others to share their views of the situation and seek to understand what others believe to be true. A useful inquiry strategy for working backward to understand the interests behind a position is called the "Five Whys" (Senge et al., 1994). When asking why five times, it is important to focus on the system and to not blame individuals. In our example, the conversation starts with something like this:

  Provider: "Evidence-based practice does not work with my patients."
  Team member: "Why is this?"
  Provider: "My patients are older and have comorbidities that do not conform to our protocols."
  Team member: "Why do our protocols not work?"
  Provider: "If I follow one protocol, it often contradicts another protocol for the same patient."
  Team member: "Why are you trying to use multiple protocols with the same person?"
  Provider: "Management requires I use evidence-based practices for each diagnosis and this does not make sense when one person has multiple problems."
  As detailed by Kline (2010), the process continues for a few more repetitions using a systematic process for capturing and categorizing

responses with a goal of achieving convergence back to a few systemic sources. (For a further description of how to implement this problem-solving technique, see http://www.suite101.com/content/the-systems-approach-to-organizational-problem-solving-a273919.)

Health care organizations need to develop a culture that encourages and focuses the ideas and ingenuity of health care professionals through commitment-based management philosophies rather than strangling providers by over-regulating them, forcing compliance, and assigning blame (Khatri et al., 2009).

- *Prepare people for teaching and learning.* Not all people are equally able or prepared to learn the same things at the same time. Research has shown that learning occurs more readily when the message is delivered in a way appropriate to the level of the learner (Hersey and Blanchard, 1984). Managers and clinicians must be able to recognize levels of readiness for learners and apply appropriate methods for teaching and coaching.

- *Integrate learning and teaching focus.* Do physicians and other clinicians ensure that everyone in the organization is supported in their efforts to teach and learn? To build a learning organization, managers and clinicians must be sure that policies and practices are aligned with incentives for people to acquire, develop, and practice their skills. For example, if the policies support learning but incentives only reward work, people will choose to work instead of attending workshops or seminars that enhance their learning. Managers must ensure that their expectations for performance are reinforced by the incentives within the system. This can be reinforced through leading by example, such as having senior clinicians with "mastery" in a skill instruct others.

- *Develop a teachable point of view.* Physicians and other clinicians need to tell their own stories that illustrate core values, beliefs, and expectations. This is an example of a successful business leadership development technique emphasized by Tichy (1997) for many years and is especially useful for training physicians. In telling their stories, individuals should consider the following: What are the key experiences that have shaped my life? How do these experiences continue to guide my own work? When leaders develop a teachable point of view, they engage people's imaginations and encourage commitment. By telling their own stories, leaders provide real and honest examples of success, failure, and learning while communicating values, behaviors, and skills that are important to the organization.

- *Be a role model.* Leaders who demonstrate a positive attitude toward high achievement encourage commitment and performance from those around them. Leaders can increase participation in decision making as employees gain familiarity with the mission, values, and goals of the organization. As people gain ownership of the organization's mission, leaders must provide them with ongoing opportunities for participation in shaping the future of the organization. Through greater participation and ownership, leaders create an open environment where big ideas can lead to big accomplishments.

Central to applying these strategies is ensuring that managers and clinicians communicate in ways that others within the organization understand. Through storytelling and shared participation, leaders work with others in building mental models that incorporate the vision of the organization that they want to create. Developing common models requires more than creating a desirable vision for the future, however. Before people can build new organizational patterns, they must have a clear understanding of what is not working, why it isn't working, and how it needs to change.

A common understanding depends upon different groups within the organization learning and becoming familiar with complementary values and norms that collectively contribute and help to ensure commitment to the organization's vision. The key is to build a shared mental model while accommodating different viewpoints and expectations that arise based upon people's varying roles and responsibilities. Clinical leaders, for example, need to have the flexibility to develop expectations for the organization that respond to improving care for individuals, while management needs mental models that represent improving organizational efficiencies. Using scientific evidence from clinical applications and research, clinicians can accumulate the necessary information they need to motivate changes in the provision of care. Implementing targeted feedback for physicians supported by continuing professional development is an emerging strategy for integrating physician assessment with performance improvement in the larger health care system (Bellande et al., 2010). Similarly, managers can improve organizational processes by gaining cooperation from clinicians in designing, implementing, and evaluating organizational changes, using relevant evidence and proven methods of improvement.

In health services, rapid change and competitive markets frequently require organizational responses and innovations that are more dramatic than what can be accomplished through incremental quality improvement efforts alone. Making big, adaptive changes and fostering a climate of innovation only occurs when people understand the changing environmental context and their roles in it, have the flexibility to make key decisions that affect their work, and are accountable to customers for their quality of service and outcomes. Managers and clinicians must articulate expectations for quality and outcomes and specify the parameters of available resources and time frames; they must then give people the opportunity to meet these expectations in a manner consistent with the needs and their knowledge of the situation. An individual with multiple, complex health problems cannot be successfully managed in a single 10-minute office visit; thus, clinicians and managers need to have both the flexibility to develop and tailor cost-efficient options for managing complex patients and the incentives that reward appropriate personalization.

Learning to provide specific information about what needs to be accomplished, supported by evidence and a rationale for making a change, will facilitate others' acceptance. By communicating how change will be accomplished using concrete and measurable terms, leaders can stimulate others to find ways to make the vision a reality. Leaders must demonstrate the same kind of energy, commitment, high standards, continuous learning, and willingness to share information that they expect from those around them (Adler et al., 2003).

By sharing stories, modeling commitment, and listening to others, it is possible to move organizations toward deeper learning. It will not happen without commitment from all participants, however, and pursuing a comprehensive organizational priority on learning demands a substantial commitment of the leader's time and attention. The reward for such commitment is a greater capacity to grow leadership within the organization (Adler et al., 2003; Tichy, 1997).

Individuals respond to a crisis by changing their behaviors; when there is no perceived crisis, little change occurs. However, Tucker and Edmondson (2003) report that many health care organizations are quick to convert "errors," which are unacceptable, into "problems," which are more tolerable, thus lessening the ability of organizations to maximize learning that could be obtained from failures, especially those that are potential crises. What is needed is a way for health care leaders to communicate a sense of crisis—not to create panic, but to create a sense of urgency around the need to make a change so that the organization, the patient, the community, and the system survive and thrive. Managers, physicians, and other key personnel must help others recognize that the traditional responses will not cure chronic organizational problems. Just as chronic health problems grow more severe the longer they remain undiagnosed and untreated, many of our current organizational problems will not be cured if treated incrementally. The organizations that survive will be those that institute revolutionary strategies and foster opportunities for quantum ideas to emerge (Tichy, 1997).

Managers and clinicians alike need to find ways to expose chronic, underlying organizational issues that are amenable to correction and invite participation in figuring out a path to success. In many instances, changing long-standing problems requires new approaches and greater organizational flexibility. Building a culture that encourages innovation will occur only if employees are rewarded and recognized for their contributions to envisioning and executing new organizational solutions. Leaders need to commit themselves and their organizations to employee training and development that promotes innovation and change, learning, and teaching (Barnsley et al., 1998).

Strategies for Physician Involvement

Within the health care organization, physician participation and involvement in organizational change and transformation are imperative. In order to secure participation from physician leaders, there are multiple strategies managers can employ.

- *Provide information about organizational goals and objectives.* Disseminating information that describes the organization's interest in change and improvement allows physician leaders to consider the impact on their work and patients. Providing explicit information about the goals that are to be accomplished is essential to gaining buy-in and participation from others. In addition, the organization must make sure that incentives for participation are clear, available, and consistent with other incentives operating within the system. Another key component of information sharing is to outline the outcomes that are expected as a result of the effort. People are more likely to participate in planning and implementing strategies when they understand the final impact expected. Edmondson (2003) refers to the way in which the change is presented as "framing." Doing it the right way provides the motivation and the acceptance of changed roles necessary for successful implementation.

- *Align leadership style and task.* By attending departmental meetings, board meetings, intraorganizational meetings, and practice meetings, managers can observe physician interactions and identify clinical leaders who have the skills and recognition needed to persuade others of the need to change. Different leadership styles are needed for different types of issues. Emotional intelligence (EQ) is increasingly recognized as an essential component of effective leadership. The leader who engages others, motivates people to change, and builds trust to accomplish shared goals is able to generate excitement that causes good things to happen (Cooper and Sawaf, 1997). By observing how physicians interact with one another and learning who the opinion leaders are for various issues, managers can better match physician leaders to the tasks that need to be accomplished.

- *Use data and partnerships.* Physicians, because of special expertise or commitment, have particular issues upon which they want to focus. By inviting physicians to take leadership on a specific issue, administrators can gain clinical participation in improving key parts of the system. Physicians' medical training prepares them to use scientific evidence as a basis for decision making; thus, they are particularly well suited to using data to identify solutions for organizational problems. Physician leaders can also be instrumental in gaining the support of their peers for organizational change. The traditional "separate but equal" hierarchies that characterize health care decision-making structures persist in keeping medical and administrative decisions apart. To overcome such artificial boundaries, health care leaders must seek out physicians who are willing to partner with administrators at multiple levels in leading organizational change (Edwards et al., 2003). Improving information and developing standard protocols will not, by themselves, lead to the improvements in health care outcomes. Health care providers and managers need to build relationships that enhance trust, mindfulness, respect, communication, and openness to diversity as they learn to improve practice (Lanham et al., 2009).

- *Minimize boundaries.* Physician participation in organizational decision making only occurs if the incentives across the organization are aligned to support their contributions outside of the clinic. Physicians and administrators need to know that the organization values and rewards participation in activities that foster team decision making. Furthermore, the organization's policies must promote integrating information from multiple sources that collectively contribute to good clinical and management decisions (Barnsley et al., 1998; Bohmer and Ferlins, 2006). One important way to accomplish this goal, which has been discussed in Chapters 2 and 4, is through greater utilization of teams, both quality improvement teams and mission-oriented teams, and providing critically important training in how to ensure effective teamwork.

Ultimately, successful health care organizations will be those that learn to communicate across formal and informal boundaries. Boundaries may be disciplinary, ideological, vertical, horizontal, geographic, external, or a result of time (Barnsley et al., 1998). Regardless of the type of boundary, these restrictions impose limits on what our health care organizations might become. The goal is to become boundaryless in seeking options to improve health care outcomes.

CONCLUSIONS

This chapter has examined some of the underlying changes occurring in the health care industry and has provided an analysis of how these changes are transforming the business of health care to focus on value and outcomes rather than services. Understanding the nature of the changes in the health care industry serves as a platform for an assessment of the changing roles for CQI within health care organizations. CQI efforts must be transformed and organizational learning systems must be strengthened in order for the organization to be prepared to successfully foster necessary incremental change *and* radical change. Organizational structures and processes must be developed that promote standardization of care but still challenge health service providers and organizations to look beyond traditional roles to learn more about how to improve outcomes and personalize services for individual customers. Professional managers and clinicians must be committed to sharing leadership in improving health care organizations, and both must adopt strategies for securing essential broad team participation and clinician leadership in organizational learning and change.

Cross-References to the Companion Casebook

(McLaughlin, C. P., Johnson, J. K., and Sollecito, W. A. [Eds.]. 2012. *Implementing Continuous Quality Improvement in Health Care: A Global Casebook.* Sudbury, MA: Jones & Bartlett Learning.)

Case Study Number	Case Study Title	Case Study Authors
5	The Intermountain Way to Positively Impact Costs and Quality	*Lucy A. Savitz*
18	Stents vs. Bypass: Expanding the Evidence Base	*Curtis P. McLaughlin and Craig D. McLaughlin*

REFERENCES

Adler, P., Riley, P., Kwon, S. -W., et al. 2003. Performance improvement capability: Keys to accelerating performance improvement in hospitals. *Calif Manage Rev*, 45(2): 12–33.

The Advisory Board Company. 1997. *The Great Product Enterprise: Future State for the American Health System.* Washington, DC: Author.

Alexander, J. A., Weiner, B. J., Shortell, S. M., et al. 2007. Does quality improvement implementation affect hospital quality of care? *Hosp Top*, 852: 3–12.

Argyris, C. 1990. *Overcoming Organizational Defense: Facilitating Organizational Learning.* Needham Heights, MA: Allyn & Bacon.

Barnsley, J., Lemieux, C. L., and McKinney, M. M. 1998. Integrating learning into integrated delivery systems. *Health Care Manage Rev*, 23(1): 18–28.

Barratt, A. 2008. Evidence-based medicine and shared decision making: The challenge of getting both the evidence and preferences into health care. *Patient Educ Counsel*, 73: 407–412.

Batalden, P. B. 1996. *Vision for Change.* Presented at the Interdisciplinary Professional Education Collaborative—Second Milestone Conference, Institute for Healthcare Improvement, Philadelphia, November 1–2.

Bellande, B. J., Winicur, Z. M., and Cox, K. M. 2010. Commentary: Urgently needed: A safe place for self-assessment on the path to maintaining competence and improving performance. *Acad Med,* 851: 16–18.

Bohmer, R. M. J. 2009. *Designing Care: Aligning the Nature and Management of Health Care.* Boston: Harvard Business Press.

Bohmer, R. M. J., and Ferlins, E. M. 2006. *Clinical Change at Intermountain Healthcare, Case 9-607-023 rev. 01/12/2008.* Boston: Harvard Business School.

Boynton, A. C., Victor, B., Joseph, B., et al. 1993. New competitive strategies: Challenges to organizations and information technology. *IBM Syst J,* 32(1): 40–64.

Carroll, J. S., and Edmondson, A. C. 2002. Leading organizational learning in health care. *Qual Safe Health Care,* 11: 51–56.

Christensen, C. M., Grossman J. H., and Hwang, J. 2009. *The Innovator's Prescription: A Disruptive Solution for Health Care.* New York: McGraw-Hill.

Cooper, R. K., and Sawaf, A. 1997. *Executive EQ: Emotional Intelligence in Leadership and Organisations.* New York: Grosset/Putnam.

Davies, H., and Harrison, S. 2003. Trends in doctor-manager relationships. *BMJ* 326: 646–649.

Deming, W. E. 1986. *Out of the Crisis.* Cambridge: Massachusetts Institute of Technology Center for Advanced Engineering Study.

Devers, K. J., and Berenson, R. A. 2009. Can accountable care organizations improve the value of health care by solving the cost and quality quandaries? *Urban Institute Research of Record.* Retrieved March 14, 2011, from http://www.urban.org/url.cfm?ID=411975

DiBella, A. J., Nevis, E. C., and Gould, J. M. 1996. Understanding organizational learning capacity. *J Manage Studies,* 33(3): 361–379.

Edmondson, A. 2003. Framing for learning: Lessons in successful technology implementation. *Calif Manage Rev,* 45(2): 35–54.

Edwards, N., Marshall, M., Mclellan, A., et al. 2003. Doctors and managers: A problem without a solution? *BMJ,* 326: 609–610.

Fawcett, K. J., Jr., Brummel, S., and Byrnes, J. J. 2009. Restructuring primary care for performance improvement. *J Med Pract Manage,* 251: 49–56.

Flood A. B., Fremont, A. M., Jin, K., et al. 1998. How do HMOs achieve savings? The effectiveness of one organization's strategies. *Health Serv Res,* 33(1): 79–99.

Gaucher, E. 1994. *World Class Health Care.* Presentation at the National Conference on Benchmarking Health Care Forum. San Diego, CA, July 17.

Gawande, A. 2009. *The Checklist Manifesto: How to Get Things Right.* New York: Metropolitan Books.

Green, L., Fryer, G., Yawn, B. et al. 2001. The ecology of medical care revisited. *N Engl J Med,* 344: 2021–2025.

Hamburg, M., and Collins, F. 2010. The path to personalized medicine. *N Engl J Med,* 363(11): 1092.

Heard, S. R., Schiller, G., Aitken, M., et al. 2001. Continuous quality improvement: Educating towards a culture of clinical governance. *Qual Health Care,* 10(II): ii70–ii78.

Heifetz, R., Grashow, A., and Linsky, M. 2009. *The Practice of Adaptive Leadership: Tools and Tactics for Changing Your Organization and the World.* Boston: Harvard Business Press.

Hersey, P., and Blanchard, K. H. 1984. *The Management of Organizational Behavior* (4th ed). Englewood Cliffs, NJ: Prentice Hall.

Hurley, R. 1997. Approaching the slippery slope: Managed care as the industrial rationalization of medical practice. In Boyle, P. (Ed.), *Rationing Sanity: The Ethics of Mental Health.* Washington, DC: Georgetown University Press.

Kaluzny, A., and McLaughlin, C. P. 2003. *Mass Customization. Encyclopedia of Health Care Management.* Thousand Oaks, CA: Sage.

Khatri, N., Brown, G. D., and Hicks, L. L. 2009. From a blame culture to a just culture in health care. *Health Care Manage Rev,* 344: 312–322.

Kline, C. 2010. The systems approach to organizational problem solving. Retrieved March 28, 2011, from http://www.suite101.com/content/the-systems-approach-to-organizational-problem-solving-a273919

Kumar, A. 2007. From mass customization to mass personalization: A strategic transformation. *Int J Flex Manuf Syst,* 19: 533–547.

Landrigan, C. P., Parry, G. J., Bones, C. B., et al. 2010. Temporal trends in rates of patient harms resulting from medical care. *N Engl J Med*, 363: 2124–2134.

Lanham, H. J., McDaniel, R. R., Jr., Crabtree, B. F. et al., 2009. How improving practice relationships among clinicians and nonclinicians can improve quality in primary care. *Joint Commission J Qual Patient Safety*, 359: 457–466.

McLaughlin, C. P. 1996. Why variation reduction is not everything: A new paradigm for service operations. *Int J Serv Ind Manage*, 7(3): 17–30.

McLaughlin, C. P., and Johnson, S. P. 1995. Inherent variability in service operations: Identification, measurement and implications. In Armistead, C. G., and Teare, G. (Eds.), *Services Management: New Directions and Perspectives* (pp. 226–229). London: Cassell.

McLaughlin, C. P., Yang, S., and van Dierdonck, R. 1995. Professional service organizations and focus. *Manage Sci*, 41: 1185–1193.

McNeese-Smith, D. 1996. Increasing employee productivity, job satisfaction, and organizational commitment. *Hosp Health Serv Adm*, 41(2): 160–175.

Moldrup, C. 2009. Beyond personalized medicine. *Personalized Med*, 6: 231–233.

Nash, D. B., and Quigley, G. D. 2008. Looking forward: The end of autonomy. *Headache*, 485: 719–724.

Pascale, R. T., Millemann, M., and Gioja, L. 1997. Changing the way we change. *Harvard Business Rev*, 75(6): 126–139.

Pfaff, H., Driller, E., Ernstmann, U., et al. 2010. Standardization and individualization in care for the elderly: Proactive behavior through individualized standardization. *Open Longevity Sci*, 4: 51–57.

Piller, F., and Tseng, M. M. (Eds.). 2010. *Handbook of Research in Mass Customization and Personalization: Strategies and Concepts/Applications and Cases*. New York: World Scientific Press.

Porter, M., and Teisberg, E. O. 2004. Redefining competition in health care. *Harvard Business Rev*, 82(6): 64–76, 136.

Schwarz, R. M. 1989. Understanding and changing the culture of an organization. *Popular Govern*, 45(2): 23–26.

Senge, P. 1990. *The Fifth Discipline*. New York: Doubleday.

Senge, P. M., Kleiner, A., Roberts, C., et al. 1994. *The Fifth Discipline Fieldbook: Strategies and Tools for Building a Learning Organization*. New York: Doubleday/Currency.

Shih, A., Davis, K., Schoenbaum, S., et al. 2008. Organizing the U.S. Health Care Delivery System for High Performance. *Report of the Commission on a High Performance Health System.* Washington, DC: The Commonwealth Fund.

Shortell, S., and Casalino, L. 2008. Health care reform requires accountable care systems. *JAMA,* 3001: 95–97.

Stroud, L., McIlroy, J., and Levinson, W. 2009. Skills of internal medicine residents in disclosing medical errors: A study using standardized patients. *Acad Med,* 8412: 1803–1808.

Svensson, C., and Jensen, T. 2003. The customer at the final frontier of mass customization. In Piller, F. T., and Tseng, M. M. (Eds.), *The Customer Centric Enterprise: Advances in Mass Customization and Personalization* (Chapter 18). New York/Berlin: Springer-Verlag.

Swensen, S., Meyer, G., Nelson, E., et al. 2010. Cottage industry to postindustrial care—The revolution in health care delivery. *N Engl J Med,* 362(5): 12.

Tichy, N. 1997. *The Leadership Engine.* New York: Harper Business.

Tucker, A., and Edmondson, A. 2003. Why hospitals don't learn from failures: Organizational and psychological dynamics that inhibit system change. *Calif Manage Rev,* 45(2): 55–72.

Weick, K., and Sutcliffe, K. 2003. Hospitals as cultures of entrapment: A re-analysis of the Bristol Infirmary. *Calif Manage Rev,* 45: 75–84.

CHAPTER 11

Classification and Reduction of Medical Errors

Joseph G. Van Matre, Donna J. Slovensky,
and Curtis P. McLaughlin

"Human fallibility is like gravity, weather, and terrain, just another foreseeable hazard."

—J. T. Reason (1997, p. 25)

A decade has passed since the publication of two Institute of Medicine studies (2000, 2001) demanding action to address medical errors, clinical quality, and patient safety. In this time, providers, researchers, and policy makers have directed much attention and resources to improving the problem. The first report, *To Err Is Human* (2000), emphasized the surprisingly large scale of the problem, while the second, *Crossing the Quality Chasm* (2001), focused more on solutions. Although the numerical findings in these reports initially were debated heavily in the professional literature, few argued that serious system-based problems and human errors were evident in health care.

While reports of unacceptable levels of medical errors have been written about occasionally since at least 1951, these early reports appear to have had little impact on the medical profession until Dr. Lucien Leape's article "Error in Medicine" appeared in 1994 in the *Journal of the American Medical Association* (Millenson, 2002). By this time, related issues of quality improvement were already receiving wide attention, and these two sets of issues blended to form a fertile ground for cultivating solutions.

Often missing from these efforts, however, was reference to the extensive research reported on the etiology and treatment of human error—especially catastrophic human error—in a number of fields, including airline and rail safety, nuclear reactor safety, and workplace accidents. Two notable exceptions are provided by Feldman and Roblin (1997) and by Eagle et al. (1992), who recommend using a failure analysis process in health care settings.

The medical profession often avoided explicit recognition of this problem, for a number of reasons, including protecting fellow professionals ("there but for the grace of God go I") and malpractice costs. Moreover, the overemphasis on blaming the individual in health care, something that quality improvement advocates have been fighting, may have subtly led otherwise knowledgeable individuals to play down the topic of human error. A close look at the literature on human error shows that it consistently emphasizes system improvement and deemphasizes blaming the individual. Stewart and Grout (2001) also suggest that academic research concerned with quality improvement may be biased toward statistical methods and away from detailed process design issues, including their cognitive dimensions. Yet even an advocate of system-based solutions like Deming suggests that human errors are a part, perhaps as much as 15%, of the problem (1986). Reducing human errors ought to be a part of the analysis and the solution (Becher and Chassin, 2001).

This chapter begins with a review of the definitions that can be used in classifying medical errors based on the work of Reason (2002) and Weick and Sutcliffe (2001), among others, and presents a taxonomy for both active and inactive human errors and for system faults. These are supported with examples and then with suggestions about how these categories of error can be matched with arrays of countermeasures for rapid and effective corrective action. We also outline how a cross-sectional analysis of errors can be useful in identifying systematic organizational problems that might be overlooked when focusing on the multiple causes of a single incident or error. The chapter concludes with thoughts on the past and the future of the patient safety movement.

MEDICAL ERRORS

An error occurs when a process does not proceed the way it was intended by its designers and managers. The most frequent error occurs when a step is omitted from a planned sequence of activities (Gawande, 2009;

Reason, 2002). Note that this definition does not relate directly to the outcome of that process. As Reason (2002) notes:

> Errors themselves are not intrinsically bad—indeed, they are often highly adaptive as in trial and error learning or the serendipitous discovery that can arise from error. However, they can have damaging and even fatal consequences, particularly in the "hands on" often uncertain activities associated with delivering health care to vulnerable patients—although these injurious outcomes are probably far fewer than their contextual opportunities would warrant. Unlike some epidemics, there is no specific countermeasure for error. Rooted as it is in the human condition, fallibility cannot be eliminated—nor is that a sensible goal—but its adverse consequences can be moderated through targeted error management techniques. (p. 40)

As concern about errors and safety has grown, some relatively specialized terms have been developed, including *adverse event* and *sentinel event*, which are defined as follows (The Joint Commission, 2011):

- *Adverse event*—An untoward, undesirable, and usually unanticipated event, such as the death of a patient, an employee, or a visitor in a health care organization. Incidents such as patient falls or improper administration of medications are also considered adverse events, even if there is no permanent effect on the patient.
- *Sentinel event*—An unexpected occurrence involving death or serious physical or psychological injury, or the risk thereof. Serious injury specifically includes loss of limb or function. The phrase "risk thereof" includes any process variation for which a recurrence would carry a significant chance of a serious adverse outcome. Such events are called "sentinel" because they signal the need for immediate investigation and response.

The World Health Organization (WHO) defines a near miss as "an incident that did not reach the patient," while The Joint Commission (TJC) defines it as "any variation during the provision of care, treatment, or services that did not affect the outcome, but for which a recurrence carries a significant risk of an adverse outcome" (Croteau, 2010).

An example of targeted management techniques is provided in Reason's article, "Combating Omission Errors Through Task Analysis and Good Reminders" (2002). In the same issue of that journal, Barber (2002) utilizes Reason's human error classification system to analyze medication noncompliance as a medical error. The continued usefulness of the reminder approach is exemplified by the checklist movement currently in the public spotlight (Gawande, 2009; Haynes et al., 2009; WHO, 2008), which builds on the earlier work of Pronovost (Szalavitz, 2009).

Organizations should include near misses and nonadverse events in their studies of errors. Weick and Sutcliffe (2001), for example, identify one of the characteristics of a reliable organization as having a focus on failures, not just successes, including highlighting and investigating near misses and nonadverse errors. They suggest a number of characteristics associated with successful, high-reliability organizations, observing that these organizations:

1. Focus on errors in their earliest manifestations, while successfully avoiding disasters

2. Try to understand processes in depth, not focus on simplification

3. Emphasize knowledge of operations and learning on the front line

4. Build in resilience to overcome the errors that do occur

5. Listen to and respect experience and expertise at the operational level

These types of organizations also build on Reason's work (2002), listing four attributes of a "mindful" culture, one that seeks out weaknesses in the system:

1. The culture values *reporting*. No adverse events are hidden. In fact, they are seen as opportunities to learn.

2. The culture is *just*. One does not shoot the messenger, and there is no scapegoating.

3. The culture is *flexible*. Information flows freely, and higher-rank individuals respect local expertise.

4. The culture values *learning*. New understanding is diligently sought and prized.

These and other sets of observations (Gibson and Prasad, 2003; Walshe and Shortell, 2004) are consistent with the CQI philosophy, including Deming's "profound knowledge." These practices can also operate beside the traditional professional social controls documented in Charles Bosk's

Forgive and Remember: Managing Medical Failure (1979). They also bring to mind the work of Thomas Kuhn (1962) on scientific revolutions, in which he noted that paradigm shifts in science occur when newcomers pay attention to discrepancies (even minor ones) between established theories and empirical observations and generate new hypotheses about system behavior that take these into account. The learning culture is also discussed at length in Chapter 10 of this text.

The cost of medical errors in the United States is acknowledged to be great, but estimates of both cost and error rates vary widely. A 1964 article based on data from Yale–New Haven Medical Center reported that 1.3% of patients died due to complications from some procedure intended for the patient's benefit (Shimmel, 1964). However, iatrogenic negative results do not equate to medical error. All procedures carry some risk of negative outcomes. Then, Lucian Leape coauthored a study that focused more on medical errors and reported that 4% of patients in the study suffered an injury that prolonged their hospital stay or resulted in measurable disability and that 69% of these injuries were caused by errors (Leape, 1994). Since 1994, the rate of research and publications concerning medical errors has increased markedly (Millensen, 2002).

WHY A CLASSIFICATION SYSTEM?

The mix of activities (products, if you will) in health care organizations is so varied that classification systems become extremely important components of any comparative analysis of health care quality issues. It is no accident that the field of quality improvement in health moved very slowly until the widespread adoption of the Diagnosis-Related Group (DRG) system, designed to evaluate and report measures of health care quality. Quality comparisons are much easier when there is a common classification system for human errors in health care that can be applied in parallel across institutions and product lines. A classification system is also necessary to encourage knowledge management efforts among institutions concerning medical error.

The existence of a classification system for errors is an important precursor of a systematic method for developing error responses. For example, TJC's *Sentinel Events Alert* is very good about citing "risk reduction" steps for each error studied. However, the next step would be to categorize those errors that are human errors and then associate them with corresponding preventive steps using a comprehensive classification structure, so that those responding to other errors could readily transfer such steps to their situations. Chang et al. (2005) have published a suggested taxonomy for TJC that includes a classification for practitioner-induced human errors. Meanwhile a WHO-sponsored drafting committee is working on another taxonomy that seems to go in a somewhat different direction. The World Health Alliance for Patient Safety, acting on behalf of the WHO, developed a Taxonomy for Patient Safety, which aims to define, harmonize, and group patient safety concepts into an internationally agreed-upon classification (Runciman et al., 2009).

Starting Points

One widely cited classification system was developed by James Reason (1990), which he called the Generic Error Modeling System (GEMS). A professor of psychology, he asserts that despite the wide range of experiences involving human error, errors "tend to take a surprisingly limited number of forms." He further states that "errors appear in very similar guises across a wide range of mental activities. Thus it is possible to identify comparable error forms in action, speech, perception, recall, recognition, judgment, problem solving, decision making, concept formation, and the like" (p. 2). He defines human error as "a generic term to encompass all those occasions in which a planned sequence of mental or physical activities fails to achieve its intended outcome, and when these failures cannot be attributed to the intervention of some chance agency" (p. 7). This definition contains three major points. First, there must be *intention* in the action sequence for an error to occur; errors cannot occur absent intention (of the actor or the organization). Secondly, the failure may occur because of *errors in the plan* or in *the execution of the plan*. In fact, this dichotomy was, and to some degree remains, a popular classification (Norman, 1988). The GEMS approach, however, separates the planning error into two parts: rule-based mistakes and knowledge-based mistakes. Finally, a tragic outcome *need not involve error* because a chance event may occur (e.g., a pulmonary embolism can occur despite taking all the steps normally necessary to avoid it).

GEMS Basic Error Types

This framework extends the popular dichotomy of slips (failure in execution) and mistakes (planning errors) and argues for four basic error types:

- Skill-based slips (and lapses)
- Rule-based mistakes
- Knowledge-based mistakes
- Violations of rules or norms

Splitting the rule-based performance from the skill-based performance was a useful contribution of Reason's work. These categories parallel those of Bosk (1979), who outlined technical errors, judgmental errors, and normative errors while analyzing the training and socialization of surgeons.

Skill-based performance is governed by stored patterns of preprogrammed instructions. For example, most clinical caregivers are taught to take blood pressure readings using a procedure that involves a specific sequence of steps. After countless repetitions, the steps become part of the knowledge base and little or no conscious "thought" is required when the caregiver fits and inflates the cuff and observes the pressure readings. Nevertheless, the individual does have to pay attention and perform certain "checks" to monitor the process, such as ensuring that the cuff is properly secured. A *lapse* occurs when the caregiver fails to check to see whether the cuff is secure. A *slip* occurs when the caregiver writes down an illegible number after reading the gauge correctly. These errors may occur due to being distracted or tired, or otherwise not giving full attention to the process.

Rule-based performance is applied to *familiar* problems in which solutions are governed by stored rules of the "if–then" type. These rules are based on previous experiences and are called into play when a trigger event or situation occurs. For example, when a patient goes into cardiac arrest, the medical team responds to a "code blue" alarm with the cardiopulmonary resuscitation protocol. Errors occur when a new situation is perceived as the same as or similar to a previous situation and the response model for the prototypical situation is wrongly applied.

Knowledge-based performance applies to *novel* problems when actions must be planned in "real time" using attentional control in conjunction with working memory. In other words, this situation calls for

---

TABLE 11–1 Health Care Examples Using the GEMS Framework

Error Type	Example
Skill-based slip	A physician orders Inderal intravenously for a patient but writes the order for the typical oral dosage.
Skill-based lapse	A physician forgets to prescribe beta-blockers following myocardial infarction, although he is aware of the strong research evidence that this helps prevent re-infarction and normally prescribes it in such cases.
Rule-based mistake	A patient presents with a high white blood cell count and lower right quadrant pain. The physician's schema defaults to the most frequently observed outcome (acute appendicitis), but confirmatory tests are not ordered, and the diagnosis proves incorrect.
Knowledge-based mistake	Confirmation bias: A physician presumes a diagnosis of cancer based on an initial blood chemistry value and dismisses subsequent counterevidence from a biopsy.

"hard thinking." The individual must assess the situation, draw relevant information from memory, and formulate a response. Knowledge-based performance often requires incremental decision making as additional information becomes available. Planning errors can occur, for example, when the relevant probabilities are incorrectly assessed, perhaps because of experience biases in decision making. Health care examples illustrating these categories of medical errors are shown in **Table 11–1**.

REPRESENTING THE SUGGESTED APPROACH

Given the four types of error shown by the GEMS model and the earlier categories of action–inaction, intention (good or bad), and planning vs. execution, we suggest the classification system for practitioner errors identified in **Figure 11–1**. Our criteria in developing it were that it be practically useful, cover a wide range of health care situations, and not support the biases that often occur—namely, blaming the victim, scapegoating the staff, or faulting the system. In complex situations, all might be partially involved, although we know that the first two are all too likely. Additional work has proposed classifications for patient-induced errors as well (Buetow et al., 2009; Woods et al., 2005).

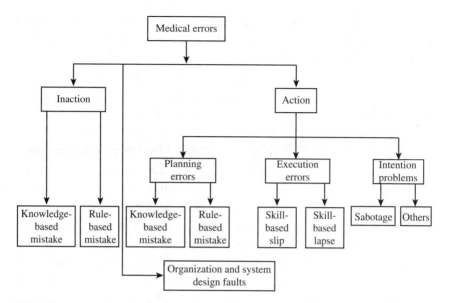

FIGURE 11–1 Potential Classification of Human Medical Errors

Action vs. Inaction

The first consideration is whether the error involves action or inaction. The nature of the analysis differs between these two categories. If no action took place, there is often no physical evidence and little opportunity to determine whether a step in a procedure was omitted. The process to be reviewed is primarily cognitive. The issue of intention is internal to the cognition of the decision maker and is difficult to separate from one's rules and knowledge states. Therefore, we have limited the intention issue to analysis of those cases where there was an action, since many health care situations have multiple actors who might have had differing intentional states that may need to be sorted out.

On the other hand, inaction events are likely to be highly significant in identifying system errors. The much reported, much reviewed, much litigated 1994 death of a patient at Dana-Farber Cancer Institute who received four times the intended daily dose of chemotherapy and soon died could have been dismissed as a single human slip of dosage entry. Yet there were many subsequent system questions raised as to why it went unnoticed over the subsequent 3 months; why the error was not caught by physicians, nurses, and pharmacists; why no postmortem was held; and so on. These inactions were all revealing of system problems later identified by accrediting and licensing bodies (Bohmer and Winslow, 1999; Crane, 2001).

Furthermore, attention to inaction may lead to refinement of what is or is not a medical error. One example is Barber's argument that patient noncompliance is a medical error (2002). Another example to consider would be the diabetic patient, obviously in some distress, who presents herself one Saturday afternoon at the local hospital emergency room. She reports having tested her glucose level and finding it unusually high. Once her findings are confirmed, the duty nurse calls her physician for an order but is unable to reach him. The patient waits and worsens for several hours until the physician finally responds. Then she is treated and released. In most cases, this inaction would not be reported as a medical error. The patient might well complain to the hospital administration, but this could be treated as a case of patient dissatisfaction rather than a medical error. Unless the quality assurance staff is alerted to the importance of inaction, they are unlikely to address the systematic issues generating such delay and unnecessary distress.

Planning and Execution Errors and Violations

The second step is to determine whether the error involved planning, execution, or motivation. If the issue is primarily related to planning or execution skills, the GEMS categories outlined previously can be applied.

Planning

Most reported medical errors are in execution, such as the wrong drug dosage administered or the wrong side operated on, but many of these errors have their genesis in the planning stage. If one operates on the wrong side of the brain, it is obvious that the physician did not read the chart or X-ray correctly and that numerous other signals were transmitted or ignored before the wrong action was taken. This may be the result of a knowledge error, such as the wrong side of an X-ray being displayed on the light box, or rule-based failure, such as not asking the patient which side they believe will be affected. In all likelihood, there was more than one mistake as well as failure of the systems intended to avert such mistakes (Steinhauer, 2001). A more clearly rule-based mistake occurred when a man was brought to the emergency room in intense abdominal pain.

Without ordering a CT scan, the surgeon assumed a kidney stone. None was found, and 18 hours later the patient died of a ruptured abdominal aortic aneurism (Gawande, 1999).

Execution

No matter how good the planning, however, the individual carrying it out may err. For example, contrary to instructions, an inexperienced surgical resident performing a tracheotomy made a horizontal cut across the patient's neck instead of the correct vertical incision (Gawande, 1999). This would have been a skill-based lapse had the resident not internalized the instructions and a rule-based mistake had the incision been the correct approach for a different surgical procedure, such as a thyroidectomy.

Violation

Other categories refer to motivational problems behind individual *violations* of the plan, stem from organizational factors, or combine both. An example of a personal motivational problem would be an aide who skips steps in a care process because he wants to sneak away early for a date. Using Reason's term, "violations," Barber (2002) notes the importance of motivational problems in his analysis of prescription medicine compliance as a medical error problem: "Violations include taking 'short cuts' that bend the rules to make life easier, such as taking several medicines together which should be taken at different times, or taking a non-steroidal anti-inflammatory drug on an empty stomach" (p. 83). Presumably the patient has been informed of the right medication procedures and internalized the appropriate rules to follow but decides to do something else for personal reasons.

Reason (1995) suggests three types of violations:

- *Routine violations*—The individual cuts corners, as described by Barber (2002).
- *Optimizing violations*—The individual pursues personal ends at the expense of the process, like the aide on the telephone, or the case of a Kansas City pharmacist who pleaded guilty to diluting chemotherapy products and perhaps thousands of other medications for profit.
- *Necessary or situational violations*—The individual sees no other way out of a bind.

The early patient safety literature emphasized the systems approach to human error and somewhat neglected the violations problem. "Fix the system, not the blame" was often heard. This occurred because (1) the majority of medical errors were indeed associated with system problems (i.e., the blunt end) and (2) the punitive culture of blaming individuals led to errors going unreported, thus allowing no opportunity for improvement. More recently, violations have moved out of the closet (Leape and Fromson, 2006). There is now concern about accountability, "where the question is not what happens to the distracted caregivers who forget to clean their hands . . . but what happens when they do so habitually and willfully, despite education, counseling, and system improvements" (Wachter and Pronovost, 2009). David Marx's "just culture" is an effort to integrate the "no blame" and accountability ideas (Wachter, 2007).

Organization and Process Design System Faults

The literature on continuous quality improvement, especially root cause analysis as it is applied to sentinel events in health care, already provides a highly developed structure for analysis of organizational issues and the design of processes. These are the blunt end of medical error, the much less visible sources, since they do not necessarily involve individual failure to implement a process or procedure properly. They are implicated in many adverse situations, since they produce appropriate or inappropriate information and training, motivate proper teamwork and personal vigilance, and stimulate appropriate or inappropriate intentions. Therefore, this classification has been included in Figure 11–1 to serve as a linkage to the existing literature of quality and process improvement.

MATCHING COUNTERMEASURES TO ERROR TYPES

The test of the effectiveness of such a classification scheme is whether it can categorize experience sufficiently to lead toward the selection of appropriate responses to human error. The schema offered here should be useful because it points one toward specific types of remedies. The easiest types of medical errors to deal with are the skill-based mistakes, followed by rule-based mistakes, then knowledge-based mistakes, and finally intentional problems.

Skill-based errors occur when an individual fails to make an attentional check during the process of executing a schema or repetitive procedure that has become habitual. These omissions occur most often because an individual is fatigued, preoccupied, or distracted. Obvious countermeasures involve:

- *Attention getters*—Reason (2002) argues that one should respond with task analysis followed up by effective reminder systems and provides 10 criteria for a "good" reminder.
- *Error detection*—Stewart and Grout (2001) review the industrial literature on methods of error detection and limitation. Monitoring systems offer many opportunities for error detection in health care.
- *In-line inspection*—Many health care professionals like working in groups because their "buddy" can inspect ongoing work and help avoid or respond early to errors (Stewart and Grout, 2001).
- *Error limitation*—This is more difficult to achieve in health care than in other settings, but computer-based transactions and records can be programmed to respond when process limits are exceeded and the system is presumed to be out of control (Stewart and Grout, 2001).
- *Checklists*—These simple tools, which were introduced in earlier chapters, can be used to ensure that attentional checks are performed. They are often similar to protocols, order sets, and clinical pathways (Winters, 2009). Haynes et al. (2009) report that they are effective in a variety of hospital settings and across cultures. Gawande (2009) points out their impact on group dynamics in surgical settings, especially where the teams are highly temporary with weak interpersonal experience of each other. (See case 9 in the companion casebook [McLaughlin et al., 2012].)
- *Resource input standards*—Donabedian (1980) observed that one of the aspects of quality health care was adequate resource inputs. These include establishing reasonable staffing levels as well as limits on the number of consecutive hours worked. Such rules already exist in the airline industry, a rich source of ideas for potential error avoidance for the health care industry.
- *Substitute a rule-based solution*—If there is concern about operating on the wrong knee, write "NO" on the incorrect limb and "YES" on the correct one (Steinhauer, 2001).

Rule-based mistakes involve the inappropriate use of an "if–then" rule. When several possible rules appear appropriate, the correct choice depends on how completely the competing rules match the situation and the strength of the rule—how many times it has been applied successfully to such situations in the past. Reason suggests that the number of contingencies that "if–then" rules cover distinguishes experts from trained novices (Reason, 1990). However, one must be careful to avoid application of a "strong, but wrong" rule. For example, Reason (1995) reports a case of a patient who died of radiation burns. He was receiving his ninth treatment of 200 rads following removal of a tumor from his shoulder. The machine had two modes of delivery, with the second using 25,000 rads and a metal plate to transform the beam into therapeutic X-rays. A technician had edited the software program to correct a typo but introduced a new error that caused the machine to correctly remove the plate, but left the setting at 25,000 rads. The radiotherapist activated the machine but received the unfamiliar and cryptic message "Malfunction 54" on her computer screen. She assumed that the treatment had not happened, which is what similar messages had meant in the past, and she set up the machine to "fire" again. She repeated the process a third time when the message reappeared—with tragic results.

Countermeasures include:

- Enhancing the search process to include more alternative responses
- Sharing what has not worked well (past errors) with others
- Decision support systems to make the preceding two alternatives more feasible
- Using simulators and simulations to build a larger rule repertoire

Simulation can provide excellent learning opportunities with realistic resource utilization and without putting patients at risk (Slovensky and Morin, 1997). Had the radiotherapist encountered the "Malfunction 54" message in a simulated environment, an observer could have pointed out the consequences of her strong (but wrong) assumption. The radiotherapist would have then learned of the need to search out the meaning of warnings rather than go on past experience.

Knowledge-based mistakes occur during problem-solving situations when one's repertoire of "if–then" rules proves inadequate. There may be a lack of information, the information may be outdated, or one's judgmental decision-making heuristics may be biased. Equating ease of recall of an event with its likelihood of occurrence is an example (Tversky and Kahneman, 1974). Another example is weighting local, personal data more heavily than distant, impersonal data. For example, a community may have had an instance when a 20- to 30-year-old female had breast cancer. This single episode, pertinent and tragic, is told and retold, causing young women to seek mammograms even though national studies show them to have a very poor benefit–cost ratio. Similarly, a physician may not prescribe a new and effective medication because one of her first patients to use the drug reported dissatisfaction due to a side effect (Russo, 1999).

Countermeasures include:

- Decision-maker education, including continuing education and academic detailing
- Increasing awareness of how biases on the availability and locality of information affect decision making
- Decision support systems to increase availability of information that meet the criteria of evidenced-based medicine
- Peer review of knowledge-based schema used in frequently seen cases
- Collaborative discussion of diagnoses and treatments involving rarely seen cases

Motivational problems include categories that are so numerous and varied that we can only scratch the surface. The best way to think of them in all but the most egregious cases is that they are the epsilon factor in safety and quality. After the indolent, the malicious, and the impaired have been removed (Weick and Sutcliffe, 2001), the inability to fix the causation with the four GEMS categories probably means that there are further organizational problems to be considered (Reason, 2000). These include:

- Overspecialization of tasks (West, 2000)
- Problems of coordination, communication, and cooperation (West, 2000). These should also show up in process analyses associated with execution performance
- Diffusion of responsibility (West, 2000), which must be addressed by establishing process ownership at the appropriate level of aggregation (McLaughlin and Kaluzny, 1999)
- Goal displacement (Carthey et al., 2001; West, 2000) in which funding, profitability, or performance measures dominate quality and safety measures and damage professional morale
- Unfair blaming of individuals (Carthey et al., 2001) for systems problems and/or denying the existence of systematic error

- Conflicts between management and staff, leading to a variety of responses, including sabotage (Reason, 1995)
- Norms and cultures supporting risk-taking and rule-bending (Reason, 1995)

Organization and process design system faults are the focus of much of the quality and safety literature. Where they are not the direct cause of medical error, each might certainly be a "latent" factor behind medical error (Berwick, 2001; Reason, 1995, 2000). Understaffing can easily be a management contribution to the fatigue and inattention that leads to an implementation error by an otherwise reliable staff nurse or, if continued, to motivational problems leading to violations. Some researchers refer to these organizational issues as the "blunt end" of safe operations (Cook and Woods, 1994; Ketring and White, 2002).

Rather than attempt to list all of the organization and process design factors, we refer the reader to the numerous existing checklists, including the following:

- TJC (2002) offers a useful resource with its "Framework for Root Cause Analysis and Action," particularly the other items in the "special cause" variations array and those in the "common cause" section.
- Carthey et al. (2001) suggest a survey for institutional-level functioning in avoiding medical errors. It involves a 20-item checklist for assessing institutional resilience. They also suggest comparing the scoring across internal professional groupings to look for problem areas. The checklist is available at http://www.rmf.harvard.edu/files/documents/Mod7doclink2.pdf.
- Another useful set of organizational scales is provided by Weick and Sutcliffe (2001). Their work is also interesting because it emphasizes the importance of organizational resilience: the ability to contain and recover from the errors that will happen despite the best-laid plans and designs.

ADOPTING THE AVIATION INDUSTRY APPROACH

In addition to the specifics, one can adopt an overall approach modeled on the aviation industry approach, conducting in-depth analyses of both actual errors and "near misses." The aviation industry's approach was identified as a useful model by most of the authors cited in this chapter, and, as described in Chapter 2, aviation's successes in improving safety continues to offer lessons to the health care community (Pronovost et al., 2009). The Maccabi Healthcare Services, a nonprofit HMO in Israel, has been applying the aviation industry investigative approach for years. They report the following features of their evolving system:

- An interdisciplinary team with doctors, psychologists, and individuals with aviation experience
- A support system for supporting the reporting caregivers, including lack of blame and immunity, with emphasis on reporting near-misses as well as adverse events
- A hotline for reporting rapidly ahead of any retrospective reviews
- A carefully constructed event debriefing methodology
- Wide dissemination of reports and recommendations throughout its dispersed ambulatory care system (Wilf-Miron et al., 2003)

Sax et al. (2009) report on the use of "aviation-based crew resource" management training involving 857 participants in two affiliated hospitals over 5 years, with steadily increasing impact over that period. They conclude that behaviors can be ingrained, but it takes considerable time and effort.

MULTICAUSATION AND THE CROSS-SECTIONAL APPROACH

Organizations do not suddenly start making mistakes. They tend to slide imperceptibly into a set of conditions that produce medical errors. People start changing the way they do things for convenience or to adapt to perceived management goals. New digital equipment that is supposed to eliminate the human element is not failsafe. New personnel replace those previously trained to respond to a situation. Pressures build that lead to inattention and reduced morale. Supplies and medications are substituted that were not included in formal procedures and so on. Often it is the concatenation of these drifts that leads to major errors. Any error classification system must adapt to this multicausal reality.

Table 11–2 outlines a way of adapting this human classification system to multicausality and to the fact that multiple events may be reported within a reasonable time period within the same institution.

TABLE 11–2 Applying the Classification System

Type of causation	Indicate # present	Detailed descriptions for each	Recommended responses to each
Inaction—knowledge-based			
Inaction—rule-based			
Planning—knowledge-based			
Planning—rule-based			
Execution—skill-based slip			
Execution—skill-based lapse			
Violations			
Organization and process design system faults			

A cross-sectional analysis of commonalities across adverse events may provide a more representative snapshot of systems problems than in-depth focus on a single event (Meurier, 2000).

The cross-sectional approach encourages the organization to look at the latent conditions behind the errors, the attitudinal and information processing differences among professionals, the patterns of communications within and across teams, and environmental factors such as management pressure to speed up procedures and improve operating suite utilization or harried nursing staff lacking time to check patient identities and prescriptions (Meurier, 2000; Steinhauer, 2001). It may also lead to greater breadth of tactics applied to such errors rather than relying on one-size-fits-all or perfunctory responses such as "nurse counseled" (Bohmer and Winslow, 1999).

CONCLUSIONS

Given the complexity of health care situations and how they produce medical errors, it is important to have a conceptual schema for their classification and analysis. We have outlined one schema, drawing heavily on the work of James Reason. It is offered because it is practical and draws on the extensive work done on the psychology of human error and human factors in health and other fields, as well as organizational antecedents of errors and more recent studies involving the introduction of check-lists. It is applicable to a wide array of situations and leads to the use of some, if not all, the techniques of continuous quality improvement, but overcomes some of the biases exhibited by both those who espouse such techniques and those who avoid them.

The next step is a continuing dialogue to improve our ability to iden-tify and further codify both individual and organizational responses asso-ciated with each category of error, keeping in mind that any system must be capable of handling the multiple individual and systemic causations behind medical errors and enhance access to relevant arrays of responses and tactics.

Past Improvement and Future Expectations

On the 10th anniversary of the publication of *To Err Is Human*, Wachter (2010) evaluated the success of the patient safety movement. Although his overall grade was a moderate B–, he noted a few areas of more sig-nificant improvement. His highest assessment of A– was in the category of national and international interventions, particularly the efforts of the Institute of Healthcare Improvement (IHI), the state of Michigan's inten-sive care units (ICUs), and the WHO. Notably, all these efforts involved the use of checklists, mentioned earlier as an effective approach.

The Michigan success was led by Peter Pronovost of Johns Hopkins. The goal was to reduce the level of central line infections, and 103 participating ICUs reported data before and after the introduction of checklists and associated changes such as safety training and the pro-visioning of key supplies, such as chlorhexidine soap (Pronovost et al., 2006). The overall median rate of central line infections for the ICUs fell from 2.7 infections per 1,000 catheter-days to zero within 3 months of implementation, and this median of zero was maintained during 18 months of follow-up. Results like this prompted Lucian Leape to comment, "It is now apparent that we can use perfection as a bench-mark" (Buerhaus, 2007). The patient safety movement has, at least in the area of hospital-acquired infections, begun "chasing zero," a goal reminiscent of the industrial quality movement's "zero defects" from the 1970s (Denham et al., 2009).

The IHI's successful 100,000 Lives Campaign focused on six initia-tives (referred to by IHI as "bundles") to save lives; three of these involved checklists: the central line bundle, the surgical site infection bundle, and the ventilator bundle (Rao and Hoyt, 2008). Finally, the WHO effort led by Gawande (2009) developed a 2-minute, 19-step surgical checklist that decreased major complications by 36% and deaths by 47% in eight widely diverse international hospitals.

On the other hand, Livingstone (2010), citing these and other efforts, suggests that harsh penalties and top-down organizational programs are less likely to improve patient safety than physician-led efforts. He also notes that the alternative driver of patient accountability is still available and suggests future consideration of adding the use of checklists and team training and other safety process measures alongside currently mandated reporting of quality-of-care measures.

Cross-References to the Companion Casebook

(McLaughlin, C. P., Johnson, J. K., and Sollecito, W. A. [Eds.]. 2012. *Implementing Continuous Quality Improvement in Health Care: A Global Casebook.* Sudbury, MA: Jones & Bartlett Learning.)

Case Study Number	Case Study Title	Case Study Authors
9	Forthright Medical Center: Social Marketing and the Surgical Checklist	*Carol E. Breland*
16	The Lewis Blackman Hospital Patient Safety Act: It's Hard To Kill A Healthy 15-Year-Old	*Julie K. Johnson, Helen Haskell, and Paul Barach*

REFERENCES

Barber, N. 2002. Should we consider non-compliance a medical error? *Quality Safety Health Care*, 11: 81–84.

Becher, E. C., and Chassin, M. R. 2001. Improving quality, minimizing error: Making it happen. *Health Aff*, 203: 69–81.

Berwick, D. M. 2001. Not again! *BMJ*, 322: 247–248.

Bohmer, R., and Winslow, A. 1999. *The Dana-Farber Cancer Institute*. Boston: Harvard Business School Publishing.

Bosk, C. L. 1979. *Forgive and Remember: Managing Medical Failure*. Chicago: University of Chicago Press.

Buerhaus, P. I. 2007. Is hospital patient care becoming safer? A conversation with Lucian Leape. *Health Aff*, 266: w687–w696.

Buetow, S., Kiata, L., Liew, T., et al. 2009. Patient error: A preliminary taxonomy. *Ann Intern Med*, 7: 223–231.

Carthey, J., de Leval, M. R., and Reason, J. T. 2001. Institutional resistance in healthcare systems. *Quality Health Care*, 10: 29–32.

Chang, A., Schyve, P. M., Croteau, R. J., et al. 2005. The JCAHO patient safety event taxonomy: A standardized terminology and classification schema for near misses and adverse events. *Int J Quality Health Care*, 17: 95–105.

Cook, R. I., and Woods, D. D. 1994. Operating at the sharp end: Complexity of human error. In Bogner, M. S. (Ed.). *Human Error in Medicine*. Hillsdale, NJ: Lawrence Erlbaum Associates.

Crane, M. 2001. Who caused this tragic medication mistake? *Med Econ*, 78(19): 49–50.

Croteau, R. J. (Ed.). 2010. *Root Cause Analysis in Health Care: Tools and Techniques* (4th ed.). Oakbrook Terrace, IL: Joint Commission Resources.

Deming, W. E. 1986. *Out of the Crisis*. Cambridge: Massachusetts Institute of Technology Center for Advanced Engineering Study.

Denham, C. R., Angood, P., Berwick, D., et al. 2009. Chasing zero: Can reality meet the rhetoric? *J Patient Safety*, 54: 216–222.

Donabedian, A. 1980. *Exploration in Quality Assessment and Monitoring: Definition of Quality and Approaches to Its Assessment* (vol. 1). Ann Arbor, MI: Health Administration Press.

Eagle, C. J., Davies, J. M., and Reason, J. 1992. Accident analysis of large-scale technical disasters applied to anaesthetic complication. *Can J Anaesth*, 39: 119–122.

Feldman S. E., and Roblin, D. W. 1997. Medical accidents in hospital care: Applications of failure analysis to hospital quality appraisal. *Joint Commission J Quality Improve*, 23: 567–580.

Gawande, A. 1999, February 1. When doctors make mistakes. *The New Yorker*, 44–55.

Gawande, A. 2009. *The Checklist Manifesto: How to Get Things Right*. New York: Metropolitan Books.

Gibson, R., and Prasad, J. 2003. *Wall of Silence: The Untold Story of Medical Mistakes That Kill and Injure Millions*. Washington, DC: Lifeline Press.

Haynes, A. B., Weiser, T. G., Berry, W. R., et al. 2009. A surgical safety checklist to reduce morbidity and mortality in a global population. *N Engl J Med*, 360: 491–499.

Institute of Medicine. 2000. *To Err Is Human: Building a Safer Health System.* Washington, DC: National Academies Press.

Institute of Medicine. 2001. *Crossing the Quality Chasm: A New Health System for the 21st Century.* Washington, DC: National Academies Press.

The Joint Commission. 2002. A framework for a root cause analysis and action in response to a sentinel event. Retrieved March 15, 2011, from http://www.ttuhsc.edu/som/clinic/forms/ACForm8.12.A.pdf

The Joint Commission. 2006. Sentinel event glossary. Retrieved January 4, 2011, from http://www.jointcommission.org/Sentinel_Event_Policy_and_Procedures/

Ketring, S. P., and White, J. P. 2002. Developing a systemwide approach to patient safety: The first year. *Joint Commission J Quality Improve*, 28: 287–295.

Kuhn, T. S. 1962. *The Structure of Scientific Revolutions.* Chicago: University of Chicago Press.

Leape, L. L. 1994. Error in medicine. *JAMA,* 272: 1851–1857.

Leape, L. L., and Fromson, L. 2006. Improving patient care: Problem doctors: Is there a system-level solution? *Ann Intern Med*, 144: 107–115.

Livingstone, E. H. 2010. Solutions for improving patient safety. *JAMA*, 3022: 159–161.

McLaughlin, C. P., Johnson, J. K., and Sollecito, W. A. (Eds.). 2012. *Implementing Continuous Quality Improvement in Health Care: A Global Casebook.* Sudbury, MA: Jones & Bartlett Learning.

McLaughlin, C. P., and Kaluzny, A. D. (Eds.). 1999. *Continuous Quality Improvement in Medicine* (2nd ed.). Gaithersburg, MD: Aspen Publishers.

Meurier, C. E. 2000. Understanding the nature of errors in nursing: Using a model to analyze critical incident reports of errors which had resulted in an adverse or potentially adverse event. *J Adv Nurs*, 32: 202–207.

Millensen, M. L. 2002. Pushing the profession: How the news media turned patient safety into a priority. *Quality Safety Health Care*, 11: 57–63.

Norman, D. A. 1988. *The Psychology of Everyday Things.* New York: Basic Books.

Pronovost, P., Needham, D., Berenholtz, S., et al. 2006. An intervention to decrease catheter-related bloodstream infections in the ICU. *N Engl J Med*, 355: 2725–2732.

Pronovost, P. J., Goeschel, C. A., Olsen, K. L., et al. 2009. Reducing health care hazards: Lessons from the commercial aviation safety team. *Health Aff*, 283: w479–w489.

Rao, H., and Hoyt, D. 2008. *Institute for Healthcare Improvement: The campaign to save 100,000 lives.* Case L-13. Stanford, CA: Stanford Graduate School of Business.

Reason, J. T. 1990. *Human Error.* Cambridge, UK: Cambridge University Press.

Reason, J. T. 1995. Understanding adverse events: Human factors. In Vincent, C. (Ed.), *Clinical Risk Management.* London: British Medical Journal Publications.

Reason, J. T. 1997. *Managing the Risks of Organizational Accidents.* Aldershot, UK: Ashgate.

Reason, J. T. 2000. Human error: Models and management. *BMJ*, 320: 768–770.

Reason, J. T. 2002. Combating omission errors through task analysis and good reminders. *Quality Safety Health Care*, 11: 40–44.

Runciman, W., Hibbert, P., Thomson, R., et al. 2009. Towards an international classification for patient safety: Key concepts and terms. *Int J Quality Health Care*, 21(1): 18–26.

Russo, F. 1999, May. The clinical trials bottleneck. *The Atlantic Monthly*, 30–36.

Sax, H. C., Browne, P., Mayewski, R. J., et al. 2009. Can aviation-based team training elicit sustainable behavior change? *Arch Surg*, 144(12): 1133–1137.

Shimmel, E. 1964. The hazards of hospitalization. *Annals of Internal Medicine*, 6: 100–110.

Slovensky, D. J., and Morin, B. 1997. Learning through simulation: The next step in quality improvement. *Quality Improve Health Care*, 53: 72–79.

Steinhauer, J. 2001, April 1. So, the tumor is on the left, right? Seeking ways to reduce operating room errors. *New York Times*, Section 1, p. 27.

Stewart, D. M., and Grout, J. R. 2001. The human side of mistake-proofing. *Production Operations Manage*, 10: 440–459.

Szalavitz, M. 2009, January 14. Study: A simple surgery checklist saves Lives. *Time*. Retrieved March 15, 2011, from http://www.time.com/time/printout/0,8816,1871759,00.html

Tversky, A., and Kahneman, D. 1974. Judgment under uncertainty: Heuristics and biases. *Science,* 185: 1124–1131.

Wachter, R. M. 2007. In conversation with David Marx. *AHRQ Web M & M Perspectives on Safety*. Retrieved March 15, 2011, from http://www.webmm.ahrq.gov/perspective.aspx?perspectiveID=49

Wachter, R. M. 2010. Patient safety at ten: Unmistakable progress, troubling gaps. *Health Aff,* 291: 165–173.

Wachter, R. M., and Pronovost, P. J. 2009. Balancing "no blame" with accountability in patient safety. *N Engl J Med,* 361: 1401–1406.

Walshe, K., and Shortell, S. M. 2004. When things go wrong: How health care organizations deal with major failures. *Health Aff,* 233: 103–109.

Weick, K. E., and Sutcliffe, K. M. 2001. *Managing the Unexpected: Assuring High Performance in an Age of Complexity.* San Francisco: Jossey-Bass.

West, E. 2000. Organizational sources of safety and danger: Sociological contributions to the study of adverse events. *Quality Health Care,* 9: 120–126.

Wilf-Miron, R., Lewenhoff, I., Benyamini, Z., et al. 2003. From aviation to medicine: Applying concepts of aviation safety to risk management in ambulatory care. *Quality Safety Health Care,* 12: 35–39.

Winters, B. D. 2009. Clinical review: Checklists—translating evidence into practice. *Crit Care,* 13: 210–211.

Woods, D. M., Johnson, J., Holl, J. L., et al. 2005. Anatomy of a pediatric safety event: A pediatric patient safety taxonomy. *Quality Safety Health Care,* 14: 422–427.

World Health Organization. 2008. World Alliance for Patient Safety: Implementation Manual Surgical Safety Checklist (1st ed.). Safe surgery saves lives. Geneva: Author.

CHAPTER 12

The Role of Health Information Technology in Quality Improvement: From Data to Decisions

Curtis P. McLaughlin and David C. Kibbe

"Information is the lifeblood of modern medicine. Health information technology (HIT) is destined to be its circulatory system."

—David Blumenthal

INTRODUCTION

Total quality management's early slogan, "In God we trust; all others send data," exemplifies the importance of information to health care quality improvement. Yet its potential is severely limited without strong health information technology (HIT) support. After years of underinvestment in HIT, the United States and many other countries are on the verge of a sea change. For example, the Health Information Technology for Economic and Clinical Health (HITECH) Act portion of the American Recovery and Reinvestment Act of 2009 (ARRA) enables the investment of some $30 billion to support electronic health records and other related functions. This legislation did not underwrite investment in software or hardware. Instead, it called for payments to practices that met the functionality standards based on "meaningful use." This method of incentivization should encourage further innovation rather than limiting development of standards to current system concepts. It also opens up alternative methods of compensation linked to performance and, ultimately, to outcomes.

This chapter outlines the ways in which this HIT investment can support current and future quality improvement efforts. Among the key concepts are data availability, reliability, and access (including interoperability and transparency); statistical analysis (including data mining); and presentation. Quality data analyses can contribute effectively at the individual (provider and patient), organizational, communal, and international levels.

Evolving Health Information Technology

Porter (2009) has outlined where HIT must go in the future to support improvements in health care value, including quality.

> Simply automating current delivery practices will be a hugely expensive exercise in futility. Among our highest near-term priorities is to finalize and then continuously update . . . HIT standards that include precise data definitions (for diagnoses and treatments, for example), an architecture for aggregating data for each patient over time and across providers, and protocols for seamless communication among systems. (p. 2)

This chapter assumes steady progress in that direction supported by availability of enhanced electronic medical records. **Appendix 12–A** outlines a number of steps to improve HIT, as recommended in 2004 by a government expert panel. While some progress has been made with this list, much remains to be implemented.

USING HIT IN CONTINUOUS QUALITY IMPROVEMENT

During the early years of continuous quality improvement (CQI) in health care, each activity required a custom data collection effort. The Plan, Do, Study, Act (PDSA) model included steps of specifying and collecting process data for statistical analysis leading toward reduction of variability. More recently, health industry organizations have encouraged "voluntary" reporting of quality data, and a number of health care payers have demanded submission of quality data. Payers and accrediting organizations are increasing their requirements for regular reporting of indicator quality variables. Therefore, the HIT systems in place in the future must have capabilities for collecting process-specific data internally as needed and for routine reporting of clinical and operational quality data as by-products of the transactions of day-to-day information systems. What has yet to become widely available is the capacity to collect process and outcome data on individual patient episodes of care from multiple sources of care and longitudinally—that is, across time. This will develop if payers are successful in requiring bundled payments for episodes of care, providing a better focal point for quality data.

The fundamental importance of data—collection, storage, protection, analysis, and use—has finally been recognized. Whatever the setting or population, the dual value imperatives of cost control and quality improvement can be met only by analyzing processes of care and their impacts on outcomes. Hence, the measurement of outcomes, the assurance of health care data quality, and access to tools for analysis of health information have become core competencies for health care organizations and professionals.

THE DATA-TO-DECISION CYCLE

The effective use of HIT requires attention to the complete data-to-decision cycle illustrated in **Figure 12–1**. In this cycle, data are transformed to information, information then becomes knowledge, and that knowledge supports decisions and actions for improved performance. The cycle suggests that in the ideal setting, data collection efforts occur alongside the routine delivery of health care and that performance improvement decisions should determine the data to be collected, providing feedback between data and decisions.

Data, information, and *knowledge* are terms commonly used as synonyms. However, information management for CQI requires that they be defined more precisely and that the distinctions between them be clarified.

Data are Facts

Data elements by themselves have no meaning: they are simply isolated facts. For example, in **Figure 12–2**, we see that in the month of April there were 14 medication errors reported from nursing unit 12BG.

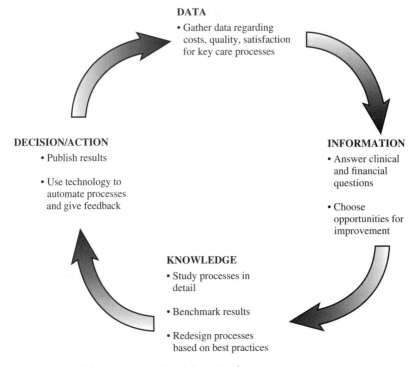

FIGURE 12–1 The Data-to-Decision Cycle

Management at the data level is concerned with the problems relating to the accuracy of the facts, their accessibility, their formatting or organization, and their storage. Data that are accurate and structured properly can be retrieved easily and combined with other data elements in a relational database for purposes of analysis. Conversely, data of poor quality, or data stored in nonstandard formats, may be next to impossible to find and therefore are useless for performance improvement.

Information is Data that have Become Meaningful

Data assembled to answer someone's question become information. At the information level, management deals with properly framing

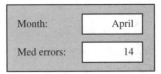

FIGURE 12–2 Data on April Medication Errors for Unit 12BG

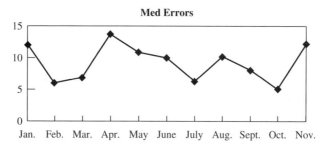

FIGURE 12–3 Information on Medication Errors for the Year

questions, identifying sources of data necessary to answer the questions, selecting and combining views of data to provide answers, and communicating the resulting information to people who want it to aid decisions. In **Figure 12–3**, enough data have been collected, assembled, and displayed to provide information about the behavior of the medication delivery processes on unit 12BG and to answer the question "What was the average monthly number of medication errors?" One very practical example of a common problem in information management involves the identification of *denominators* when rates or percentages are needed. A denominator requires that the question "How large is the whole population from which the numerator was selected?" be answered.

Knowledge Implies Prediction

Management utilizes information to predict and, insofar as possible, control the future performance of processes of care. When our information is robust and plentiful enough to permit predictions about performance, individuals and organizations possess knowledge that can be used to intervene, as required. In **Figure 12–4**, statistical process control methods have been applied to the information about medication errors on unit 12BG to ask, "Is the behavior of the process predictable? Should we intervene? What kind of intervention is required?" Statistical process control techniques can provide knowledge about the causes of variation in a process. Other methods of interpreting and synthesizing information may provide knowledge about the appropriateness of specific treatments for individual patients or populations or identify patients at risk. (See Chapter 3.)

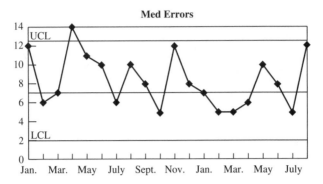

FIGURE 12–4 Knowledge About the Medication Error Process

Decisions Lead to Action or Inaction

Feedback about likely results of our actions based on knowledge of processes and systems is the best possible motivation for improvement. Some organizations threaten and punish individuals who are "noncompliant"; however, it is preferable to seek improvement based on knowledge and collaboration based on shared goals and an appeal to evidence. In **Figure 12–5**, a quality improvement team has used data, information, and knowledge of the medication delivery process to make specific decisions about how to improve the processes. The subsequent data collection efforts shown here illustrate that the desired results (i.e., consistently fewer medication errors) have been achieved.

Finally, the data-to-decision cycle points directly to the issues of data management and data quality as a place to begin discussing information systems and quality improvement. It leads us toward issues of standards,

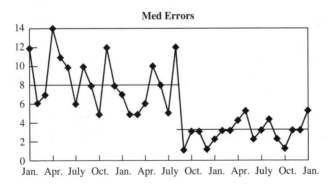

FIGURE 12–5 Decisions Have Been Taken to Improve the Medication Delivery Process

interfaces, and community networks that expand quality improvement efforts beyond institutional walls.

More data is not necessarily a blessing. To become useful information, data must be reliable, relevant to the task at hand, and accessible at a reasonable cost. Data must be in a form that can be analyzed statistically and then presented effectively—first to the improvement team and then to management for its approval of any planned changes.

Data Availability

Health care processes must produce, code, and record relevant data. Where paper records are still used, data must be reentered in digital form to facilitate analysis. Other chapters of this text cover the design of quality improvement efforts, which involves consideration of what is available from existing information systems and what is to be collected (often at considerable cost) for a given study.

INFORMATION TYPES

Routine Service Information

Current U.S. health insurance payers require a specific array of uniformly coded information pertaining to the type of service and discharge diagnosis in a predetermined format. Unfortunately, patient identifiers tend to be provider and/or payer specific.

Single-payer systems in other countries do not have the identifier problem and may or may not adopt widely accepted diagnostic coding systems. However, they have considerable latitude in how they code their process variables, including cost and labor utilization measures. Fee-for-service systems tend to have detailed charge data, while capitated systems are likely to be less detailed. Unfortunately, the more anyone customizes their routine service reporting systems to study topics of special interest, the harder it may become to make meaningful interorganizational and international comparisons.

Purposefully Collected Information

When desired data elements are not produced by the routine transaction processing systems, quality efforts must establish special data collection routines. This often involves extracting data from the ongoing system and then entering selected supplementary variables. Where the information is organized by diagnosis or disease, these specialized systems are called *registries* and often include information from multiple providers. While registries are often thought of in terms of large multicenter studies, it is important that each provider entity have the software capacity to build their own registries in order to follow their own performance and to compare it with their peers. Increasingly, subspecialty societies are insisting on internal and comparative studies of outcomes and improvement efforts that require an inexpensive in-house registry capability.

DATA SYSTEM CHARACTERISTICS

Data Reliability

Electronic medical records, decision support systems, survey reporting systems, executive information systems, cost accounting systems, and quality management/performance systems all utilize data elements that come from somewhere to be stored in electronic databases. For example, the data most hospitals collect for profiling and administrative analysis comes from standard forms (produced when patients are admitted and discharged from the hospital or receive professional services in an outpatient setting). They usually contain demographic data about the patient (birth date, sex, race, discharge status), codes for several diagnoses and procedures, and total charges aggregated by type of service, such as pharmacy, laboratory, and radiology. These data typically contain no clinical results, nor do they include any measures of the patient's satisfaction or functional status before or after treatment.

How good is the quality of claims data? Not very. Investigators have consistently found serious quality problems in large federal and insurance claims databases, including error rates and rates of discrepancy between similar databases. In a study of almost 13,000 patients hospitalized for cardiac catheterization, Jollis et al. (1993) found that "claims data failed to identify more than one-half of patients with prognostically important conditions." The authors concluded that "insurance claims data lack important diagnostic and prognostic information when compared with concurrently collected clinical data in the study of ischemic heart disease" (1993). A review of the 2006 durable medical equipment claims by the Inspector General of the Department of Health and Human

Services (HHS) indicated double-digit error rates in the claims involved, although the estimated rates varied widely depending on perceptions of the documentation required (Levinson, 2008). Overall, the review of fee-for-service Medicare claims for 2005 reported an error rate of 5.2% (a substantial improvement over prior years), although only 1.6% and 1.5%, respectively, were related to medical necessity or coding. Most of the rest related to quality of documentation (CMS, 2009).

Clinical trials have all kinds of built-in safeguards to ensure that the information produced is reliable. Similar considerations apply to quality improvement efforts, but hopefully with considerably less investment in control systems. Several types of reliability problems exist.

Observer (Measurement) and Recorder Error

Quality improvement teams are temporary systems whose members may or may not be skilled observers and data recorders. Teams may also have to depend on observers who are not team members. Management must make sure that the appropriate team members are trained to observe and record the relevant events and variables. They also should make sure that all those likely to become involved understand the CQI process and the importance of reliable data. This may also be backed up with validation of those data that are most critical in determining which alternative procedure to adopt.

All participants remain primarily involved with the demands of their usual duties. Therefore, management must make sure that current and potential team members understand that continuous improvement efforts will be a component of future performance evaluations (Zmud and McLaughlin, 1989).

Timeliness

Team leaders need to make sure that the data being used are timely. This is not likely to be a problem with data collected specifically for the study. However, caution is necessary when historical data are used. They must be associated with the current version of the process or they could be misleading.

Checking for Biases in Specification

Existing data are often collected for an intended use. They may be biased to favor the perceived interests of a group of individuals or institutions or for ease of collection. For example, "cost" data may be highly inflated to justify the prices charged and cost shifting. This is done in part by providing the average posted cost of a service rather than its incremental (or marginal) cost of production and by loading the estimates with very heavy overhead allocations. Negative results such as infection or readmission rates may be defined or manipulated to reduce their apparent frequency and to make everyone look better. Quality and process analyses will work effectively only if the data providers are both rigorous and unbiased.

Data Access

Even when data exist and are reliable, the team may have problems accessing them at the appropriate point of comparison. If all data come from within a specific work unit, this should not be as much of a problem as it is for interorganizational, intercommunity, and international comparisons. Yet many of the long-term payoffs in quality, efficiency, and effectiveness improvement require just such interorganizational comparisons (Herzlinger, 2007; Porter and Teisberg, 2006).

Comparability

Different organizations and national programs may use different definitions of seemingly identical variables. For example, comparison of the effectiveness of national folic acid supplementation programs to avoid neural tube defects in newborns had to recognize that reported incidence rates for spina bifida and other neural tube defects differed depending on the country's classification of pregnancy terminations and stillbirths (McLaughlin and McLaughlin, 2008). (See Case 13 in the companion casebook [McLaughlin et al., 2012].)

Transparency

If value improvement at the regional and national levels is to rest on more than avoiding medical errors and some duplicated costs, patients and payers must have access to de-identified, episode-of-care–based clinical and cost data. This will require a huge change from the culture of obfuscation that has dominated health care. We have referred earlier to biased data, but bigger problems relate to the general unavailability of relevant data and of sufficient information to interpret what is made available. Let's face it: both the enhancement of the professional mystique and the environment of cost shifting have been supported by the absence of reliable information. Transparency of cost and clinical quality are keys to effective and affordable care regardless of the means of organization or financing of care.

Interoperability

Care of an illness, even an acute one, seldom takes place under the control of a single entity. Patients move from primary care to specialty care and then back to community-based care and finally to personal care. Assessing the effectiveness of and improving any disease treatment or prevention process is best based on data from the whole episode of care. Records will exist in the pharmacy, office practice, hospital, home health agency, and so on. Outcomes cannot be assessed until one knows about subsequent medical events, often in a number of different settings. Intra-organizational movement of data is critical to coordination of acute care, but interorganizational movement of data is essential to chronic disease care and to health system improvement.

One of the most frustrating aspects of U.S. health care quality improvement is the lack of record linkages for interorganizational searching. Although virtually all quality improvement efforts that cross organizational lines can work well with de-identified data, linkage is still a problem. Until this problem is solved, there will be resistance to interorganizational searches that must now rely on identifiers such as patient name or Social Security number. While these may be legal under the Health Insurance Portability and Accountability Act (HIPAA), patient privacy advocates are legitimately concerned. This privacy problem has been frequently cited as an impediment to the survival of Regional Health Information Organizations (RHIOs) and certainly stands in the way of an effective National Health Information Network (NHIN).

National health systems elsewhere did not need to seek much information interorganizationally and avoided this problem. This may explain why the widespread implementation of HIT in many countries is ahead of the United States. Such systems can be justified not only on the basis of their impact on current clinical care but also on the use of the data for process oversight and improvement based on multisite and episode-of-care comparisons.

Whether it is accountability for decision making by consumers, payers, or large government agencies, patients and providers cannot be evaluated for their behavior or performance until we can aggregate data across relevant care settings and relate these to outcomes. The marketplace or even a nationalized system like the U.K. National Health Service can make appropriate decisions on provider selection, treatment recommendations, designing of decision support systems, and performance-based compensation only when data are available for valid comparisons.

STATISTICAL ANALYSIS

The purpose of collecting or extracting data in quality improvement is to analyze it for variation and help identify the root causes of undesired outcomes. The quality improvement team must develop early its specifications for data collection including the sampling strategy and analytical approaches to be applied.

Sampling

Critical to any sampling strategy is identification of the sampling frame, defined as the source of data for the key elements that are to be analyzed and from which a sample is to be taken in order to make inferences about the larger population of interest, such as the medical care database from the institution whose quality we are assessing. Likewise, the strategy should include the specific sampling methodology that is to be used and how often sample elements will be collected. Also critical to successful sampling strategies is careful determination of sample size. Sample size is always important because it plays a role in determining precision of estimates of quality metrics and also directly affects study cost estimates (Levy and Lemeshow, 2008). Our experience is that the first thing that often happens is that the designers overestimate the prevalence of the phenomenon being studied and hence underestimate the cost of finding enough affected individuals. When the recruitment of participants lags, the perception that the budget is fixed leads to a reduction in those cases surveyed, often jeopardizing what conclusions might be reached. The team must test those prevalence assumptions early on and plan realistically; one of the ways this can be accomplished is through the use of smaller "pilot" studies prior to carrying out the final survey. Interorganizational access to data could make the task of assessing prevalence much easier as well.

Analytical Approaches

There are a number of possibilities for data analysis using transactional data as well as specialized registries. The gold standard of the quality world has been statistical quality control, often epitomized by control charts. There are several options for carrying out quality control and quality improvement analyses, starting with classical statistics.

Classical Statistics

Biostatistics, epidemiology, systems analysis, and quality control are all rooted in classical statistical methods and have measurement and analysis of variation as a central component. As Deming (1986) pointed out, there are two types of variation: inherent variation due to the underlying process when under control, and unnecessary variation. Wennberg and colleagues have often used the term *unwarranted variation* in referring to the latter type (Mullan, 2004). Health care has a much higher level of inherent variation than most sectors because patients vary so much due to natural factors and there is much underlying lack of knowledge about causal factors (Bohmer, 2009). Moreover, great variation is introduced by patient preferences, physician training and preferences, service availability, and financial incentives (Wennberg et al., 1982), all of which are malleable over time. A further detailed discussion of causes of variation is presented in Chapter 3.

Event Analysis

Much of what observers call control charts are really run charts—charts reporting events and their frequency over time to see whether they coincide with an intervention. Even when control limits are reported, they tend to be symmetrical and set to an arbitrary level of three sigma, as a measure of "acceptable" variation, whereas most health care variables have asymmetrical consequences and may warrant more sophisticated calculations of their applicable control limits. However, it is very useful to follow trends in data and identify the time of pattern changes to see what is affecting them and by how much, and control charts serve that purpose. Examples of these types of analyses are presented in Chapter 3.

Data Mining

Large databases can be studied in a number of ways, including case finding and analysis of correlations between treatments and outcomes, interventions and process changes, and so on. While the gold standard of health care is the randomized double-blind clinical trial, access to very large databases involving relevant data from much of the population can ultimately serve many of the same quality improvement purposes at much lower costs. This is especially important in the currently weakly motivated arena of postmarketing surveillance for therapies and procedures. The potential of data mining using available information is currently presaged by the use of shared data at the national and international levels for purposes of biosurveillance.

For example, on November 12, 2008, Google announced development of an early warning system, Flu Trends. This system analyzed the geographic origins of Google search requests from the general public for information about flu-like symptoms and reported significant changes in levels of search behavior by state. The Google system was reported to offer a 2-week lead-time advantage over the Centers for Disease Control and Prevention (CDC) bioterrorism intelligence system based on reports from hospitals, laboratories, public health departments, and clinics (Helft, 2008). Google's system apparently took less than 2 years to develop.

Data mining is already used by many actors in health care, including the Centers for Medicare and Medicaid Services (CMS) and state governments for fraud and abuse studies; by health plans to evaluate providers and care approaches; by Quality Improvement Organizations (QIOs) to identify outliers (see Chapter 15); by corporate human resources departments to indentify high-risk employees; and by hospitals to determine how to personalize services for customer satisfaction (Gerver and Barrett, 2006; Giannangelo, 2007; Youngstrom, 2010). However, it is still in its infancy with respect to identifying population-specific responses to treatment alternatives and other efforts to provide the evidence for evidence-based clinical action.

PRESENTATION

Having results is not the final step in process improvement. Many good recommendations end up on the shelf because the implementers have been unable to convince management and their peer implementers to change the way care is delivered (Tufte, 2007). Other chapters of this text deal extensively with the efforts necessary to set the stage for and motivate change based on a team's findings or reports of improved outcomes elsewhere. Some individuals will be impressed with tables, some with graphs, and some with diagrams. Study data should be maintained in a data structure that can be addressed readily by the organization's standard data presentation packages. This encourages team members to experiment with presentation modes without extensive investments in training. Where time permits, the organization's basic CQI training packages should include exercises in effective presentation.

PATIENT PRIVACY

The many benefits of HIT are usually accompanied by concerns about potential loss of privacy, even when permitted by the HIPAA legislation. Certainly, efforts to allow aggregation of records across organizations will increase the concern levels of privacy advocates. Any attempts to limit use of even de-identified data by requiring specific patient permission for each use would be a major threat to data mining and similar efforts. Ownership of health information is still debated. For example, **Table 12–1** shows one active proposal for a patient's Data Bill of Rights. The fourth point might or might not preclude use without specific authorization.

TABLE 12–1 A Declaration of Health Data Rights

In an era when technology allows personal health information to be more easily stored, updated, accessed, and exchanged, the following rights should be self-evident and inalienable. We the people:

1. Have the right to our own health data
2. Have the right to know the source of each health data element
3. Have the right to take possession of a complete copy of our individual health data, without delay, at minimal or no cost; if data exist in computable form, they must be made available in that form
4. Have the right to share our health data with others as we see fit

These principles express basic human rights as well as essential elements of health care that is participatory, appropriate, and in the interests of each patient. **No law or policy should abridge these rights.**

Source: Retrieved September 18, 2009, from http://www.HealthDataRights.org.

A group of experts assembled by the Markle Foundation and others has suggested the following policy in conjunction with the enhanced privacy requirements of ARRA-HITECH.

> The likelihood of failure for different security systems is often unknown because the system can be attacked by a variety of means. A determined attacker with massive computational power may find a gap in the defenses. The most robust security systems will use a layered approach to data security that incorporates hashing, encryption, and limits on the amount of data that is disclosed. Data at rest should be encrypted or hashed, and the digital connection along which the data is shared should also be encrypted. Whenever possible, PHI (patient health information) should be subjected to a one-way hash prior to being shared with another party. Parties that seek data, like researchers, should specify the purpose to which the data will be put and collect only data needed to accomplish that purpose. (Connecting for Health, 2009)

That requirement for prior specification might create considerable problems for those contemplating data mining efforts, for example, to find medical errors or identify unanticipated long-term side effects of treatments.

HIT IMPACT AT VARIOUS AGGREGATION LEVELS

Individual Applications

Gawande (2007) suggests that the keys to maintaining the highest quality in one's own practice are to select a process, measure its progress over time, and then share the results with others. Comparing one's work with one's peers is also considered a most effective way of motivating process change. Johnson and Batalden (see Chapter 13) argue for training professionals to measure and evaluate the performance of their own microsystems. Hopefully, those trained will find such efforts supported by their local HIT systems.

Some subspecialty certification boards now mandate participation in ongoing quality improvement efforts as a requirement for achieving and maintaining certification (www.abms.org/Maintenance_of_Certification/ MOC_competencies.aspx). (See Case 12 in the companion casebook [McLaughlin et al., 2012].) If this is to be facilitated by the HIT system, that system must include the capacity to readily follow a set of cases abstracted from the practice's routine records, augmented by additional variables and observations. Therefore, the HIT systems at each level of the organization, from the individual practice on up, must have an easily established and accessed registry capability.

Registries

As introduced earlier, a registry is a list of patients with a specific set of attributes, usually a disease or a predisposition to a disease. It can be used for comparative analysis and for the improvement of care. Ortiz (2006) reports on how to build and use a simple registry, using the example of following a practice's diabetics using Microsoft Excel, assuming one lacks an electronic health record (EHR) system with that capability. He notes that the motivation for developing a diabetes registry was to meet his central organization's requirements for improvements in chronic disease monitoring and care.

Ortiz reports that the "conditional formatting" function of Excel is to generate "what if" conditions. For example, if the diabetic's A1c values are above a defined level, the cell for that patient in the A1c column changes color, signaling a call for action.

Ortiz points out that while this system is simple, its most difficult task is case-finding from existing patient records and then entering the initial patient data. He discusses the special motivational efforts taken to involve the staff in registry design and gradually building the database. An EHR system that extracts this information automatically and responds to cues such as lab reports operates more easily and reliably. The application that he describes, however, underlines the importance of registries to the improvement of care at the individual level and at the organizational level.

Organizational Applications

Most market-based recommendations for health care reform rely on competition to force delivery organizations to become more effective and efficient. Often they point to integrated delivery organizations as the ideal model. One advantage of integrated delivery organizations is that their information systems can often access many aspects of an episode of care without special record linkage efforts. The further assumption of many of these recommendations is that there is a management structure employing the providers, one which can use the information system to compare processes and outcomes and take action accordingly.

As Bohmer (2009) notes, the more scientific certainty applicable to a health care process, the more an empowered management can apply an industrial model. One aspect of that industrial model is built-in process control. According to Bohmer:

> This change . . . has been accompanied by a change in the role of the "artist." Once central to the creation of the product, professionals now design and oversee processes and manage exceptions—new roles requiring no less expertise. Pilots, for example, once responsible for flying the plane by hand-manipulating the control, now oversee the "automated cockpit." In many industries, the demands by regulators and consumers for increased reliability, safety, and efficiency—coupled with increased technological capability and increased stage-of-production knowledge—was a key drive of this transition. Exactly the same forces are currently at work in the health care industry, and it is therefore possible that the health care professionals will not be exempt from such a transition in roles and responsibilities. (p. 184)

However, Bohmer notes that what passes for "certainty" in health care processes is also transitory, and therefore, the organization must expend a great deal of energy on developing and maintaining its unlearning and learning processes. One indicator of the need for change can be the organization's continuing standing in the league tables of clinical quality and cost.

Communal Applications

Intra-organizational measurement and comparison have a key potential role in the control of health care costs. The group at Dartmouth that has mined the Medicare database to show very wide variations among the utilization and costs of care in the United States has calculated that reduced variation in physician judgment in discretionary settings could have a profound impact on U.S. health care costs, perhaps sufficient to make Medicare financially viable (Fisher et al., 2009; Sirovich et al., 2008).

Similar local databases would have considerable potential for studying intraregional differences and responses of other populations and subpopulations to specific treatment approaches. At some point, it may be possible to think of such data mining approaches as alternatives to double-blind clinical trials, if they include sufficiently large and representative populations.

A National Program

Concerns about quality and cost led the White House to issue a policy statement on HIT in April 27, 2004. In it, President Bush called for widespread adoption of interoperable EHRs within 10 years and established the Office of the National Coordinator for Health Information Technology (ONCHIT) in HHS by Executive Order 13335. ONCHIT funded a number of demonstration projects of RHIOs, which then might interact to form an NHIN. More than a hundred such organizations have been formed, but relatively few have found a viable long-term business model. Most such health information exchanges have relied primarily on grant funds and have been constrained by issues of privacy, funding, and cooperation by local institutions. Little is known about their actual impact in their communities, although they do have the opportunity to increase transparency and provide aggregate community performance data, heretofore available only from the CMS and other databases, which provide only limited data on limited populations or specific providers.

The act ties incentive payments (and ultimately reimbursement reductions) to physician adoption and use of certified, connected EHRs. The ONCHIT was permanently established and funded in 2009 as part of the ARRA–HITECH legislation and is continuing to fund efforts to establish and expand local, state, and national networks.

Electronic Health Records

The focus since the passage of the ARRA–HITECH legislation has been on the promotion of "meaningful use" of EHRs in both hospital and office practice settings that are interoperable. The federal government's interests in such systems are multiple and significant. David Blumenthal, MD, appointed to head ONCHIT in 2009, has outlined how the activities under the HITECH act are to contribute to health improvement. **Figure 12–6** illustrates a variety of efforts designed to promote adoption of EHRs and encourage or mandate exchange of information leading to meaningful use to accomplish the following (Blumenthal, 2009):

- Improve individual health outcomes
- Improve population health outcomes
- Increase transparency and efficiency
- Improve our ability to study and improve health care

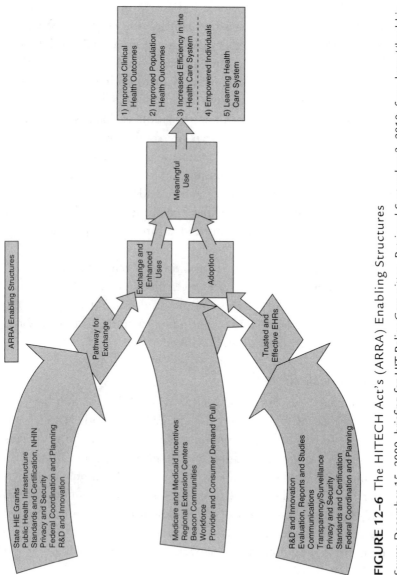

FIGURE 12–6 The HITECH Act's (ARRA) Enabling Structures

Source: December 15, 2009, briefing for HIT Policy Committee. Retrieved September 3, 2010, from http://healthit.hhs.gov/portal/server.pt/document/909919/blumenthaloncoverview121509.pt.

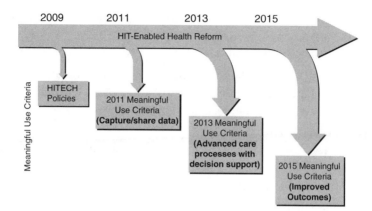

FIGURE 12–7 HIT-Enabled Health Care Reform

Source: Meaningful Use Workgroup Presentation to HIT Policy Committee on July 16, 2009. As presented by Paul Tang, Palo Alto Medical Foundation, Committee Chair, and George Hripcsak, Columbia University, Committee Co-Chair. Retrieved July 21, 2009, from http:// healthit.hhs.gov/portal/server.pt/document/876941/application_vnd_ms-powerpoint.

Clearly these all point toward CQI on a large scale backed up by expanded comparative effectiveness research and then by pay for performance expanded well beyond current levels. The "meaningful use" justification of compensation should encourage new entrants who offer modular, plug-and-play solutions as well as the vendors of customized systems and services based on earlier hospital information system technologies.

The newly formed HIT Policy Committee under ONCHIT has had the task of defining *meaningful use*, which is a prerequisite for HIT incentive payments. Their strategy as communicated in 2009 and 2010 was to let the use evolve over three stages as presented in **Figure 12–7** (Tang and Hripcsak, 2009).

Stage 1, planned for 2011, includes implementation of or capabilities for the following quality-related objectives, 15 of which are core and must be met, and another 10 are on a menu from which 5 must be met during stage 1. A partial list of core requirements includes the following (Kibbe, 2010):

- Electronically capturing health information in a coded format, including:
  - Electronic order entry and e-prescribing (starting with 30%, with some medications ordered using computerized physician order entry), and drug–drug and drug–allergy interaction checks

- Current active problem, medication, and medication allergy lists
- Demographic information
- Vital signs and smoking status
- Implementing at least one clinical decision support rule
- Reporting ambulatory clinical quality measures to CMS or the states
- Providing electronic clinical visit summaries and electronic copies of patient health records on request
- Being able to exchange key clinical information electronically with other providers
- Conducting or reviewing a security risk analysis and maintaining system security

Some of the menu set of objectives are (Kibbe, 2010):

- Sending reminders to patients
- Providing patients with timely electronic access to their medical records
- Providing patient-specific education resources
- Providing summary of care records when referring patients out and medication reconciliation for those coming in
- Incorporating test results as structured data and implementing drug-formulary checks
- Enabling the reporting of public health information
  - Immunizations reported to registries
  - Syndromic surveillance

The final rule incorporating the stage 1 objective and measures was published in the *Federal Register* on July 28, 2010 (DOC 75 FR 44314).

Stage 2, as originally planned for 2013, aims for electronic capture of health information and its use to track key clinical conditions automatically. The HIT information would be used for disease management, clinical decision support, medication management, patient access to health information, quality measurement and research, and bidirectional communication with health agencies. This would include:

- Computerized physician order entry for all orders
- Evidence-based data sets
- Decision support for many chronic conditions
- More registries for specialists

- Electronic prescribing with hospital discharge
- Prescription refill reminders and control
- Additional quality measure reporting including some relating to appropriateness of utilization

By the introduction of stage 3 in 2015, there would be much wider use of IT-driven clinical outcome measures, efficacy and safety measures, and more extensive automated quality reports, population-based performance measures, and HIT-enabled surveillance efforts. This stage would also involve greater patient access to self-management tools.

Overcoming Barriers

Much has been written about the slow uptake of HIT systems by providers. Some of this is due to the need for system improvement (Fernandopulle and Patel, 2010), but it is also clear that organizational change efforts are required along the lines required for CQI. For example, DeVore and Figlioli (2010) report the following:

- Processes must match the demands of the task at hand. They specifically cite the need to integrate and evaluate alerts and reporting requirements.
- Senior leadership is required for cultural change to be effective.
- Clinical champions are important to success.
- Medical staff training is needed to support the effort.
- Clear policies on how decisions are to be documented must be established.
- Budgeting must be flexible to support the changes.

Regional and National Networks

One issue that has yet to be addressed is whether the regional data should reside with one or more regional providers or in a freestanding data warehouse along the lines of those offered by Google and Microsoft, or whether the RHIO should supply the capacity to search out data on cue from regional providers using Web-based bridge software with a service-oriented architecture, such as dbMotion, which is in use in Israel and some U.S. medical centers. As time has gone by, the lack of a viable business model and technical problems with the warehouse approach seem to point toward Web-based solutions. Then there is the need for standards so that RHIOs are able to communicate with each other as components of any national network.

These networks have special relevance to biosurveillance. States and some communities as well as the federal government have been participating in a number of experiments with Web-based information systems to identify epidemics and other health threats as early as possible. The CDC has led the federal government efforts by connecting state laboratories and evaluating the intelligence information they produce and integrating it with intelligence from other sources. New York City has also been developing an extensive system to monitor data coming out of its facilities and a number of local practices.

Pay for Performance

Information technology plays a major role in the implementation of pay for performance (P4P). Activity levels have to be captured and reported. Ultimately, so will comparative outcomes. Given the current state of interoperability and multiple payers in the United States, it is difficult to implement a successful P4P system unless it is driven by a locally dominant payer. The importance attached to P4P as a value improvement tool is a major driver of the business case for HIT.

Most U.S. P4P systems are based on meeting internally set targets, although the U.K. P4P system within its unitary National Health Service, including EHR in primary care, is based on incremental levels of process improvement (McDonald and Roland, 2009). The same research indicates that P4P impact is quite sensitive to the availability of and design and implementation of the HIT system. One issue that McDonald and Roland raise is that the information system can present so many tasks to the provider that it begins to divert attention from the patient's concerns. What is possibly lost is the "doorknob" moment when the real reason for the visit or a significant snippet of information is allowed to surface. (See Case 14 in the companion casebook [McLaughlin et al., 2012].)

International Cooperation

So far international transfer of quality and cost information has been limited to highly aggregated information like that provided by the Organisation for Economic Co-operation and Development (OECD) for developed countries and by the World Health Organization (WHO).

There has, however, been much proprietary transfer of information for clinical trials and in specific international registries.

One area of considerable cooperation using Web-based technology has been in the area of biosurveillance. U.S. infectious disease surveillance systems, while embryonic, are still ahead of similar efforts in most other countries—particularly in the developing world—even though, as of 2007, some 23 U.S. states did not use national disease tracking standards. The CDC has employees working in more than 46 countries and is expanding its Global Disease Detection and Response Centers in China, Egypt, Guatemala, Kenya, and Thailand.

In 2000, the WHO launched the Global Outbreak Alert and Response Network (GOARN), which compiles global disease surveillance information from a wide range of official and unofficial sources. GOARN also includes a response network of more than 140 partner organizations around the world that move rapidly to contain disease outbreaks in their respective regions. Computerized, interoperable medical records anywhere could greatly facilitate the management of large-scale outbreaks of infectious disease.

The WHO relies on individual countries for information about outbreaks of infectious disease. In 2005, the member states negotiated a major revision of the International Health Regulations (IHR). These 2007 regulations affected how countries are to report and respond to major epidemics. The revised IHR contained three major innovations:

1. First, instead of having to report only three communicable diseases (plague, cholera, and yellow fever), the participating countries have to notify the WHO within 24 hours of *any* event that has the potential to become a public health emergency of international concern (PHEIC).

2. The term *PHEIC* has been more broadly defined to cover accidental or deliberate releases of biological, chemical, or radiological agents that could harm more than one country.

3. The WHO may draw on informal sources of information when identifying and investigating a possible PHEIC, in addition to official governmental sources.

The revised IHR also provided that within 5 years after the regulations would go into effect, all of the participating countries must establish the national surveillance capabilities needed to identify and report disease outbreaks of international concern (Grotto and Tucker, 2006).

Other multinational (often regional) tracking systems also follow influenza-like outbreaks, polio, immunization rates, enteric diseases, malaria, acute hemorrhagic fevers, antibiotic resistance, and sexually transmitted diseases (Hitchcock et al., 2007).

CONCLUSIONS

Effective quality improvement depends on quality data. This chapter has reviewed the steps in the data-to-decision cycle and its importance to national and international improvement efforts. There are great expectations for HIT, but there is still a long way to go before it is robust, representative, and accessible enough to reach that potential. Fortunately, many governments, including those of the United States, Australia, and the United Kingdom, are finally willing to make the investments necessary to reach the bulk of the population with such systems. Undoubtedly there will be mistakes and waste along the way, but understanding the role of information and information technology is becoming a requirement for professional effectiveness as well as the cornerstone of improved delivery efficacy throughout health care.

Cross-References to the Companion Casebook

(McLaughlin, C. P., Johnson, J. K., and Sollecito, W. A. [Eds.]. 2012. *Implementing Continuous Quality Improvement in Health Care: A Global Casebook*. Sudbury, MA: Jones & Bartlett Learning.)

Case Study Number	Case Study Title	Case Study Author
5	The Intermountain Way to Positively Impact Costs and Quality	*Lucy A. Savitz*
12	Quality in Pediatric Subspecialty Care	*William A. Sollecito, Peter A. Margolis, Paul V. Miles, Robert Perelman, Richard B. Colletti*
13	The Folic Acid Fortification Decision Bounces Around the World	*Curtis P. McLaughlin and Craig D. McLaughlin*
14	Continuing Improvement for the National Health Service Quality and Outcomes Framework	*Curtis P. McLaughlin*

REFERENCES

Blumenthal, D. 2009. Briefing meaningful use working group. Retrieved December 15, 2009, from http://healthit.hhs.gov/portal/server.pt/document/909918/blumenthalonc review121509.ppt

Bohmer, R. M. J. 2009. *Designing Care: Aligning the Nature and Management of Health Care.* Boston: Harvard Business Press.

Centers for Medicare and Medicaid Services. 2009. National Medicare FFS error rate. Retrieved March 30, 2011, from https://www.cms.gov/apps/er_report/preview_er_report.asp?from=public&which=long&reportID=15&tab=3

Connecting for Health. 2009. Guidance specifying the technologies and methodologies that render protected health information unusable, unreadable, or indecipherable to unauthorized individuals for purposes of breach notification requirements under the American Recovery and Reinvestment Act. Retrieved March 15, 2011, from http://www.connectingforhealth.org/resources/20090522_breach_methodologies.pdf

Deming, W. E. 1986. *Out of the Crisis.* Cambridge: Massachusetts Institute of Technology Center for Advanced Engineering Study.

DeVore, S. D., and Figlioli, K. 2010. Lessons premier hospitals learned about implementing electronic health records. *Health Aff,* 29(4): 664–667.

Fernandopulle, R., and Patel, N. 2010. How the electronic health record did not measure up to the demands of our medical home practice. *Health Aff,* 29(4): 622–628.

Fisher, E. S., Bynum, J. P., and Skinner, J. S. 2009. Slowing the growth of health care costs: Lessons from regional variation. *N Engl J Med,* 360(9): 849–852.

Gawande, A. 2007. *Better: A Surgeon's Note on Performance.* New York: Picador.

Gerver, H. M., and Barrett, J. 2006. Data mining-driven ROI: Health care cost management. *Benefits Compensation Web Exclusives,* 43(6): 1–5.

Giannangelo, K. 2007. Mining Medicare and Medicaid data to detect fraud. *J AHIMA,* 78(7): 66–67.

Grotto, A. J., and Tucker, J. B. 2006. Biosecurity: A comprehensive action plan. Retrieved March 15, 2011, from http://www.americanprogress.org/kf/biosecurity_a_comprehensive_action_plan.pdf

Helft, M. 2008, November 12. Google uses searches to track flu's spread, *New York Times*. Retrieved March 15, 2011, from http://www.nytimes.com/2008/11/12/technology/internet/12flu.html

Herzlinger, R. 2007, July 19. Where are the innovators in health care? *Wall Street Journal.* Retrieved March 15, 2011, from http://www.manhattan-institute.org/html/_wsj-where_are_the_innovators_in_health_care.htm

Hitchcock, P., Chamberlain, A., Van Wagoner, M., et al. 2007. Challenges to global surveillance and response to infectious disease outbreaks of international importance. *Biosecur Bioterror*, 5(3): 206–227.

Jollis J. G., Ancukiewicz, M., DeLong, E. R., et al. 1993. Discordance of databases designed for claims payment versus clinical info systems: Implications for outcomes research. *Ann Intern Med*, 119(8): 844–850.

Kibbe, D. C. 2010. A physician's guide to the Medicare and Medicaid EHR incentive program: The basics. *Fam Pract Manage*, 17(5): 17–21.

Levinson, D. R. 2008. *Medical Review of Claims for the Fiscal Year 2006 Comprehensive Error Rate Testing Program.* Washington, DC: Office of Inspector General, Department of Health and Human Services, A-01-07-00508.

Levy, P. S., and Lemeshow, S. 2008. *Sampling of Populations: Methods and Applications* (4th ed.). New York: John Wiley & Sons.

McDonald, R., and Roland, M. 2009. Pay for performance in primary care in England and California: Comparison of unintended consequences. *Ann Fam Med*, 7: 121–127.

McLaughlin, C. P., Johnson, J. K., and Sollecito, W. A. (Eds.). 2012. *Implementing Continuous Quality Improvement in Health Care: A Global Casebook.* Sudbury, MA: Jones & Bartlett Learning.

McLaughlin, C. P., and McLaughlin, C. D. 2008. *Health Policy Analysis: An Interdisciplinary Approach.* Sudbury, MA: Jones & Bartlett Publishers.

Mullan, F. 2004. Wrestling with variation: An interview with Jack Wennberg. *Health Aff Web Exclusive*, DOI 10.1377/hlthaff.var.73, pp. VAR-73–VAR-80.

Ortiz, D. D. 2006. Using a simple patient registry to improve your chronic disease care. *Fam Pract Manage*, 13(4): 47–48, 51–52.

Porter, M. E. 2009. A strategy for health care reform: Toward a value-based system, *N Engl J Med*, 361(2): 109–112.

Porter, M. E., and Teisberg, E. O. 2006. *Redefining Health Care: Creating Value-Based Competition on Results.* Boston: Harvard Business School Press.

Sirovich, B., Gallagher, P. M., Wennberg, D. E., et al. 2008. Discretionary decision making by primary care physicians and the cost of U.S. health care. *Health Aff,* 27(3): 813–823.

Tang, P., and Hripcsak, G. 2009. Meaningful use workgroup presentation (slide 6). HIT Policy Committee. Retrieved March 30, 2011, from http://healthit.hhs.gov/portal/server.pt?open=512&objID =1269&parentname=CommunityPage&parentid=5&mode=2

Tufte, E. R. 2007. *Visual Explanations: Images and Quantities, Evidence and Narrative.* Cheshire, CT: Graphics Press.

Wennberg, J. E., Barnes, B. A., and Zuboff, M. 1982. Professional uncertainty and the problem of supplier-induced demand. *Soc Sci Med,* 16: 811–824.

Youngstrom, N. 2010. AHIMA: Physician query constraints should be same for coders and clinical documentation improvement specialists. Atlantic Information Service reprinted from *Report on Medicare Compliance,* March 26.

Zmud, R., and McLaughlin, C. P. 1989. "That's not my job": Managing secondary tasks effectively. *Sloan Manage Rev,* 10(2 Winter): 29–37.

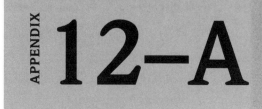

Example of HIT CQI Recommendations: Measuring Health Care Quality—Obstacles and Opportunities[1]

SPECIFIC FINDINGS AND RECOMMENDATIONS

1: Test Results

Create a mechanism for reporting selected inpatient and outpatient laboratory results in a standard transaction.

2: Vital Signs/Objective Data

Create a mechanism for reporting selected vital signs (e.g., blood pressure) and objective data measurements (height/weight and body mass index) on inpatient encounters and outpatient visits in a standard transaction.

---

1 *Source*: Proposed in May 2004, *Workgroup on Quality, National Committee on Vital and Health Statistics*. Retrieved March 15, 2011, from http://www.ncvhs.hhs.gov/040531rp.pdf.

3: Secondary Admission Diagnosis Flag

Facilitate the reporting of a diagnosis modifier to flag diagnoses that were present on admission on secondary diagnosis fields in all inpatient claims transactions.

4: Operating Physician

Require the existing data element for operating physician to be reported for the principal inpatient procedure.

5: Dates and Times for Admission and Procedures

Modify the requirements for reporting the admission date/time and procedure date/time data elements to include both date and time for admission and for selected procedures on the institutional claim transaction. Encourage NQF and others to identify the procedures for which these data elements would be required.

6: Episode Start and End Dates for Global Procedure Codes

Encourage payers to modify their billing instructions to providers to align procedure start and end dates with services included in selected global procedure codes in standard HIPAA claims transactions.

7: Functional Status Coding

Review the available options for coding patients' functional status in administrative transactions, electronic health records (EHRs), and other clinical data sets, and recommend standard approaches.

8: Functional Status Reporting

Create a mechanism for reporting functional status codes in a standard transaction.

9: Adequate Benchmarking Data

Develop survey-sampling approaches that can ensure the availability of adequate benchmarking data at the state and metropolitan area levels and for racial and ethnic subpopulations.

10: Standard Survey Items for the Same Quality Measures

Standardize currently inconsistent items that are used to report the same measure of quality (e.g., immunization and screening rates, functional status) across federal surveys. Coordinate with states and private sector quality measurement/oversight organizations on the adoption of common items across federal, state, and private sector surveys.

REDUCING DISPARITIES IN HEALTH AND HEALTH CARE

11: Race/Ethnicity Data for All Insured

Modify existing mechanisms for reporting race and ethnicity of subscribers and dependents on the HIPAA enrollment transaction.

12: Race/Ethnicity Data for Patients

Investigate how best to capture race and ethnicity on a standard provider transaction.

13: Primary Language

Modify existing mechanisms for reporting the primary language of both subscribers and dependents on the HIPAA enrollment transaction.

BUILDING THE DATA AND INFORMATION INFRASTRUCTURE TO SUPPORT QUALITY

14: Standard Clinical Terminologies

Adopt standard clinical terminologies, including a "crosswalk" or meta-thesaurus of clinical synonyms that can be used to consistently identify and describe clinical conditions, procedures, treatments, and outcomes across electronic health records, administrative data, and provider and patient surveys.

15: Common Patient Vocabulary

Promote the identification of lay terms that represent synonyms for standard clinical terms and that are easily comprehensible to patients of different cultures and educational attainment. Include these lay terms in the "crosswalk" or meta-thesaurus of clinical synonyms described above.

16: Expansion of Standard Clinical Codes for Diagnoses

Adopt *ICD-10-CM* for coding and classification of diagnosis and health conditions in administrative transactions.

17: Mapping of Standard Clinical Codes for Procedures

Create a mechanism for efficiently mapping procedure codes across current and proposed HIPAA standard coding systems to facilitate querying and aggregating procedure information across care settings.

18: Clinical Decision Support

Standard functionality requirements for electronic health records should include clinical decision support (e.g., guideline-driven data entry templates, reminders, prompts, and alerts), to facilitate the planning and delivery of evidence-based care to individual patients and groups.

19: Population-Based Query and Reporting

- EHRs should employ uniform data standards for core content and data storage formats to facilitate population health surveillance and reporting functions.
- EHRs should include functionality that "supports continuous quality improvement, utilization review, risk management, and performance monitoring."

20: Interoperability of Clinical Data Systems

Develop standards for interoperability of electronic clinical data systems and EHRs, and adopt a core set of output record formats that EHRs should be capable of exporting and importing to support care coordination and QA/QI.

21: Standard Provider Identifiers

HHS should recommend the adoption of the NPI as a consistent provider identifier in clinical data systems, EHRs, provider surveys, and clinical record and reporting formats, as well as in HIPAA transactions. HHS should implement this recommendation within all federally funded health information systems.

22: Voluntary Patient Identifier or Identifier Logic

Develop a voluntary, standardized patient identifier or patient identifier logic that, when authorized by the patient, can be used to link health care records for the same patient across payers, providers, and care settings.

BALANCING PATIENTS' INTERESTS IN QUALITY AND CONFIDENTIALITY

23: Clarify Privacy Protections

- Examine privacy protections under existing federal law that inhibit access to and linkage of patient records across payers, providers, and care settings for the purposes of care coordination and management and quality assessment and improvement.
- Revise and/or clarify current regulations to reduce these obstacles, while effectively balancing the best interests of patients and populations.

Applications

CHAPTER 13

Educating Health Professionals to Improve Care Within the Clinical Microsystem

Julie K. Johnson and Paul B. Batalden

"All health professionals should be educated to deliver patient-centered care as members of an interdisciplinary team, emphasizing evidence-based practice, quality improvement approaches, and informatics."

—A vision for health professions education, articulated by the Institute of Medicine, 2003

In 2003, the Institute of Medicine (IOM) in the United States articulated a landmark vision for health professions education (IOM, 2003). This guiding vision is in contrast to the growing realization that preparing learners to function within an interdisciplinary team stops short of the more accurate statement of the need, which is for learners to function within the "clinical microsystem."

The purpose of this chapter is to define frameworks for how best to educate and train professionals to work within the evolving delivery system as well as to improve the quality and safety of patient care. This chapter begins with a brief background on health professions education and then explores health professional development from the perspective of three quality improvement strategies—organization-centered, issue-centered, and clinical microsystem–centered strategies.

BACKGROUND

In 2001, the IOM published a report, *Crossing the Quality Chasm: A New Health System for the 21st Century*. This report was a culmination of the work of the Committee on the Quality of Health Care in America, which was formed in 1998 (IOM, 2001). Among many points, the committee acknowledged that most health professionals have had limited education in extracting information directly from their own practice experience and using it to redesign their everyday care systems. The committee recommended that strategies be developed for:

> (1) restructuring clinical education to be consistent with the prin-
> ciples of the 21st century health system throughout the continuum
> of undergraduate, graduate, and continuing education for medical,
> nursing, and other professional training programs and (2) assessing
> the implications of these changes for provider credentialing programs,
> funding, and sponsorship of education programs for health profes-
> sionals. (IOM, 2001)

The committee also recommended that an interdisciplinary summit be held to develop next steps for the reform of health professions education to enhance patient care quality and safety. This summit was convened in June 2002.

The calls for educational reform and the work of the interdisciplinary summit were based on several points (IOM, 2003):

- Health professionals (e.g., physicians, nurses, health administrators) are not adequately prepared—in either academic or continuing education venues—to address shifts occurring in the U.S. patient population such as changes in diversity, aging of the population, increasing incidence of chronic illnesses, and improved access to health information.
- Once in practice, health professionals are expected to work as part of interdisciplinary teams, yet they have not been trained as part of an interdisciplinary team and often lack team-based skills. (See Case 1 in the companion casebook [McLaughlin et al., 2012].)

- There is a rapidly expanding evidence base for making health care decisions, but there is a lack of consistency in training about how to search and evaluate the evidence base and how to apply it to practice.
- There is a mismatch between what is known about quality and safety of care and the coursework that is available to health professions students regarding how to assess quality and safety-of-care information and how to design and test solutions.
- There is no basic foundation of training on informatics.

The committee concluded by recommending a set of "core competencies" that all health professionals should acquire during training, regardless of their discipline. These competencies include (1) providing patient-centered care, (2) working in interdisciplinary teams, (3) employing evidence-based practice, (4) applying quality improvement, and (5) using informatics.

Many organizations in the United States that govern medical education—from medical schools through the medical specialty boards—and nursing education focused on identifying these core competencies and what they mean for professional education in their field. For instance, the Accreditation Council for Graduate Medical Education, in increasing its focus on educational outcome assessment in residency programs, identified and endorsed six general competencies that residents must demonstrate—patient care, medical knowledge, practice-based learning and improvement, professionalism, interpersonal skills and communication, and systems-based practice (Accreditation Council for Graduate Medical Education, 2007). Physician specialty boards (e.g., the American Board of Pediatrics and the American Board of Internal Medicine) under the auspices of the American Board of Medical Specialties followed suit, recognizing the need for physicians to demonstrate core competencies both as part of their initial specialty certification and for ongoing maintenance of that time-limited certification. (See Case 12 in the companion casebook [McLaughlin et al., 2012].) Specifically, competency would be measured through an evaluation of clinical practice according to specialty-specific standards for patient care and by demonstrating an ability to assess the quality of care provided compared to peers and national benchmarks. Physicians would then apply the best evidence or consensus recommendations to improve care using follow-up assessments (American Board of Medical Specialties, 2006).

In 2005, the Robert Wood Johnson Foundation funded a project, Quality and Safety Education for Nurses (QSEN), to address the challenges in preparing prelicensure nurses with the core competencies to graduate with the knowledge, skills, and attitudes necessary to continuously improve the quality and safety of the health care systems within which they work (Cronenwett et al., 2007). The effects of these efforts are more fully described in Chapter 17.

Until recently, the concept of acquiring, demonstrating, and maintaining core competencies presented new challenges to health professions education. For example, although most residency programs focused on providing physicians with substantial training in patient care and medical knowledge, only a few exposed residents to systems-based practice and practice-based learning and improvement (Eliastam and Mizrahi, 1996; Mohr, Randolph, et al., 2003; Ogrinc et al., 2004; Weingart, 1996, 1998). Developing these two competencies challenged residency programs to find innovative ways to integrate quality improvement and systems thinking into training and evaluation. More recent literature suggests that academic leaders have risen to this challenge by actively engaging residents in clinical quality improvement initiatives (Batalden and Davidoff, 2007; Berwick and Finkelstein, 2010; Boonyasai et al., 2007; Patow et al., 2009). On the whole, it appears that many of these efforts have been more effective in teaching quality improvement skills than in improving patient outcomes.

Another challenge has been how best to address the "silos" of organizational quality improvement and residency education. In 2007, the Alliance of Independent Medical Centers started an 18-month program for 19 organizational members to organize quality improvement teams focused on individual quality improvement projects strategically aligned with their hospital's specific improvement goals (Daniel et al., 2009; Patow, 2009). A unique approach was to develop a new residency program, as demonstrated by the Dartmouth-Hitchcock Medical Center (DHMC) Leadership Preventive Medicine residency, which combines 2 years of leadership preventive medicine with another DHMC residency training program. The aim of the program is to train physicians to lead change and improvement of the systems they work within (Foster et al., 2008).

THE PROCESS OF PROFESSIONAL PREPARATION AND DEVELOPMENT

Health professionals have long been proud of their personal commitment to lifelong learning and to their role as leaders in the design and delivery of health care. The exact process varies for each professional discipline, but at a high level, the processes resemble one another and can be illustrated with the case of medicine. The process can be described by the categories of formal educational preparation:

- *Basic health professional preparation* leading to an MD degree
- *Graduate health professional preparation* leading to time-limited specialty certification
- *Postgraduate health professional preparation* for continuing medical education and maintenance of certification

Each step of the process has a defined content of learning. That definition of content has been based on some expert assessment of what is known, what is appropriate for the learner at this stage of his or her preparation, and what the profession in general has established as knowledge needed for competency as a professional at that stage of development. State, national, and professional exams have been designed to assess the candidate's knowledge and skills at that level. Although training is focused on the individual within the profession, in reality it has been a long time since we have had a model of care in which a patient is cared for by only one professional; multiple professionals interact to meet the patient's needs. Essentially, we have gone from a ratio of one professional to one patient to a ratio of many professionals to one patient (Batalden et al., 2006). This evolution has implications for the quality and safety of patient care as well as for the training of the health professional.

While everyone seeking professional training goes through the same formal education process, each person also progresses through an individually unique process of skill and knowledge development. The Dreyfus model, developed by brothers Stuart Dreyfus and Hubert Dreyfus, suggests five stages—novice, advanced beginner, competent, proficient, and expert. This model was developed based on work commissioned by the U.S. Air Force to describe the development of the knowledge and skill of a pilot. They later identified a similar process of development in the chess

Explorer:	What is the role all about?
Novice:	What are the rules that can help me?
Advanced beginner:	What do I need to remember about the setting/context for care?
Competent:	What goes into a good plan for the care of this patient?
Proficient:	How can I get some of the waste out of my life?
Expert:	What complex cases do you have for me?
Master:	What can I learn from the surprise that just happened to me?

FIGURE 13-1 The Modified Dreyfus Model of Skill Acquisition

player, the adult learning a second language, the adult learning to drive an automobile, and many other scenarios (Dreyfus and Dreyfus, 1986). We adapted the model to reflect lifelong professional development and added two additional stages: explorer and master. (See **Figure 13-1**.)

For example, when applied to medicine in the *explorer stage*, the premedical student is making decisions about whether to pursue medicine as a career. In the *novice stage*, the freshman medical student begins to learn the process of taking a history and memorizes the elements, chief complaint, and history of the present illness, review of systems, and family and social history. In the *advanced beginner stage*, the junior medical student begins to see aspects of common situations, such as those facing hospitalized patients (e.g., admission, rounds, discharge) that cannot be defined objectively apart from concrete situations and can only be learned through experience. Maxims emerge from that experience to guide the learner. In the *competent stage*, the resident physician learns to plan the approach to each patient's situation. Risks are involved, but supervisory practices are put in place to protect the patient. Because the resident has planned the care, the consequences of the plan are knowable to the resident and offer the resident an opportunity to learn. In the *proficient stage*, the specialist physician early in practice struggles with developing routines that can streamline the approach to the patient. Managing the multiple distracting stimuli in a thoughtful way is intellectually and emotionally absorbing. In the *expert stage*, the midcareer physician has learned to recognize patterns of discrete clues and to move quickly, using what he or she might call "intuition" to do the work. The physician is attuned to distortions in patterns and knows to slow down when things don't fit an expected pattern. The *master* works explicitly, and with curiosity, on the system of expertise (Batalden et al., 2002).

Initial professional formation occurs within disciplinary channels, even though health professionals of varying disciplines usually work together. Furthermore, health professions education does not occur in isolation. It occurs within a particular context—the organization in which formative professional development occurs. In combining the existing process of preparation of the health professional with the newly defined core competencies of health professionals, we must consider how the formative processes of health professional development and the *context* of the setting—that is, the organization and delivery of patient care—can interact and adapt to deployment strategies for the continual improvement of health and health care.

The relevance of the context cannot be overlooked. Heclo suggests that we operate as if individuals act without context and as if the context does not matter. Furthermore, he says that we think of professional work as "role-playing" rather than "office occupying." He goes back to the now somewhat archaic idea that priests, rabbis, physicians, nurses, and so on have all occupied certain "offices" and that such offices were designed in relation to the work. "Occupying" such an office meant that the whole person—head, hand, and heart—was part of the proposition. It is not enough to "play" a role or a part, or to wear a costume or mask (Heclo, 2008). These concepts relate to the following sections on specific strategies for improving quality and safety at different levels of the organization.

TAKING ACTION FOR IMPROVED QUALITY AND SAFETY—ORGANIZATION-CENTERED, ISSUE-CENTERED, AND MICROSYSTEM-CENTERED STRATEGIES

Traditionally, there has been an organization-centered and an issue-centered deployment strategy for continual improvement of quality and value of health care. Both have specific implications for health professional development—and each has strengths as well as important vulnerabilities (Batalden, 1998). This chapter explores these strategies. We also add a third strategy to the mix by considering the role of the clinical microsystem and outlining the contribution that it can make in training health professionals for quality improvement.

Organization-Centered Strategies

Organization-centered improvement in health care has been alive in the United States for several decades, ever since the American College of Surgeons began accrediting hospitals (Brennan and Berwick, 1996). The macro-organization became the unit of attention when health care organizations, particularly hospitals, began to explore the lessons of continual improvement that were being learned concurrently in other sectors. In 1980, new visibility for organization-wide efforts to improve quality came from the public television documentary *If Japan Can, Why Can't We?* (Dobyns and Crawford Mason, 1991). Early visibility in the United States for "company-wide quality" (Mizuno, 1988) or "total quality" came in manufacturing settings, most prominently in the automotive sector. By the mid-1980s, efforts were underway in health care in the Alliant Hospital System in Kentucky and the Hospital Corporation of America in Nashville, Tennessee (McEachern and Neuhauser, 1989; Walton, 1990). Many more in health care became interested as the Joint Commission on the Accreditation of Healthcare Organizations and subsequently the National Committee on Quality Assurance incorporated this thinking into accreditation processes. Important characteristics of the organization-centered strategy include a focus on the context for work; knowledge of work as a system/process; attention to patients, payers, and communities as beneficiaries or customers; the leader's role in promoting learning; and organizational networks. These features are described next.

Focus on the Context for Work

Efforts were made to clarify what it meant to engage quality as a business or organizational strategy, including work on organizational policy statements of mission, values, and vision to create visibility for the objectives of continual improvement of services and products. These efforts were aimed at fostering a work environment that recognized and celebrated the value of learning at work. Deming wrote a set of guidelines for Western management, widely known as "Deming's fourteen points," (see Chapter 1), that were extensively studied as descriptive of a workplace that was to be encouraged (Deming, 1986). Health care versions of these points were made, referred to as "adaptation of the 14 points to medical service," and they facilitated study by health professionals and their organizations (Deming, 1986). Deming's system of "profound knowledge" (or, as we have known it, "improvement knowledge") couples subject matter with disciplinary knowledge, and together they work to enable continual improvement (Batalden and Stoltz, 1993; Deming, 1993).

Knowledge of Work as a System/Process

Building on and complementing the work of many general systems thinkers (Ackoff, 1981; Bertalanffy, 1968; Brockman, 1977; Checkland, 1981; Churchman, 1971; Forrester, 1990; Mitroff and Linstone, 1993), Deming offered a view of the work of organizations as a system that explicitly involved the recipient of service as part of the system of production and, as proposed, was a system capable of continual improvement (Deming, 1986). Adaptations of this model were made and used in health care (Batalden and Stoltz, 1993; Batalden and Mohr, 1997). With the focus on health care as a system and process came adaptations of process and system change strategies in the form of projects where, in many cases, the people leading the change had never been active in those roles. This newfound opportunity gave them additional pride in their work. Tribes grew up around particular improvement methods and approaches. The language of one approach was sometimes difficult for others to understand; it was easier to classify the label than to understand its relationship to the underlying phenomenon. Sometimes the proprietary interests of authoring individuals and organizations got in the way of dissemination and critical methods analysis. Some evaluation efforts were aimed at assessing what happened when people were engaged in "doing quality improvement" rather than seeing "improving the quality of what you do" as a key aspect of work. Despite these limitations, these new methods and skills for understanding and changing health care in usual practice settings gained visibility.

Attention to Patients, Payers, and Communities as "Beneficiaries" or "Customers"

The focus on the design and delivery of patient care required better understanding of personal preferences, values, and aims of the person receiving that care. This requirement is aligned with Deming's model of a system that includes the customer or recipient of the service. Many methods for creating the new knowledge and understanding were offshoots from the customer focus in sectors other than health care (Batalden and Nelson, 1990; Joint Commission on Accreditation of Healthcare Organizations, 1992; Nelson and Batalden, 1993). It was no longer a matter of patient relations or patient satisfaction, as it became clear that we needed more insight into our efforts to design care. Coping with the reality of multiple—and sometimes apparently conflicting—customer requirements placed health care alongside many other sectors with similar struggles. Including customers (i.e., patients) as part of the caregiving system along with the health care professionals invites a new understanding of what it means to be professional.

The Leader's Role in Promoting Learning

To bring these changes about, leaders had to move beyond "command and control" understandings of their own work (Taylor and Taylor, 1994). Work done by Argyris and Schön (Argyris, 1991; Argyris and Schön, 1996) expanded our understanding of what it meant to learn in the work setting. As introduced in Chapter 10, the work of Peter Senge and his colleagues at the Massachusetts Institute of Technology provided great visibility to the idea of a learning organization, identifying five disciplines as fundamental to the creation of such organizations (Senge, 1990; Senge et al., 1994).

Organizational Networks

The desire for opportunities to share learning that was under way in similar organizations led to the creation of multiple networks of organizations. For example, the Institute for Healthcare Improvement's Quality Management Network (QMN), the Group Practice Improvement Network (GPIN), the Healthcare Forum's Quality Improvement Networks (QINs), and the Hospital Corporation of America's Healthcare Quality Technology Network (HQTN) all had active, regular meetings and cross-network learning. These networks provided settings in which organizations and their leaders came together to share and accelerate their own efforts at organization-wide improvement.

Such organization-centered efforts led to positive changes in how we organize and deliver health care, but at the same time, other changes occurred in health care organizations that were toxic to the organization. Organizational definitions changed weekly with the flurry of new partnerships, mergers, acquisitions, divestitures, joint ventures, and so on, which added confusion and complexity at the level of the caregiving personnel, as new procedures for connecting their services emerged continuously. Old patterns of working wherever one wanted as a graduated medical specialist were supplanted by the need to go where there was work, as layoffs, cutbacks, and hiring freezes targeted oversupplied medical specialties. As documented in the Dartmouth Atlas of Health Care, there were huge variations in caregiving and health resource capacity, as measured by the number of beds, doctors, nurses, and caregiving practices per thousand population (Wennberg, 2010; Wennberg et al., 1996). These variations prompted many to ask why they were bearing the additional costs and morbidity experienced in their geographic region.

Furthermore, as comparable clinical outcomes were being documented, purchasers accelerated their pressures for cost reductions. With minimal agreement about measures of quality, assumptions that "all care is about the same, only the costs are different" led purchasers to engage in demand- or target-pricing strategies, whereby the purchaser tells the health plan how much less they will pay for their health care premiums the next year. These pressures further contributed to the disconnect between the senior leaders and the frontline caregivers who were being asked to work harder to achieve these external demands. This would have been of little consequence if real changes in the value and quality of care were not desired. However, real changes were sought by recipients of care and by those paying for care. They perceived that provider "unresponsiveness" was a matter of will, and they sought political, regulatory, or "contractual" relief.

At the same time, in fields unrelated to health care, we witnessed changes in the way manufacturing and service enterprises were led. Expectations about customer-driven design, process and system analysis, and improvement were built into the public's assumption structure. While the leaders in other sectors were often able to make these changes, it has been difficult for many leaders in health care to consider such changes as relevant and deserving of the same priority. Though we have learned the names and terms, we have had difficulty learning and incorporating the basic insights offered by Deming and others (Batalden and Stoltz, 1993; Deming, 1993). Some in health care recognize this requirement for new knowledge and its application (McLaughlin and Kaluzny, 1999). Market pressures and regulatory pressures have helped increase the recognition of the terms and the pace of such change.

Few macro-organizations engaged in both organization-wide improvement of patient care and health professions education combined the two initiatives. Each initiative seemed to have its own "home" within the organization. Strategic initiatives for improvement of care were much more common than strategic initiatives for professional education and development, and few common initiatives linked the improvement of patient care with professional development. Line leaders were more comfortable asking for accountability around patient care improvement than around professional development.

In summary, organization-centered strategies for the improvement of health care gave new emphasis and energy to many features of organization life that were helpful in improving quality. However, the fundamental realities that organizations of all kinds were becoming less stable, organization-wide efforts of all kinds were becoming less dependable, and "quality" was becoming only another theme for the harried top leaders left the unmistakable impression that complete dependency on organization-centered strategies for the improvement of health care quality left these efforts vulnerable. In addition, health care delivery is highly fragmented in ownership and control. In most hospitals, physicians are not employees, and in some communities, they can move their business among institutions at will. The reality is that at the macro-organization level, there is a limited ability to directly improve quality and value of care. Organizations do not provide the care; individual professionals do. It is the same phenomenon with professional education and development—macro-organizations do not "educate physicians and nurses"; people do. Furthermore, most individual health care professionals working in complex organizations do not provide care as individuals; they work together as part of interdependent systems.

Issue-Centered Strategies

Improving health care by finding topics or conditions that could be improved, conducting tests of change, and disseminating those efforts is as old as the application of empiricism to health care. What seemed new was the public identification of gaps between what was known and what was usually done coupled with strategies to accelerate closing those gaps. In his 1994 keynote address to the annual National Forum of the Institute for Healthcare Improvement, Donald Berwick, MD, challenged the group by naming specific conditions and clinical situations where the scientific evidence suggested one path for practice, and the increasingly available data about our common practices suggested that another path was in use, indicating a real performance gap. Later, these observations were prominently featured in a widely circulated medical journal (Berwick, 1994).

These observations arose from increasingly available comparative practice data made public by purchasers, private data companies, and public sources, including states. These data invited comparisons across provider settings and revealed wildly varying care processes and outcomes. Variation in care across small areas had been known for years (Wennberg and Gittlesohn, 1973). What was new was the extent of the variation and its significance for both clinical outcomes and costs (Wennberg et al., 1996).

Under the auspices of the Institute for Healthcare Improvement, a series of issue-specific efforts began in May 1995. This model brought together a panel of knowledgeable subject matter experts and a panel of people who had been able to make change in their practices. Together they developed a set of "change concepts" worth trying. Other teams of subject matter practitioners were invited to join a cooperative effort to rapidly test these concepts in their home settings and to compare experiences through closely networked communications and follow-up meetings. Their collective experiences were then made public in publications and a national congress for the larger interested public. The gains were impressive. Stretch goals of change showed that more than a 40% change in practice was achieved by more than 25% of participants, and more than a 20% change in practice was achieved in 78% of the first 147 organizational participants (C. M. Kilo, personal communication, 1997). The rush of issue-centered activity sharpened the focus for improvement. Many changes were made and networking increased among similarly motivated clinicians and other health care leaders.

At the same time, it became clear that all this highly visible activity masked real unevenness in execution—sometimes within the same organization. The idea that improvement could occur without explicit attention to the context for work grew. The popularity of "naming the issues" caught on, and the impatience to name the next issue seemed to take precedence over deployment of systematic change. The longevity for an issue seemed to be getting shorter. Improving patient care, issue by issue, became the same as creating a "quick-fix skunkworks"—delegating the responsibility for improvement to that group and assuming that they would accomplish all that was needed. Privately, some wondered about the sustainability of the larger numbers, faster issues, and activity vortex that seemed to obscure unresolved deployment challenges and threatened to exhaust dedicated (but finite) professional resources. Some also wondered about the cost of this late education and wondered why the acquisition of this knowledge and these skills could not become a part of the regular preparation of health professionals.

It did not occur to many to actively couple the professional learning and development with issue-centered improvement. Students were busy learning the "tried and true" ways, which—somewhat paradoxically— were the focus of change and of the "improvement hot houses" within organizations. Graduate-level learners could only be helpful players in these efforts if their faculty were actively engaged in these efforts. Yet faculty were rarely recruited to join improvement teams. As a result, it seemed appropriate to keep professional education and issue-centered improvement separate.

With the vulnerability of organization-centered strategies and the questions about the sustainability and overall impact of issue-centered programming, the future for the improvement of health care seemed less than certain. Furthermore, the two strategies were not seeking explicit linkages to professional development. Fortunately, another option began to emerge. More recent research on quality improvement efforts suggest that "project-based" improvement efforts do not result in safer hospitals (Landrigan et al., 2010), which adds further credibility to the system-sensitive strategies presented in the following section.

Microsystem-Centered Strategies

Systems of care exist at multiple levels—the individual patient involved in a self-care system; the physician/clinician–patient dyad; the clinical microsystem that recognizes the multiple people, activities, technology, and information involved in providing patient care; the larger macro-organization that provides an institutional home for multiple microsystems; and, finally, the external environment surrounding the macro-organizations. These multiple systems can be depicted as the series of concentric circles shown in **Figure 13–2**.

The focus on the clinical microsystem provides a conceptual and practical framework for thinking about the organization and delivery of care.

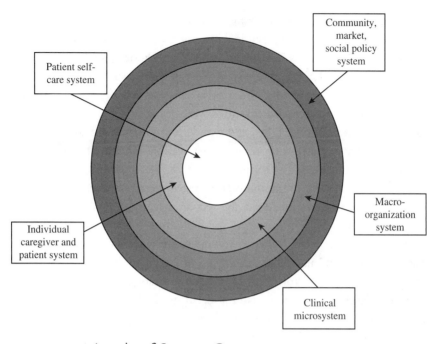

FIGURE 13-2 Levels of System Care

The clinical microsystem is also discussed briefly in several other chapters (see Chapters 4, 9, and 14). A clinical microsystem is a group of clinicians and staff working together with a shared clinical purpose to provide care for a population of patients (Batalden et al., 1997; Mohr, 2000; Nelson et al., 1998). The clinical purpose and its setting define the essential components of the microsystem. These include the clinicians and support staff, information and technology, the specific care processes, and the behaviors that are required to provide care to its patients. Microsystems evolve over time, responding to the needs of their patients, providers, and external pressures. They most often coexist with other microsystems within a larger (macro) organization. Academic clinical microsystems—microsystems that exist within academic health centers—face the challenge of a dual mission to provide excellent patient care and excellent professional development/learning. While academic clinical microsystems clearly have these dual missions, in fact, all clinical microsystems are about both patient care and professional formation.

The conceptual theory of the clinical microsystem is based on ideas developed by Deming (1986), Senge (1990), Wheatley (1992), and others who have applied systems thinking to organizational development, leadership, and improvement. The seminal idea for the clinical microsystem stems from the work of James Brian Quinn (1992). Quinn's work is based on analyzing the world's best-of-best service organizations such as FedEx, Mary Kay Cosmetics, McDonald's, and Nordstrom. He focused on determining what these extraordinary organizations were doing to achieve high quality, explosive growth, high margins, and wonderful reputations with customers. He found that these leading service organizations organized around, and continually engineered, the frontline relationships that connected the needs of customers with the organization's core competency. Quinn called this frontline activity that embedded the service delivery process the "smallest replicable unit" or the "minimum replicable unit." This smallest replicable unit, or the microsystem, is the key to implementing effective strategy, information technology, and other key aspects of intelligent enterprise.

In the late 1990s, Mohr and Donaldson investigated high-performing clinical microsystems (Donaldson and Mohr, 2000; Mohr, 2000). This research was based on a national search for the highest-quality clinical microsystems. Forty-three clinical units were identified using a theoretical sampling methodology. Semistructured interviews were conducted with leaders from each of the microsystems. Analysis of these interviews suggested that several dimensions are associated with effective microsystems. Additional research built on the Mohr and Donaldson study conducted 20 case studies of high-performing microsystems and included on-site interviews with each member of the microsystem and analysis of individual microsystem performance data (Batalden et al., 2003; Godfrey et al., 2003; Huber et al., 2003; Kosnik and Espinosa, 2003; Mohr, Barach, et al., 2003; Nelson et al., 2002; Nelson et al., 2003; Wasson et al., 2003). The "microsystem assessment tool" included in **Figure 13–3** was first published in 2002 and is based on the dimensions described in the research (Mohr and Batalden, 2002).

As we continue to move beyond conceptual theory and research to application in clinical settings, the emerging fields of chaos theory, complexity science, and complex adaptive systems have influenced how these concepts have been applied to improving microsystems (Arrow et al., 2000; Peters, 1987; Plsek and Greenhalgh, 2001; Plsek and Wilson, 2001). This is evident in the work seeking to bring together microsystems from around the world to learn and share best practices. Updates on these efforts are available at the Clinical Microsystems Web site

CLINICAL MICROSYSTEM ASSESSMENT TOOL

Instructions: Each of the "success" characteristics (e.g., leadership) is followed by a series of three descriptions. For each characteristic, *please check* the description that *best describes* your current microsystem and the care it delivers or use a microsystem you are *most familiar with*.

Characteristic and Definition		Descriptions		
Leadership	**1. Leadership:** The role of leaders is to balance setting and reaching collective goals, and to empower individual autonomy and accountability, through building knowledge, respectful action, reviewing, and reflecting.	☐ Leaders often tell me how to do my job and leave little room for innovation and autonomy. Overall, they don't foster a positive culture.	☐ Leaders struggle to find the right balance between reaching performance goals and supporting and empowering the staff.	☐ Leaders maintain constancy of purpose, establish clear goals and expectations, and foster a respectful positive culture. Leaders take time to build knowledge, review and reflect, and take action about microsystems and the larger organization.	☐ Can't Rate
	2. Organizational Support: The larger organization looks for ways to support the work of the microsystem and coordinate the handoffs between microsystems.	☐ The larger organization isn't supportive in a way that provides recognition, information, and resources to enhance my work.	☐ The larger organization is inconsistent and unpredictable in providing the recognition, information, and resources needed to enhance my work.	☐ The larger organization provides recognition, information, and resources that enhance my work and makes it easier for me to meet the needs of patients.	☐ Can't Rate
Staff	**3. Staff Focus:** There is selective hiring of the right kind of people. The orientation process is designed to fully integrate new staff into culture and work roles. Expectations of staff are high regarding performance, continuing education, professional growth, and networking.	☐ I am not made to feel like a valued member of the microsystem. My orientation was incomplete. My continuing education and professional growth needs are not being met.	☐ I feel like I am a valued member of the microsystem, but I don't think the microsystem is doing all that it could to support education and training of staff, workload, and professional growth.	☐ I am a valued member of the microsystem, and what I say matters. This is evident through staffing, education and training, workload, and professional growth.	☐ Can't Rate
	4. Education and Training: All clinical microsystems have responsibility for the ongoing education and training of staff and for aligning daily work roles with training competencies. Academic clinical microsystems have the additional responsibility of training students.	☐ Training is accomplished in disciplinary silos, for example, nurses train nurses, physicians train residents, and so on. The educational efforts are not aligned with the flow of patient care, so that education becomes an "add-on" to what we do.	☐ We recognize that our training could be different to reflect the needs of our microsystem, but we haven't made many changes yet. Some continuing education is available to everyone.	☐ There is a team approach to training, whether we are are training staff, nurses, or students. Education and patient care are integrated into the flow of work in a way that benefits both from the available resources. Continuing education for all staff is recognized as vital to our continued success.	☐ Can't Rate
Patients	**5. Interdependence:** The interaction of staff is characterized by trust, collaboration, willingness to help each other, appreciation of complementary roles, respect, and recognition that all contribute individually to a shared purpose.	☐ I work independently, and I am responsible for my own part of the work. There is a lack of collaboration and a lack of appreciation for the importance of complementary roles.	☐ The care approach is interdisciplinary, but we are not always able to work together as an effective team.	☐ Care is provided by an interdisciplinary team characterized by trust, collaboration, appreciation of complementary roles, and a recognition that all contribute individually to a shared purpose.	☐ Can't Rate
	6. Patient Focus: The primary concern is to meet all patient needs—caring, listening, educating, and responding to special requests, innovating to meet patient needs, and smooth service flow.	☐ Most of us, including our patients, would agree that we do not always provide patient-centered care. We are not always clear about what patients want and need.	☐ We are actively working to provide patient-centered care and we are making progress toward more effectively and consistently learning about and meeting patient needs.	☐ We are effective in learning about and meeting patient needs—caring, listening, educating, and responding to special requests, and smooth service flow.	☐ Can't Rate

© 2001, Julie K. Johnson, MSPH, PhD

Side A

Please continue on Side B

FIGURE 13-3 Clinical Microsystem Assessment Tool

Source: Johnson, 2001.

CLINICAL MICROSYSTEM ASSESSMENT TOOL
- CONTINUED -

Characteristic and Definition	Descriptions			
Patients				
7. Community and Market Focus: The microsystem is a resource for the community; the community is a resource to the microsystem; and the microsystem establishes excellent and innovative relationships with the community.	☐ We focus on the patients who come to our unit. We haven't implemented any outreach programs in our community. Patients and their families often make their own connections to the community resources they need.	☐ We have tried a few outreach programs and have had some success, but it is not the norm for us to go out into the community or actively connect patients to the community resources that are available to them.	☐ We are doing everything we can to understand our community. We actively employ resources to help us work with the community. We add to the community, and we draw on resources from the community to meet patient needs.	☐ Can't Rate
Performance				
8. Performance Results: Performance focuses on patient outcomes, avoidable costs, streamlining delivery, using data feedback, promoting positive competition, and frank discussions about performance.	☐ We don't routinely collect data on the process or outcomes of the care we provide.	☐ We often collect data on the outcomes of the care we provide and on some processes of care.	☐ Outcomes (clinical, satisfaction, financial, technical, safety) are routinely measured, we feed data back to staff, and we make changes based on data.	☐ Can't Rate
9. Process Improvement: An atmosphere for learning and redesign is supported by the continuous monitoring of care, use of benchmarking, frequent tests of change, and a staff that has been empowered to innovate.	☐ The resources required (in the form of training, financial support, and time) are rarely available to support improvement work. Any improvement activities we do are in addition to our daily work.	☐ Some resources are available to support improvement work, but we don't use them as often as we could. Change ideas are implemented without much discipline.	☐ There are ample resources to support continual improvement work. Studying, measuring, and improving care in a scientific way are essential parts of our daily work.	☐ Can't Rate
Information and Information Technology				
10. Information and Information Technology: Information is THE connector—staff to patients, staff to staff, needs with actions to meet needs. Technology facilitates effective communication, and multiple formal and informal channels are used to keep everyone informed all the time, listen to everyone's ideas, and ensure that everyone is connected on important topics.				
A. Integration of Information with Patients	☐ Patients have access to some standard information that is available to all patients.	☐ Patients have access to standard information that is available to all patients. We've started to think about how to improve the information they are given to better meet their needs.	☐ Patients have a variety of ways to get the information they need, and it can be customized to meet their individual learning styles. We routinely ask patients for feedback about how to improve the information we give them.	☐ Can't Rate
B. Integration of Information with Providers and Staff	☐ I am always tracking down the information I need to do my work.	☐ Most of the time, I have the information I need, but sometimes essential information is missing and I have to track it down.	☐ The information I need to do my work is available when I need it.	☐ Can't Rate
Given the complexity of information and the use of technology in the microsystem, assess your microsystem on the following three characteristics: (1) integration of information with patients, (2) integration of information with providers and staff, and (3) integration of information with technology.				
C. Integration of Information with Technology	☐ The technology I need to facilitate and enhance my work is either not available to me or it is available but not effective. The technology we currently have does not make my job easier.	☐ I have access to technology that will enhance my work, but it is not easy to use and seems to be cumbersome and time-consuming.	☐ Technology facilitates a smooth linkage between information and patient care by providing timely, effective access to a rich information environment. The information environment has been designed to support the work of the clinical unit.	☐ Can't Rate

© 2001, Julie K. Johnson, MSPH, PhD

Side B

FIGURE 13-3 Clinical Microsystem Assessment Tool

Source: Johnson, 2001.

(http://clinicalmicrosystem.org). Lessons learned from more than a decade of translating microsystem research into practice are also available (Nelson et al., 2007; Nelson et al., 2011).

What were the implications of the clinical microsystem on health professionals? Most patients get health care from health professionals who work in very complex organizations. Patients interact with multiple microsystems as they navigate through the health care system. The handoffs between microsystems, even for the savviest consumers of health care, can be difficult and confusing. Similarly, health care professionals rotate through multiple microsystems as they receive their initial clinical training. They often receive little orientation to the way an individual microsystem works; indeed, they are often members of that microsystem only for a few weeks before rotating to a different microsystem. As students and trainees, they are "rewarded" for finding ways to work around the system to accomplish patient care activities (Mohr and Arora, 2004). As they are immersed in the daily work of caring for patients as part of a microsystem, students, trainees, and the fully trained health care professional experience the system issues that impede high-quality care, yet they lack the tools and resources needed to make changes in that work environment. Not surprisingly, they become frustrated with their own ability to respond to the macro-organization and societal pressures to remove cost while maintaining or improving the quality of care. After graduation, these students assume practitioner roles and continue their professional formation and development. Unless the work settings are explicitly aimed at good patient care *and* good professional development, the results will reflect the shortages and frustrations currently being experienced widely in U.S. health care.

Recognizing the role of the microsystem both in training health professionals and in providing patient care offers several advantages. Training within the clinical microsystem allows for cross-profession development. Traditionally, health professionals have been prepared within their disciplinary, professional silo. However, once practicing in a professional setting, they work together in processes that require them to reach common understandings about the design of change and improvement of care. Moreover, models of professional development that offer a theory of knowledge and skill acquisition that crosses disciplines have the added attraction of offering special opportunities for those faculty who understand the new information and skills and who can integrate them into their own way of teaching the current subject matter. Such an integrated model of frontline work offers health professions faculty the opportunity to demonstrate what the continual improvement of care and systems-based practice means in the daily work of the faculty and other learners. Learners acquire the knowledge and skill as part of their experiential learning.

This model emphasizes the context within which students and trainees learn and are assessed, and it suggests how to link the development of learner competencies to the specific environment. Improvement efforts—educational as well as clinical—may be more effective when designed and implemented at the microsystem level and supported by the larger organization. Clearly, there is a role for the organization-centered strategy and the issue-centered strategy. By explicitly including students and trainees in designing and testing interventions, we can enhance our efforts to achieve the mission of teaching and assessing specific core competencies within the academic clinical microsystem.

An example of this idea at work can be seen on unit 1 East at Dartmouth Hitchcock Medical Center—a busy inpatient general medicine clinical microsystem that determined it wanted to do better with pneumonia immunization in the adult patients it cares for and with providing earlier treatment of adult patients with community-acquired pneumonia. A resident learner in the Dartmouth Hitchcock Leadership Preventive Medicine program began to work with the faculty and nursing leadership. New practices for discharge and admission were co-developed by the resident, medical faculty, and nursing leadership, resulting in higher levels of immunization and more prompt administration of antibiotics on admission.

Linking health professions development and improved patient care with the macro-organization policy and practice, issue-centered innovation and change, and enhanced frontline operations in the clinical microsystems where patients and providers regularly meet offers many challenges. Faculty need to be encouraged and recognized for leading in these ways. Infrastructure—such as information and human resource policy and practices—that has improved patient care needs to serve professional development. Educational requirements that have celebrated frequent rotations in and out of frontline systems of care need to be reexamined for their effect on the total system of patient care and professional development. Learning about professional work depends on role models who are able to integrate providing and improving care. Accreditation practices must explore both learning and patient care. Fortunately, such changes invite a more satisfying professional life and are likely to be attractive to many, though many existing systems and operational habits are likely to need reexamination and probably modification.

CONCLUSIONS

Health care improvement that is undertaken with a single strategy as the major driver will meet with limited success. Improvement that is part of the fundamental processes of health professional development and able to attract the synergy of an integrated approach—organization-centered, issue-centered, and microsystem-centered—may create a more robust strategy. Such an effort offers the health care sector a potentially transforming and more durable model for the continual improvement of health care.

Cross-References to the Companion Casebook

(McLaughlin, C. P., Johnson, J. K., and Sollecito, W. A. [Eds.]. 2012. *Implementing Continuous Quality Improvement in Health Care: A Global Casebook.* Sudbury, MA: Jones & Bartlett Learning.)

Case Study Number	Case Study Title	Case Study Authors
1	West Florida Regional Medical Center	Curtis P. McLaughlin
12	Quality in Pediatric Subspecialty Care	William A. Sollecito, Peter A. Margolis, Paul V. Miles, Robert Perelman, and Richard B. Colletti
16	The Lewis Blackman Hospital Patient Safety Act: It's Hard to Kill a Healthy 15-Year-Old	Julie K. Johnson, Helen Haskell, and Paul Barach

REFERENCES

Accreditation Council for Graduate Medical Education. 2007. Accreditation Council for Graduate Medical Education Outcomes Project: General Competencies. Retrieved April 6, 2011, from http://www.acgme.org/outcome/comp/GeneralCompetencies Standards21307.pdf

Ackoff, R. L. 1981. *Creating the Corporate Future.* New York: John Wiley & Sons.

American Board of Medical Specialties. 2006. About ABMS maintenance of certification. Retrieved May 17, 2010, from http://www.abms.org/Maintenance_of_Certification/

Argyris, C. 1991. Teaching smart people to learn. *Harvard Business Rev,* 69(3): 99–109.

Argyris, C., and Schön, D. A. 1996. *Organizational Learning II: Theory, Method and Practice.* Reading, MA: Addison-Wesley.

Arrow, H., McGrath, J., Berdahl, J. L., et al. 2000. *Small Groups as Complex Systems.* Thousand Oaks, CA: Sage Publications.

Batalden, P., and Davidoff, F. 2007. Teaching quality improvement: The devil is in the details. *JAMA,* 298(9): 1059–1061.

Batalden, P., and Mohr, J. 1997. Building a knowledge of health care as a system. *Quality Manage Health Care,* 5(3): 1–12.

Batalden, P., Mohr, J., Nelson, E. C., et al. 1997. Continually improving the health and value of health care for a population of patients: The panel management process. *Quality Manage Health Care,* 5(3): 41–51.

Batalden, P., Nelson, E., Edwards, W. H., et al. 2003. Microsystems in health care: Part 9. Developing small clinical units to attain peak performance. *Joint Commission J Quality Safety,* 29(11): 575–585.

Batalden, P., Ogrinc, G., Batalden, M., et al. 2006. From one to many. *J Interprof Care,* 20(5): 549–51.

Batalden, P., and Stoltz, P. 1993. Performance improvement in health care organizations. A framework for the continual improvement of health care: Building and applying professional and improvement knowledge to test changes in daily work. *Joint Commission J Quality Improve,* 19: 424–452.

Batalden, P. B. 1998. Why focus on health professional development? *Quality Manage Health Care,* 6(2): 52–61.

Batalden, P. B., Leach, D., Swing, S., et al. 2002. General competencies and accreditation in graduate medical education. *Health Aff,* 21(5): 103–111.

Batalden, P. B., and Nelson, E. C. 1990. Hospital quality: Patient, physician and employee judgments. *Int J Health Care Quality Assurance,* 3(4): 7–17.

Bertalanffy, L. V. 1968. *General System Theory: Foundations, Development, Applications.* New York: George Braziller.

Berwick, D. M. 1994. Eleven worthy aims for clinical leadership of health system reform. *JAMA*, 272(10): 797–802.

Berwick, D. M., and Finkelstein, J. A. 2010. Preparing medical students for the continual improvement of health and health care: Abraham Flexner and the new public interest. *Acad Med*, 85(9): S56–S65.

Boonyasai, R. T., Windish, D. M., Chakraborti, C., et al. 2007. Effectiveness of teaching quality improvement to clinicians: a systematic review. *JAMA*, 298(9): 1023–1037.

Brennan, T. A., and Berwick, D. M. 1996. *New Rules: Regulation, Markets, and the Quality of American Health Care*. San Francisco: Jossey-Bass.

Brockman, J. 1977. *About Bateson: Essays on Gregory Bateson*. New York: E. P. Dutton.

Checkland, P. 1981. *Systems Thinking, Systems Practice*. New York: John Wiley & Sons.

Churchman, C. W. 1971. *The Design of Inquiring Systems: Basic Concepts of Systems and Organization*. New York: Basic Books.

Cronenwett, L., G. Sherwood, Barnsteiner, J., et al. 2007. Quality and safety education for nurses. *Nurs Outlook*, 55(3): 122–131.

Daniel, D. M., Casey, D. E., Jr., Levine, J. L., et al. 2009. Taking a unified approach to teaching and implementing quality improvements across multiple residency programs: The Atlantic Health experience. *Acad Med*, 84(12): 1788–1795.

Deming, W. E. 1986. *Out of the Crisis*. Cambridge: Massachusetts Institute of Technology Center for Advanced Engineering Study.

Deming, W. E. 1993. *The New Economics for Industry, Government, Education*. Cambridge: Massachusetts Institute of Technology Center for Advanced Engineering Study.

Dobyns, L., and Crawford Mason, C. 1991. *Quality or Else: The Revolution in World Business*. Boston: Houghton Mifflin.

Donaldson, M. S., and Mohr, J. J. 2000. Improvement and innovation in health care microsystems. A technical report for the Institute of Medicine Committee on the Quality of Health Care in America. Princeton, NJ: Robert Wood Johnson Foundation.

Dreyfus, H., and Dreyfus, S. 1986. *Mind over Machine*. New York: Free Press.

Eliastam, M., and Mizrahi, T. 1996. Quality improvement, housestaff, and the role of chief residents. *Acad Med*, 71(6): 670–674.

Forrester, J. W. 1990. *Principles of Systems*. Portland, OR: Productivity Press.

Foster, T., M. Regan-Smith, Murray, C., et al. 2008. Residency education, preventive medicine, and population health care improvement: The Dartmouth-Hitchcock Leadership Preventive Medicine approach. *Acad Med*, 83(4): 390–398.

Godfrey, M. M., Nelson, E. C., Wasson, J. H. et al. 2003. Microsystems in health care: Part 3. Planning patient-centered services. *Jt Comm J Qual Saf*, 29(4): 159–170.

Heclo, H. 2008. *On Thinking Institutionally*. Boulder, CO: Paradigm Publishers.

Huber, T., Godfrey, M., Nelson, E. C., et al. 2003. Microsystems in health care: Part 8. Developing people and improving worklife: What front-line staff told us. *Joint Commission J Quality Safety*, 29(10): 512–522.

Institute of Medicine. 2001. *Crossing the Quality Chasm: A New Health System for the 21st Century*. Washington, DC: National Academies Press.

Institute of Medicine. 2003. *Health Professions Education: A Bridge to Quality*. Washington, DC: National Academies Press.

Joint Commission on Accreditation of Healthcare Organizations. 1992. *Striving Toward Improvement: Six Hospitals in Search of Quality*. Oakbrook Terrace, IL: Author.

Kosnik, L., and Espinosa, J. 2003. Microsystems in health care: Part 7. The microsystem as a platform for merging strategic planning and operations. *Joint Commission J Quality Safety*, 29(9): 452–459.

Landrigan, C. P., Parry, G. J., Bones, C. B., et al. 2010 Temporal trends in rates of patient harm resulting from medical care. *N Engl J Med*, 363(22): 2124–2134.

McEachern, J. E., and Neuhauser, D. B. 1989. The continuous improvement of quality at the Hospital Corporation of America. *Health Matrix*, 7: 5–11.

McLaughlin, C., and Kaluzny, A. (Eds.). 1999. *Continuous Quality Improvement in Health Care*. Gaithersburg, MD: Aspen Publications.

McLaughlin, C. P., Johnson, J. K., and Sollecito, W. A. (Eds.). 2012. *Implementing Continuous Quality Improvement in Health Care: A Global Casebook*. Sudbury, MA: Jones & Bartlett Learning.

Mitroff, I. I., and Linstone, L. A. 1993. *The Unbounded Mind: Breaking the Chains of Traditional Thinking*. New York: Oxford University Press.

Mizuno, S. 1988. *Company-Wide Total Quality Control.* Tokyo: Nordica International Limited.

Mohr, J. 2000. *Forming, Operating, and Improving Microsystems of Care* (p. 250). Hanover, NH: Center for the Evaluative Clinical Sciences, Dartmouth College.

Mohr, J., and Arora, V. 2004. Break the cycle: Rooting out the workaround. *ACGME Bulletin*, November.

Mohr, J., Barach, P., Cravero, J. P., et al. 2003. Microsystems in health care: Part 6. Designing patient safety into the microsystem. *Joint Commission J Quality Safety* 29(8): 401–408.

Mohr, J., and Batalden, P. 2002. Improving safety at the front lines: The role of clinical microsystems. *Quality Safety Health Care*, 11(1): 45–50.

Mohr, J., Randolph, G., Laughon, M. M., et al. 2003. Integrating improvement competencies into residency education: A pilot project from a pediatric continuity clinic. *Ambulatory Pediatr*, 3(3): 131–136.

Nelson, E., Batalden, P., and Godfrey, M. M. (Eds.). 2007. *Quality by Design: A Clinical Microsystems Approach.* San Francisco: Jossey-Bass.

Nelson, E., Batalden, P., Godfrey, M. M., et al. (Eds.). 2011. *Value by Design: Developing Clinical Microsystems to Achieve Organizational Excellence.* San Francisco: Jossey-Bass.

Nelson, E., Batalden, P., Homa, K., et al. 2003. Microsystems in health care: Part 2. Creating a rich information environment. *Joint Commission J Quality Safety* 29(1): 5–15.

Nelson, E., Batalden, P., Huber, T. P., et al. 2002. Microsystems in health care: Part 1. Learning from high-performing front-line clinical units. *Joint Commission J Quality Improve*, 28(9): 472–493.

Nelson, E., Batalden, P., Mohr, J. J., et al. 1998. Building a quality future. *Frontiers Health Serv Manage*, 15(1): 3–32.

Nelson, E. C., and Batalden, P. B. 1993. Patient-based quality measurement systems. *Quality Manage Health Care*, 2(1): 18–30.

Ogrinc, G., Headrick, L. A., Morrison, L. J., et al. 2004. Teaching and assessing resident competence in rractice-based learning and improvement. *J General Intern Med*, 19: 496–500.

Patow, C. 2009. Making residents visible in quality improvement. *Acad Med*, 84(12): 1642.

Patow, C. A., Karpovich, K., Riesenberg, L. A., et al. 2009. Residents' engagement in quality improvement: A systematic review of the literature. *Acad Med*, 84(12): 1757–1764.

Peters, T. 1987. *Thriving on Chaos: Handbook for a Management Revolution.* New York: Harper & Row.

Plsek, P. E., and Greenhalgh, T. 2001. Complexity science: The challenge of complexity in health care. *BMJ*, 323(7313): 625–628.

Plsek, P. E., and Wilson, T. 2001. Complexity, leadership, and management in healthcare organisations. *BMJ*, 323(7315): 746–749.

Quinn, J. B. 1992. *The Intelligent Enterprise.* New York: Free Press.

Senge, P. 1990. *The Fifth Discipline.* New York: Doubleday.

Senge, P. M., Kleiner, A., Roberts, C., et al. 1994. *The Fifth Discipline Fieldbook: Strategies and Tools for Building a Learning Organization.* New York: Doubleday/Currency.

Taylor, R. J., and Taylor, S. B. 1994. *The AUPHA Manual of Health Services Management.* Gaithersburg, MD: Aspen Publishers.

Walton, M. 1990. *Deming Management at Work.* New York: G. P. Putnam's Sons.

Wasson, J., Godfrey, M., Nelson, E. C., et al. 2003. Microsystems in health care: Part 4: Planning patient-centered care. *Joint Commission J Quality Safety*, 29(5): 159–170.

Weingart, S. 1996. House officer education and organizational obstacles to quality improvement. *Joint Commission J Quality Improve*, 22(9): 640–646.

Weingart, S. 1998. A house officer-sponsored quality improvement initiative: Leadership lessons and liabilities. *Joint Commision J Quality Improve*, 24(7): 371–378.

Wennberg, J. 2010. *Tracking Medicine: A Researcher's Quest to Understand Health Care.* New York: Oxford University Press.

Wennberg, J. E., Cooper, M. M., and Bubolz, T. A. 1996. *The Dartmouth Atlas of Health Care.* Chicago: American Hospital Association.

Wennberg, J. E., and Gittlesohn, A. M. 1973. Small area variations in health care delivery. *Science*, 183: 1102–1108.

Wheatley, M. 1992. *Leadership and the New Science: Learning About Organization from an Orderly Universe.* San Francisco: Berrett-Koehler.

CHAPTER 14

Quality Improvement in Primary Care: The Role of Organization, Systems, and Collaboratives

Leif I. Solberg

"Occupational organization . . . constitutes a dimension quite as distinct and fully as important as its knowledge."

—Eliot Freidson (1970, p. xi)

After a great national debate about health care reform in the United States that focused mainly on covering most of the uninsured, there is even greater concern about unsustainable increases in health care costs and how to improve the quality of both care and patient experience. Private purchasers of all types are desperate for relief, and government, which has just become the main purchaser/payer of care, is worried that health care costs are consuming a steadily larger portion of the budget, forcing out other kinds of services. At the same time, both the overall quality of care and disparities in quality among different populations continue to be a source of concern.

These cost and quality problems, highlighted in reports from the Institute of Medicine (IOM) at the turn of the century and documented in concurrent national studies of quality, have continued to be unresolved. The first IOM report, *To Err Is Human*, quantified the frequency and severity of errors in hospital care, while the second, *Crossing the Quality Chasm*, put those errors in a broad perspective and set six national goals for improvement (IOM, 2000, 2001). These goals added safety, timeliness, equity, efficiency, and patient centeredness to the more long-standing goal of effectiveness. As the later report so memorably states, "Between the health care we have and the care we could have lies not just a gap, but a chasm." Studies by the RAND Corporation showed that, on average, guideline-recommended acute, chronic, and preventive care was received by adults only 55% of the time in 12 metropolitan areas of the United States (McGlynn, 2003). Later studies showed similar findings for child health care (Mangione-Smith et al., 2007). Subsequent biannual reports from the Agency for Healthcare Research and Quality (2008, 2009) have shown only small incremental improvements in both overall quality and in disparities among different populations.

Nearly all of these indicators measured care that is provided largely in primary care, so that setting in particular is getting greater attention. However, as the need for primary care redesign and improvement increases, the condition of that area of care is instead continuing to deteriorate. Fewer young doctors are going into primary care, most primary care practices are financially insecure, and primary care doctors are being forced to focus primarily on productivity—what Bodenheimer (2006) describes as running faster in the hamster wheel just to stay in place. It is widely believed by policy makers that one reason developed countries other than the United States spend a much lower proportion of their gross domestic product on health care and enjoy better quality than we do is because their care systems are built on a strong primary care base. Confirmation of that assumption comes from the regional variation studies of the Dartmouth Institute, which show that regions with higher numbers of subspecialists have both lower quality and higher costs (Fisher et al., 2009).

Thus, there is a sense of urgent need to address what has been called the triple aim (improving health, patient experience of care, and costs), as well as to redesign primary care and readjust the balance between it and more specialized care (Berwick et al., 2008). This quest for *value*—higher quality and experience at lower cost—has also clarified the need to change the payment system from fee-for-service to one that pays for value rather than individual services. It is clearly necessary to redesign the payment structure before or as part of the redesign of care. This chapter will be limited to the redesign and quality improvement of primary care, although that has become shorthand for the broader goals of improving experience and value as well as quality and health.

INTERNAL KEYS TO IMPROVEMENT

Organization of Primary Care

Before describing the keys to redesigning care that will meet the triple aim and the six goals of the IOM, it is important to understand the evolving structure and function of primary care delivery organizations in the United States. Many policy makers and most researchers seem to lack this understanding, so their policies and studies often miss the mark.

Organizations that provide primary care have been evolving from largely solo doctor practices to small single-specialty groups and now to ever-larger medical groups, many of which have become multispecialty organizations able to provide almost every type of medical service. Some of this evolution has been hastened by the need to create negotiating power with managed care plans, but it was being fostered in any case by technological changes in medicine, cost pressures, changing physician attitudes about work, and heightened consumer and purchaser expectations.

When doctors first banded together, it was to share after-hours calls, billing systems, and other infrastructure in a common office or clinic site. These sites usually consisted of 2 to 10 doctors, typically of the same specialty, with 3 to 5 being the most efficient unit size. Later, and particularly in regions with high penetration and pressure from managed care plans, many of these single-site groups merged or were bought out by large care systems or hospitals that were hoping to create a captive referral network and/or gain negotiating power with insurance plans. While some of these larger aggregations continue to contain largely a single primary care specialty, many have become multispecialty as well as multisite. Larger organizations are referred to as medical groups, some of which continue to practice at a single site, but most have multiple sites or clinics; some establish smaller satellites, particularly in rural areas.

Another factor of tremendous importance for care redesign and quality improvement (QI) is the historical lack of integration within most of these medical groups, even large multispecialty groups. Formed primarily for economic or cross-coverage reasons, the physicians in early medical groups tended to maintain separate medical practices with individual autonomy in approach to care. This meant that unless an individual physician was unusually interested in organizing care patterns, there was little consistency, coordination, or outreach involved in patient care. Each patient and each visit was unique, and any care actions had to be recalled or created anew. Over time, this individualization of practice (which can be characterized as the "motel syndrome" to illustrate the shared solo-ness) tended to decline as it became clearer that both efficiency and effectiveness could be improved by systems that cross individual physician or specialty boundaries or that added non-physician clinicians. Nevertheless, this integration continued to vary enormously among different medical groups, and sometimes even at different sites within an individual group.

These increasingly complex organizations also required leadership, so medical groups found a need for a medical director, a chief administrator, committees, and boards of directors. As they became larger, multisite groups also usually created medical and administrative leaders for individual clinic sites. And as the pressure for QI and cost-efficiency increased, medical groups usually found it necessary to develop greater integration of their various sites and departments and to create an infrastructure that could develop and maintain common systems to support consistent and even standardized care. To be most effective, this infrastructure includes a specific approach to QI as well as a coordinator and a physician leader who can connect the QI efforts to organizational priorities, plans, and resources. Recently, more groups have incorporated the responsibility for QI into their overall leadership structure, since it has become increasingly apparent that it is impossible to drive real improvement (i.e., care redesign) from a separate department. The entire leadership team and often large organizational resources are needed to support these kinds of changes.

Of course, there are still many solo or small medical practices in many parts of the country, especially in rural areas. If they are to survive, many will follow the historical pattern of merger or buy-out by larger groups, and all will need effective internal leadership.

QI Requires an Organizational Focus

The extensive discussion of organizational structure in the previous section illustrates that real QI requires an organizational focus. Continuing medical education has little effect on the medical care behaviors of participants and is clearly incapable of producing the large practice redesign changes that are now required—changes that are at the level of the organization above individual clinicians. What does that mean in practical terms? It means developing, implementing, and maintaining practice systems that make care consistent for the common aspects of many acute, chronic, and preventive conditions. Examples of such systems include the following:

- Registries of patients with chronic conditions
- Routine identification of risk factors during office visits
- Paper or electronic systems to monitor whether patients are up-to-date on preventive services and whether consistent care is being provided for chronic conditions
- Delegation of orders or delivery of many preventive and screening services to nursing staff
- Coordination of care transitions between inpatient and outpatient settings and between primary and subspecialty care services
- Care managers for patients with stable chronic conditions

These practice systems and others that ensure comprehensive, continuous, and coordinated care are at the heart of the primary care practice redesign currently called "medical homes" (Rosenthal, 2008; Rosser et al., 2010). The presence of these systems, built to implement the domains of the Chronic Care Model, also form the core of the assessment being used by the National Committee on Quality Assurance (NCQA) for recognition of medical homes at three levels of competence (American Academy of Family Physicians, 2009). The real challenge that is highly pertinent to this chapter is how to transform traditional primary care medical practices into medical homes (Carrier et al., 2009; Rosser et al., 2010). The American Academy of Family Physicians (AAFP) funded the National Demonstration Project in 2006 as a controlled trial of external facilitation of this transformation (Loxterkamp and Kazal, 2008). Early evaluation of this project concluded that transformation is a very difficult process, one that requires physicians to reconsider their own roles as well as the ways in which they deliver care (Nutting et al., 2009). It is precisely this practice transformation process that this chapter is focused on. How can practices best move beyond incremental changes to a whole new design for primary care, and how can that be most efficiently achieved?

There is extensive literature now attesting to the need for major QI changes in practice, but the need was abundantly clear in a study that my colleagues and I published in 2000. In order to better understand how to foster QI, we identified the most experienced and insightful physicians and coordinators for QI in our region among the medical groups with the most success in improving quality. We led them through a series of interviews and a formal group process-rating exercise aimed at first identifying and then ranking the factors and strategies that they considered most important for QI (Solberg et al., 2000a).

There were several important lessons from these experienced leaders of change in medical groups of all sizes. One was the need to consider a great many factors while attempting to improve quality; they thought that 38 of the 87 factors they identified were either extremely or very important to be considered in any effort to improve quality or implement guidelines. Another 42 factors were thought to be quite a bit important. **Table 14–1** displays the 21 factors that received the highest ratings. Most of these 21 are directly or indirectly related to practice systems and organizational change.

TABLE 14–1 Factors Ranked in Order of Rated Importance to Ability to Improve Quality

Rank	Factor
1	**Presence of Organized Systems** in the clinic
2	**Commitment to Change** by leadership
3	**Voluntary Leadership** by enthusiastic volunteers
3	**Internal Clinician Champions** for the guideline
3	**Priorities** for quality vs. finance by the group
6	**Resources Available** for guideline implementation
6	**CQI Understanding and Skills** in the organization
6	**Collaborative Psychological Working Environment**
6	**Clinician Cohesiveness** to shared mission/policies
6	**Relative Advantage** of the new care process
6	**Importance** of the guideline topic to clinicians
12	**Standardized Organizational Process** for making change
12	**Change Management Infrastructure** well developed
12	**Internal Clinician Interest** in making the changes
12	**Internal Turmoil** present from internal changes
12	**Leadership Support** for steps to fulfill their vision
17	**Management Authorization** of resources for guidelines
17	**Strategic Plan Inclusion** of implementation in annual goals
17	**Resource Agreement Process** at all organizational levels
17	**Active Leadership Involvement** personally in the change
17	**Organizational Culture** supportive of planned change

Another lesson from these practical experts was the need to use multiple strategies rather than the single strategies that have been the focus of much of the research literature on QI. They identified 25 strategies and rated 20 of them as needing to be used at least frequently, believing that when used, they would be extremely or very effective. The top 10 strategies were:

1. Using system supports like reminders, registries, and task delegation

2. Focusing on changes that would make physician work easier

3. Reducing or removing barriers

4. Measuring for improvement periodically

5. Providing information or training

6. Delegating authority to the implementation planners

7. Providing comparative feedback of relevant measurements

8. Pretesting change through pilots and rapid cycling

9. Tailoring implementation to each practice setting

10. Focusing on changes that make the system better for patients

Both Complexity and Simplicity Are Needed

It is not enough to understand the factors affecting the ability to improve quality and the most effective strategies for change. Each organization must also adopt a particular approach to QI, one that fits its culture and is feasible for its internal leaders and change agents. When QI was first imported from other industries into medical care in the late 1980s (mostly in hospitals), it usually adopted an approach of creating specific projects, managed by special QI teams that applied a formal process with many separate steps (Berwick, 1989; Laffel and Blumenthal, 1989). These steps began with extensive data collection efforts to understand the process needing improvement and progressed through developing an entirely new and detailed process, which was then implemented en masse after a year or more of development work. National QI leaders recommended evaluating the change through more measurement after implementation and then cycling back through the QI steps for further improvement.

In practice, this part usually did not occur because of participant and organizational fatigue with the long time the development process had taken. The culture of medical practice, the tendency to focus on administrative rather than clinical problems, an insufficient appreciation for the importance of leadership support and resources, and other problems also contributed to discouragement about this QI model by the mid-1990s (Early and Godfrey, 1995; Goldberg et al., 1998; Shortell et al., 1995).

At about the same time, a new model of QI was being developed through leaders connected with the Institute for Healthcare Improvement (IHI). This model is described in detail in *The Improvement Guide* and many articles (Berwick, 1996, 1998; Langley et al., 1994; Langley et al., 2009; Nolan, 1997). Instead of many steps, this model proposed that QI teams first answer three questions:

1. What are we trying to accomplish?

2. How will we know that a change is an improvement?

3. What changes can we make that will result in improvement?

QI teams then start making small tests of change, using the Plan, Do, Study, Act (PDSA) cycle as they gradually develop the pieces of a new system. As they do this, a solid understanding and application of systems thinking, measurement, variation, and change management are needed, no matter what change they are trying to accomplish.

A more recent modification in this approach is to focus on microsystems, "the small, functional, frontline units that provide most health care to most people" (Nelson et al., 2008; Wasson et al., 2008). Although this term is also used for the units that provide frontline specialized or inpatient care, the concept is particularly important in primary care because it focuses on the strong, multidisciplinary teamwork that appears necessary to improve quality (Grumbach and Bodenheimer, 2004). Microsystems are discussed extensively in Chapters 9 and 13.

Finally, it is becoming increasingly apparent that successful QI needs to be incorporated into the normal management of the primary care organization rather than being conducted as special projects using ad hoc teams of volunteers. Many of the latest strategies described previously still apply, but if a QI effort is led by or reports to senior management and is conducted by existing relevant leaders, it is more likely to be implemented thoroughly and much more likely to be sustained. Again, that applies just as much to a one- or two-physician practice as it does to larger clinics and medical groups.

In order to make practical use of the preceding information, it is help-ful to have a simplified conceptual framework for what is needed for a clinic or medical group to improve the effectiveness and efficiency of its care. **Figure 14–1** provides such a framework (Solberg, 2007). This framework suggests that improvements depend mainly on three factors and that if any of those three are absent or only minimally present, there will not be much improvement:

1. High priority for the specific improvement by leaders, higher than their need to undertake most other changes in the organization

2. High capability to manage the change process, including knowl-edge and experience with a particular approach to change as well as adequate resources and leadership

3. Choice of care process changes that are highly likely to be effective for the improvements desired

Of course, there are other factors, both internal and external, that can facilitate or inhibit these three. For example, a group's priority for change is greatly affected by external incentives, competition, and key customers, as well as internal competing changes and problems. Both the change and care processes can be greatly affected by the organization's culture and the existence of other practice systems like having a good clinical informa-tion system. Nevertheless, focus on these three main factors can simplify the job of practice redesign and help in assessing whether a particular improvement effort is likely to succeed.

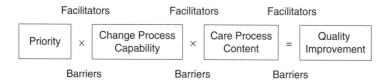

FIGURE 14–1 Conceptual Framework for Practice Improvement

Source: Reproduced from Solberg, L. I. 2007. Improving medical practice: A conceptual framework. *Ann Fam Med*, 5(3): 251–256.

EXTERNAL FACILITATORS
OF IMPROVEMENT

Payers, Purchasers, and Public Accountability

The founders of the health maintenance organization (HMO) concept that later evolved into managed care health plans believed that HMOs would have "a vested interest in regulating output, performance, and costs in the public interest" through better organization, integration, and coordination of care (Ellwood et al., 1971). When that belief was only partly realized, the newly founded NCQA was developed to apply pressure on health plans for pushing QI by requiring inspection and certification as well as public reporting of performance measures among their members through the Health Plan Employer Data Information Set (Corrigan and Nielsen, 1993). As the limited impact this approach had on quality and costs became apparent, purchasers began to get into the act more directly, through pressure by both large national companies and various business coalitions for real improvement in both care and costs. Later, more heterogeneous associations such as the National Quality Forum and the Leapfrog Group developed and included unions, professional associations, consumer groups, and even health plans. Many of these groups as well as individual health plans have tried various pay-for-performance programs, hoping thereby to stimulate improvements. However, the incentives have usually not been large, and most payers are only responsible for a small portion of the patients of any individual practice, so this approach tends to have small impact; moreover, there is much concern about unintended consequences, especially for the sickest patients.

The next step in external pressures for improvement was the development of performance measures focused on the individual medical groups and clinics that provide care rather than on their aggregated performance at the level of health plans. This was pioneered in Minnesota through the development of Minnesota Community Measurement, an organization sponsored by all the health plans that developed standardized ways of measuring quality at the group or site level and reported this information publicly on a Web site available to anyone (http://www.mnhealthscores.org) (Amundson and Frederick, 2003; Bershow, 2006). Subsequently, other regions have developed similar public accountability measures through a variety of mechanisms (e.g., the Wisconsin Association for Healthcare Quality and the Massachusetts Health Care Quality and Cost Council).

While providing some stimulus for improvement, these various groups have reinforced the impression that performance measures, incentives, and penalties that are only focused on or used by health plans are not likely to be very effective. External bodies have limited ability to foster the redesign of care unless there is a change in the payment system, and the failure of capitation with return to fee-for-service payment to physicians and their organizations has only reinforced that reality. At least we now know that physicians and care delivery organizations must take a leading role in any serious improvement in care and costs, and that will only happen when payment systems require and reward such changes (Ellwood and Lundberg, 1996; Guterman et al., 2009). Continuing to base physician payment on the volume of services provided neither incentivizes significant changes in care approach nor covers the costs of making such changes.

Practice Improvement Facilitators

Assuming that some kind of external pressure leads primary care practices to want to transform themselves, the question becomes whether they can do it on their own using the best available concepts, techniques, and tools, or whether they will need assistance from some kind of external group or consultant. It is widely believed, even among primary care leaders, that assistance will be needed, at least for the small practices that still characterize primary care in most of the United States. Most of the randomized controlled trials of QI have utilized such external facilitators to help practices implement the intervention to be tested (Dietrich et al., 1992; Dietrich et al., 1998; Goodwin et al., 2001; McBride et al., 2000; Solberg et al., 2000b; Wei et al., 2005). The National Demonstration Project of the AAFP (described earlier) was also based on such facilitators. The assumption seems to have been that if the results were positive (only some have been), then this type of external help could be applied in a large-scale way. However, that assumption has so far not been realized, because few primary care practices have the resources to pay for such consultative help and no external organizations have been willing to support it for more than a few sites. However, there is currently increasing interest in a government-supported resource similar to the agricultural extension agent program that played such a large part in the transformation of American agriculture (Rogers, 1995).

QUALITY IMPROVEMENT COLLABORATIVES

As an alternative or in addition to external facilitators, one of the most promising ways to help clinics and medical groups to improve may be through their participation in local, regional, or national quality improvement collaboratives (QICs), which were introduced in Chapter 1. The most well-known QICs are those short-term ones that have been run for specific topics by the IHI in the so-called Breakthrough Series (IHI, 2003; Kilo, 1998). This approach grew out of an IHI reappraisal of the lack of demonstrable impact of its previous focus on courses and an annual national forum on quality. In the Breakthrough Series model, IHI hosts collaborative efforts by teams from 20 to 40 organizations that work together on a particular quality topic for 9 to 12 months through three 2-day "learning sessions" and a final presentation at a national congress, with work at home in between. These series have been popular, but they are very expensive for participants and tend to attract mainly large care delivery organizations or those paid for by the government.

A wide variety of other QICs have developed on a regional basis or within a large organization like the Department of Veterans Affairs. One of the oldest and most successful has been the Institute for Clinical Systems Improvement (ICSI) in Minnesota, now cosponsored by all the managed care plans in the state, and with medical group and hospital members now consisting of 80% of the state's physicians (Allen, 2008; Farley et al., 2003). Founded in 1993, ICSI began as a way to develop local buy-in for evidence-based guidelines (available at http://www.icsi.org) and soon moved on to emphasize implementation and improvement of broad quality topics beyond any particular guideline. Evaluations of the ICSI program have suggested that participating medical groups and clinics tend to evolve in their understanding and work on quality through four stages as they participate in the ICSI collaborative:

1. Implementation of specific guidelines, one at a time

2. Implementation of combinations of guidelines that use similar systems (e.g., all preventive services) or relate in a specific condition

3. Development or remodeling of the group's general systems and infrastructure for improvement of care

4. Redesign of the entire approach the group takes to providing health care as well as the culture of the group

Enough separate QICs have been implemented in the United States that they now have their own national association, the Network for Regional Healthcare Improvement, and efforts are being made to identify the characteristics that are important for QIC effectiveness (Ayers et al., 2005; Solberg, 2005). In a systematic review of the evidence for the impact of QICs in 2008, Schouten et al. (2008) concluded that "[t]he evidence underlying quality improvement collaboratives is positive but limited and the effects cannot be predicted with great certainty. . . . Further knowledge of the basic components' effectiveness, cost effectiveness, and success factors is crucial to determine [their] value." However, this evidence is limited by the same problem that has limited all studies of QI in medical practice—there is still inadequate financial advantage for high-quality performance, much less for the prodigious effort needed to make substantive organizational changes.

What is needed for QI in primary care may be best illustrated by an example from a current ongoing major improvement initiative in Minnesota called DIAMOND, which stands for Depression Improvement Across Minnesota: Offering a New Direction (Jaeckels, 2009; Korsen and Pietruszewski, 2009).

DIAMOND: AN EXAMPLE OF MAJOR QUALITY IMPROVEMENT

The goal of DIAMOND, which was initiated in 2008, is to greatly improve the care and outcomes for adult patients with depression in primary care clinics. This goal is being addressed by changes in both the payment system and the care systems in participating clinics. All health plans in Minnesota have agreed to provide a new monthly payment for depression care management services that would not normally be covered, as long as the clinics billing for these services have been trained and certified for providing them through a well-defined model of care. This new care model has a very strong evidence base of more than 35 randomized controlled trials, but it was tailored specifically to resemble that used in one of those trials (IMPACT) (Gilbody et al., 2006; Unutzer et al., 2002; Williams et al., 2007). It consists of seven integrated components:

1. Consistent use of a validated instrument for assessing and monitoring depression (the PHQ9), both initially and at most contacts thereafter (Kroenke and Spitzer, 2002; Lowe et al., 2004)

2. Systematic patient follow-up tracking and monitoring with a registry

3. Evidence-based stepped care for treatment intensification for all patients failing to improve adequately

4. Relapse prevention planning for all patients whose depression has gone into remission

5. A care manager in the practice to educate, monitor, and coordinate care in collaboration with the primary care physician

6. A psychiatrist to provide scheduled weekly caseload supervision and consultation for the care manager and treatment recommendations for the primary care clinicians

7. Monthly reports for specified measures of patients activated into the program, including PHQ9 scores at baseline and at 6 and 12 months

The new payment covers these services as a group, unrelated to the number of contacts or effort involved in the care of individual patients, until a patient has been in remission for 2 months or in the program for a maximum of 12 months, whichever comes first. Primary care clinics are expected to make their own arrangements and payments for the psychiatrist and the internal care manager, whose duties are specified but whose profession and training are not. Most clinics have hired a nurse or medical assistant for this job, but others have chosen to use a social worker, nurse practitioner, or others. Most have also taken advantage of a low-cost registry provided by the University of Washington, but others have developed their own electronic system or adapted their electronic medical record to document and report on the necessary elements of care.

As of this writing, 85 primary care clinics with more than 500 primary care physicians from 24 separate medical groups throughout the state have chosen to participate in DIAMOND and have been trained and certified for the new payments by ICSI. As members of this regional QIC, most of these clinics already had some experience with internal QI techniques, but none had many of the seven care process components in place. Thus, they all had to participate in a 6-month training program involving both workshops and conference calls and to verify that they had implemented each of the seven components of the new care management program. To make this training program feasible, it was conducted in five clusters of clinics at 6-month intervals from March 2008 to March 2010.

Data collected and analyzed at ICSI from reports by these clinics show that DIAMOND has been very effective. More than 4,000 patients have been activated into the program, with 6-month remission rates of 45% among those followed to that point (60% of activated patients). For comparison, randomized controlled trials in the literature of a similar intervention have attained a 35–40% remission compared to a usual care rate of about 20%. Thus, this initiative has led to substantially better outcomes than usual care and appears to be doing even better than research studies that involve much greater control over the care changes.

Lessons Learned from DIAMOND

Such a remarkable QI effort did not just happen. It was built on ICSI's 15 years of experience in developing evidence-based guidelines by consensus among member medical groups and with facilitating the implementation of both specific guidelines and more general quality improvements and care redesign. Member groups also have developed considerable expertise in implementing the organizational changes necessary for major QI. This success was also built on the high degree of trust and common mission created during that history, both among medical groups and between those groups and the sponsoring health plans. Finally, it was built on several years of collectively trying to improve depression care by other means, both internal QI efforts and external incentives, care management programs, and facilitation through the ICSI equivalent of breakthrough series like those of IHI nationally.

After prior efforts by payers, medical groups, and ICSI had seen little change in depression care or outcomes, there was substantial readiness to try something else ("A New Direction"). Thus, when ICSI called its members and sponsors together to plan a new approach, they responded quickly. After a literature review demonstrated a strong evidence base for a collaborative care model, a steering committee and multiple subcommittees were established to work out the details of a local adaptation of this care model as well as a newly created payment model thought to be a feasible answer to the problem of lack of financial support for that care.

Despite the many successes of DIAMOND, there have been problems that have led to much less extensive use of the care model. Some of the clinics participating in DIAMOND were only able to activate 10–20% of their depressed patients into the program. There was limited spread of the model into other groups and other clinics in participating medical groups. Extensive interactions and site visits with participating clinics suggest that this limited engagement is primarily related to financial issues. Despite the support of all health plans in the state, a sizable proportion of the patients in participating clinics are not eligible for coverage of the DIAMOND care because they have Medicare or Medical Assistance fee-for-service insurance that is not participating, their self-insured employers have not agreed to coverage, they have high-deductible health insurance products, or they lack insurance altogether. The lack of coverage for many patients is compounded by a widespread feeling that the existing coverage is marginally adequate for clinic costs of this new care.

CONCLUSIONS

The DIAMOND example illustrates many of the points raised earlier in this chapter. First and foremost, it shows the absolutely critical importance of aligning payment with desired care. Second, it shows the great value of a local QIC, especially one that has developed credibility and trust among both medical groups and payers. Third, it illustrates the importance and relevance of the previously described conceptual framework for improvement: DIAMOND implementation benefited from the widespread high prioritization for improving depression, from medical groups and clinics with high levels of capability to manage change, and from identification of a feasible new care process that had proven potential to greatly improve patient outcomes.

This chapter illustrates that large-scale transformational QI has become essential for the survival of primary care, and a thriving primary care system is essential for any nation's medical care system to meet the triple aim of health, cost, and experience. It will no longer suffice for a few physicians or clinics to undertake small QI projects that may not affect the care of many patients and will not be sustained without the continued attention of a few champions. All of the components of a care system must learn to collaborate, to undertake complementary fundamental changes, and to do so in such a way as to be sustainable for patients, staff, clinicians, and indeed entire countries.

REFERENCES

Agency for Healthcare Research and Quality. 2008. *National healthcare quality and disparities reports: 2007*. Retrieved April 1, 2011, from http://www.ahrq.gov/qual/qrdr07.htm

Agency for Healthcare Research and Quality. 2009. *National healthcare quality and disparities reports: 2008*. Retrieved April 1, 2011, from http://www.ahrq.gov/qual/qrdr08.htm

Allen, J. 2008. Crossing the quality chasm: Taking the lead as ICSI turns 15. *Minnesota Physician*, XXII(2): 1, 12–13.

American Academy of Family Physicians. 2009. *Road to Recognition: Your Guide to the NCQA Medical Home*. Leawood, KS: Author.

Amundson, G. M., and Frederick, J. 2003. Making quality measurement work. *Minn Med*, 86(10): 50–52.

Ayers, L. R., Beyea, S. C., Godfrey, M. M., et al. 2005. Quality improvement learning collaboratives. *Qual Manag Health Care*, 14(4): 234–247.

Bershow, B. 2006. MN Community Measurement: Helping physicians rise to the top. *Minnesota Physician*, XIX(11): 1, 12–13.

Berwick, D. M. 1989. Continuous improvement as an ideal in health care. *N Engl J Med*, 320(1): 53–56.

Berwick, D. M. 1996. A primer on leading the improvement of systems. *BMJ*, 312(7031): 619–622.

Berwick, D. M. 1998. Developing and testing changes in delivery of care. *Ann Intern Med*, 128(8): 651–656.

Berwick, D. M., Nolan, T. W., and Whittington, J. 2008. The triple aim: Care, health, and cost. *Health Aff (Millwood)*, 27(3): 759–769.

Bodenheimer, T. 2006. Primary care—Will it survive? *N Engl J Med*, 355(9): 861–864.

Carrier, E., Gourevitch, M. N., and Shah, N. R. 2009. Medical homes: Challenges in translating theory into practice. *Med Care*, 47(7): 714–722.

Corrigan, J. M., and Nielsen, D. M. 1993. Toward the development of uniform reporting standards for managed care organizations: The Health Plan Employer Data and Information Set (Version 2.0). *Jt Comm J Qual Improv*, 19(12): 566–575.

Dietrich, A. J., O'Connor, G. T., Keller, A., et al. 1992. Cancer: Improving early detection and prevention. A community practice randomised trial. *BMJ*, 304(6828): 687–691.

Dietrich, A. J., Tobin, J. N., Sox, C. H., et al. 1998. Cancer early-detection services in community health centers for the underserved. A randomized controlled trial. *Arch Fam Med*, 7(4): 320–327, discussion 328.

Early, J. F., and Godfrey, A. B. 1995. But it takes too long. *Qual Prog*, 28(7): 51–55.

Ellwood, P. M., Jr., Anderson, N. N., Billings, J. E., 1971. Health maintenance strategy. *Med Care*, 9(3): 291–298.

Ellwood, P. M., Jr., and Lundberg, G. D. 1996. Managed care: A work in progress. *JAMA*, 276(13): 1083–1086.

Farley, D. O., Haims, M. C., Keyser, D. J., et al. 2003. *Regional Health Quality Improvement Coalitions: Lessons Across the Life Cycle*. Santa Monica, CA: RAND Health.

Fisher, E. S., Bynum, J. P., and Skinner, J. S. 2009. Slowing the growth of health care cost—Lessons from regional variation. *N Engl J Med*, 360(9): 849–852.

Freidson, E. 1970. *Profession of Medicine: A Study of the Sociology of Applied Knowledge*. New York: Dodd, Mead.

Gilbody, S., Bower, P., Fletcher, J., et al. 2006. Collaborative care for depression: A cumulative meta-analysis and review of longer-term outcomes. *Arch Intern Med*, 166(21): 2314–2321.

Goldberg, H. I., Wagner, E. H., Fihn, S. D., et al. 1998. A randomized controlled trial of CQI teams and academic detailing: Can they alter compliance with guidelines? *Jt Comm J Qual Improv*, 24(3): 130–142.

Goodwin, M. A., Zyzanski, S. J., Zronek, S., et al. 2001. A clinical trial of tailored office systems for preventive service delivery. The Study to Enhance Prevention by Understanding Practice (STEP-UP). *Am J Prev Med*, 21(1): 20–28.

Grumbach, K., and Bodenheimer, T. 2004. Can health care teams improve primary care practice? *JAMA*, 291(10): 1246–1251.

Guterman, S., Davis, K., Schoen, C., et al. 2009. *Reforming Provider Payment: Essential Building Block for Health Reform.* New York: The Commonwealth Fund.

Institute for Healthcare Improvement. 2003. *The Breakthrough Series: IHI's Collaborative Model for Achieving Breakthrough Improvement.* Boston: Author.

Institute of Medicine. 2000. *To Err Is Human.* Washington, DC: National Academies Press.

Institute of Medicine. 2001. *Crossing the Quality Chasm: A New Health System for the 21st Century.* Washington, DC: National Academies Press.

Jaeckels, N. 2009. Early DIAMOND adopters offer insights. *Minnesota Physician*, April: 28–29, 34.

Kilo, C. M. 1998. A framework for collaborative improvement: Lessons from the Institute for Healthcare Improvement's Breakthrough Series. *Qual Manag Health Care*, 6(4): 1–13.

Korsen, N., and Pietruszewski, P. 2009. Translating evidence to practice: Two stories from the field. *J Clin Psychol Med Settings*, 16(1): 47–57.

Kroenke, K., and Spitzer, R. L. 2002. The PHQ-9: A new depression and diagnostic severity measure. *Psychiatric Annals*, 32(9): 509–521.

Laffel, G., and Blumenthal, D. 1989. The case for using industrial quality management science in health care organizations. *JAMA*, 262(20): 2869–2873.

Langley, G. J., Nolan, K. M., and Nolan, T. W. 1994. The foundation of improvement. *Qual Prog*, 27: 81–86.

Langley, G. L., Nolan, K. M., Nolan, T. W., et al. 2009. *The Improvement Guide: A Practical Approach to Enhancing Organizational Performance* (2nd ed.). San Francisco: Jossey-Bass.

Loxterkamp D., Kazal L. A., Jr. 2008. Changing horses midstream: the promise and prudence of practice redesign. *Ann Fam Med*, 6(2): 167–170.

Lowe, B., Kroenke, K., Herzog, W., et al. 2004. Measuring depression outcome with a brief self-report instrument: Sensitivity to change of the Patient Health Questionnaire (PHQ-9). *J Affect Disord*, 81(1): 61–66.

Mangione-Smith, R., DeCristofaro, A. H., Setodji, C. M., et al. 2007. The quality of ambulatory care delivered to children in the United States. *N Engl J Med*, 357(15): 1515–1523.

McBride, P., Underbakke, G., Plane, M. B., et al. 2000. Improving prevention systems in primary care practices: The Health Education and Research Trial (HEART). *J Fam Pract*, 49(2): 115–125.

McGlynn, E. A., Asch, S. M., Adams, J., et al. 2003. The quality of health care delivered to adults in the United States. *N Engl J Med*, 348(26): 2635–2645.

Nelson, E. C., Godfrey, M. M., Batalden, P. B., et al. 2008. Clinical microsystems, part 1. The building blocks of health systems. *Jt Comm J Qual Patient Safety*, 34(7): 367–378.

Nolan, T. 1997. Accelerating the pace of improvement: An interview with Thomas Nolan. Interview by Steven Berman. *Jt Comm J Qual Improv*, 23(4): 217–222.

Nutting, P. A., Miller, W. L., Crabtree, B. F., et al. 2009. Initial lessons from the first national demonstration project on practice transformation to a patient-centered medical home. *Ann Fam Med*, 7(3): 254–260.

Rogers, E. M. 1995. Lessons for guidelines from the diffusion of innovations. *Jt Comm J Qual Improv*, 21(7): 324–328.

Rosenthal, T. C. 2008. The medical home: Growing evidence to support a new approach to primary care. *J Am Board Fam Med*, 21(5): 427–440.

Rosser, W. W., Colwill, J. M., and Kasperski, J. 2010. Patient-centered medical homes in Ontario. *N Engl J Med*, 362(3): e7.

Schouten, L. M., Hulscher, M. E., van Everdingen, J. J., et al. 2008. Evidence for the impact of quality improvement collaboratives: Systematic review. *BMJ*, 336(7659): 1491–1494.

Shortell, S. M., Levin, D. Z., O'Brien, J. L., et al. 1995. Assessing the evidence on CQI: Is the glass half empty or half full? *Hosp Health Serv Adm*, 40(1): 4–24.

Solberg, L. I. 2005. If you've seen one quality improvement collaborative. *Ann Fam Med*, 3(3): 198–199.

Solberg, L. I. 2007. Improving medical practice: A conceptual framework. *Ann Fam Med*, 5(3): 251–256.

Solberg, L. I., Brekke, M. L., Fazio, C. J., et al. 2000. Lessons from experienced guideline implementers: Attend to many factors and use multiple strategies. *Jt Comm J Qual Improv*, 26(4): 171–188.

Solberg, L. I., Kottke, T. E., Brekke, M. L., et al. 2000. Failure of a continuous quality improvement intervention to increase the delivery of preventive services. A randomized trial. *Eff Clin Pract*, 3(3): 105–115.

Unutzer, J., Katon, W., Callahan, C. M., et al. 2002. Collaborative care management of late-life depression in the primary care setting: A randomized controlled trial. *JAMA*, 288(22): 2836–2845.

Wasson, J. H., Anders, S. G., Moore, L. G., et al. 2008. Clinical microsystems, part 2. Learning from micro practices about providing patients the care they want and need. *Jt Comm J Qual Patient Safety*, 34(8): 445–452.

Wei, E. K., Ryan, C. T., Dietrich, A. J., et al. 2005. Improving colorectal cancer screening by targeting office systems in primary care practices: Disseminating research results into clinical practice. *Arch Intern Med*, 165(6): 661–666.

Williams, J. W., Jr., Gerrity, M., Holsinger, T., et al. 2007. Systematic review of multifaceted interventions to improve depression care. *Gen Hosp Psychiatry*, 29(2): 91–116.

CHAPTER 15

Quality Improvement Organizations and Continuous Quality Improvement in Medicare

Anna P. Schenck, Jill McArdle, and Robert Weiser

"In health care, quality means getting the right care at the right time— safely and effectively."

—Excerpt from the QIO Mission Statement, published by the American Health Quality Association

When Medicare, the health insurance program for older Americans, was implemented in the United States in 1966, continuous quality improvement (CQI) had not yet been introduced in the health care arena. More than half a century later, the Medicare program is recognized as a leader in the field of quality improvement. The Medicare program, which is administered by the Centers for Medicare and Medicaid Services (CMS) within the U.S. Department of Health and Human Services, has implemented a number of innovative approaches to drive quality improvement at the national level. These include adopting the use and promoting the development of standard quality measures, public reporting of quality measures, and pay-for-performance efforts to reward physicians for providing better quality care. Quality Improvement Organizations, or QIOs, are Medicare's primary tool for quality improvement. With a presence in every state and most federal territories, QIOs have been called "the nation's main infrastructure for quality improvement" (Hsia, 2003). In this chapter, we describe the history and evolution of QIOs, provide examples of how QIOs apply CQI in the Medicare program, and examine potential future roles for QIOs. The methods described provide an overview of CQI techniques that are applicable on a national level. (Please see Appendix 15–A for a further description of the Medicare program and Appendix 15–B for an explanation of commonly used abbreviations that are found throughout this chapter relative to Medicare and QIOs.)

HISTORY AND ROLE OF THE QIO PROGRAM

The history of the Medicare QIO program in many ways mirrors the history of the development of quality improvement in health care (see **Figure 15–1**) (IOM, 2006). In the early stage of the Medicare program, concerns about quality were addressed through physician licensure and hospital accreditation. In 1972, Professional Standards Review Organizations (PSROs) were established to provide oversight of the care provided to Medicare beneficiaries. Each state had multiple PSROs, responsible for regions within the state. PSROs conducted retrospective case review in an effort to identify poor quality of care.

Peer Review Organizations (PROs) were created by the Medicare Utilization and Quality Control Peer Review Program, enacted nationally by Congress in 1982. The PRO statute required Medicare to contract with one organization in each state and territory to monitor quality of care provided to Medicare enrollees. The initial contracts, called statements of work (SOWs), were 2 years in length; subsequent SOWs have been 3 years. Like its PSRO predecessor program, the PRO program initially used the retrospective review of hospital medical records to perform quality assurance and utilization management. However, between the time the enabling legislation was passed and the first contracts were awarded, Medicare implemented the Prospective Payment System (PPS) in October 1983. PPS, which essentially pays hospitals a fixed amount per admission based on diagnosis-related groups (DRGs), introduced new quality and utilization

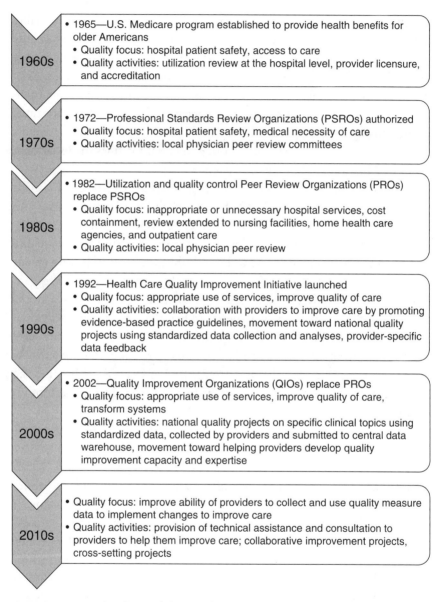

1960s
- 1965—U.S. Medicare program established to provide health benefits for older Americans
- Quality focus: hospital patient safety, access to care
- Quality activities: utilization review at the hospital level, provider licensure, and accreditation

1970s
- 1972—Professional Standards Review Organizations (PSROs) authorized
- Quality focus: hospital patient safety, medical necessity of care
- Quality activities: local physician peer review committees

1980s
- 1982—Utilization and quality control Peer Review Organizations (PROs) replace PSROs
- Quality focus: inappropriate or unnecessary hospital services, cost containment, review extended to nursing facilities, home health care agencies, and outpatient care
- Quality activities: local physician peer review

1990s
- 1992—Health Care Quality Improvement Initiative launched
- Quality focus: appropriate use of services, improve quality of care
- Quality activities: collaboration with providers to improve care by promoting evidence-based practice guidelines, movement toward national quality projects using standardized data collection and analyses, provider-specific data feedback

2000s
- 2002—Quality Improvement Organizations (QIOs) replace PROs
- Quality focus: appropriate use of services, improve quality of care, transform systems
- Quality activities: national quality projects on specific clinical topics using standardized data, collected by providers and submitted to central data warehouse, movement toward helping providers develop quality improvement capacity and expertise

2010s
- Quality focus: improve ability of providers to collect and use quality measure data to implement changes to improve care
- Quality activities: provision of technical assistance and consultation to providers to help them improve care; collaborative improvement projects, cross-setting projects

FIGURE 15-1 Timeline of the Medicare Quality Program, Focus, and Activities

issues that needed to be addressed by the PRO program. Whereas previous utilization issues focused on reducing the length of stay of an admission by identifying unnecessary days or unneeded services, issues of unnecessary admissions, premature discharge, failure to provide needed services, and preventable readmissions were a major focus of utilization and quality assurance efforts by PROs under the PPS. The program pursued quality assurance by assigning responsibility for identified instances of poor quality care to hospitals or physicians, assigning scores based on the seriousness of the problem identified, and requiring corrective action dependent upon the score for an individual case or the aggregate score over a period of time. Serious quality issues could involve the initiation of sanction activity against either a physician or a hospital, with the potential for fines or disbarment from the Medicare and/or Medicaid programs.

A congressionally mandated study by the Institute of Medicine (IOM) in 1990 recommended that PROs begin examining patterns of care and offer feedback to providers (Lohr, 1990). The IOM report also recommended that more emphasis be placed on quality. The shift to true quality improvement began in 1992 with the Health Care Quality Improvement Initiative, later called the Healthcare Quality Improvement Program (HCQIP). Under HCQIP, emphasis was placed on examining patterns of care for the population of patients rather than reviewing individual cases. PROs were directed to develop and undertake local- and state-level quality improvement projects while reducing the amount of case review performed (Jencks and Wilensky, 1992). In 1994, HCQIP became the major activity for the program with case review reduced to the minimum required by statute.

The emphasis on quality improvement by the PRO program coincided with the creation of the agency that is now called the Agency for Healthcare Research and Quality (AHRQ). AHRQ in the early 1990s had begun developing and publishing evidence-based practice guidelines on several disease topics. These guidelines served as a basis for many of the early PRO quality improvement projects by providing the norms against which provider patterns of care could be compared. In designing their initial quality improvement projects, PROs sought input from committees of hospital representatives and physicians to identify clinical topics for projects, used AHRQ and other available guidelines to establish measures and goals, collected data primarily through the abstraction of medical records, and provided feedback to hospitals who voluntarily participated in these projects. Feedback of an individual hospital's data combined with comparative data from other participating hospitals was the primary quality improvement intervention used. Data feedback was sometimes combined with educational sessions by topic experts both to explain the data and to offer suggestions on implementing systemic changes to improve measures. After allowing time for hospitals to implement changes, a second medical record abstraction was conducted; these data were used to determine the degree of improvement achieved both by individual hospitals and by the group.

Allowing PROs to work with the physicians and hospitals in their states to select and design quality improvement projects enabled PROs to develop expertise and credibility in quality improvement and encouraged the voluntary participation of the hospitals. However, it did not readily allow for the evaluation of the program on a national basis. Beginning in 1996, PROs were required to work on national quality improvement projects with standardized measures along with locally developed projects. The Cooperative Cardiovascular Project, focusing on care for Medicare patients hospitalized with heart attacks, was the first of such CMS-led national projects (Marciniak et al., 1998). The transition to national topics and measures was completed by 1999. Since that time, only rarely have locally developed projects been conducted under the QIO contracts.

Beginning in 1999, the settings in which QIOs conducted quality improvement began to expand. The expansion started with Medicare managed care plans. By 2002, nursing homes and home health agencies were included in the SOW, with physician offices added later in that same SOW. In 2002, PROs were officially renamed Quality Improvement Organizations, although many of them had already adopted the name.

Clinical Areas of Focus

The aim of the QIO contract is to focus on clinical areas and topics of great importance to the Medicare population, usually high-cost, high-impact topics such as leading causes of hospitalization among the Medicare population (heart attack, heart failure, pneumonia). Other criteria used to determine topics of QIO focus include known gaps in performance, improvement possibilities, and scientific evidence or expert consensus regarding improvement methods. In the years since improvement became the primary activity of the QIOs, the clinical topics addressed by the program, and the settings in which QIOs have worked, have changed (see **Figure 15–2**).

In the ninth SOW, which began in 2008, all QIOs were tasked with improving specific care processes and outcomes for clinical areas that

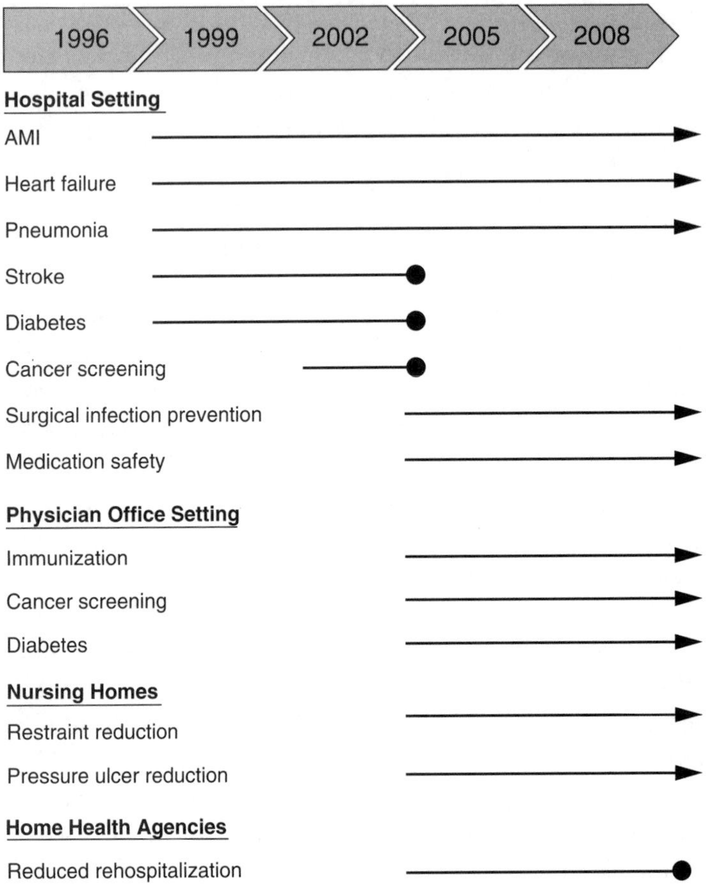

FIGURE 15-2 Timeline of Clinical Topics Included in Medicare QIO Contracts, by Setting

span two general themes: patient safety and prevention (see **Table 15–1**). In addition, there was an optional theme, care transitions, that was addressed by selected QIOs. The care transitions theme was designed to help improve the coordination of care across health care settings, transitions from the hospital to home, home health care, or skilled nursing care. Fourteen QIOs were selected by CMS through a competitive proposal process to conduct this work, which is focused on reducing unnecessary hospital readmissions and identifying ways to improve care transitions (http://www.cfmc.org/caretransitions/).

TABLE 15–1 Quality of Care Objectives for QIOs Under the Ninth SOW

Theme	Clinical Area of Focus	Objectives
Patient Safety	Surgical care infection prevention/heart failure	Increase timely administration and discontinuation of appropriate prophylactic antibiotics
		Increase appropriate hair removal for surgery patients
		Increase appropriate and timely VTE prophylaxis for surgery patients
		Increase appropriate beta-blocker administration and glucose monitoring for cardiac patients undergoing surgery
		Increase discharge on appropriate medications for heart failure patients
	Pressure ulcers in hospitals and nursing homes	Reduce pressure sores acquired in the hospital and among long-stay nursing home residents
	Physical restraints	Reduce the use of physical restraints among long-stay nursing home residents
	Methicillin-resistant *Staphylococcus aureus* (MRSA)	Increase hospital reports of MRSA infection and transmission rates
	Drug safety	Reduce drug–drug interactions and use of potentially inappropriate medications
	Nursing homes in need	Provide technical assistance to selected nursing homes to improve processes of care and outcomes for reducing pressure ulcers and physical restraints
Prevention	Breast cancer screening	Work with physician practices to use electronic health records to report data and increase breast cancer screening
	Colorectal cancer screening	Work with physician practices to use electronic health records to report data and increase colorectal cancer screening
	Immunizations	Work with physician practices to use electronic health records to report data and increase immunizations for influenza and pneumonia
	Disparities (limited to 33 states)	Improve diabetes measures within the underserved populations
	Chronic kidney disease (optional theme)	Increase timely testing to reduce the rate of kidney failure due to diabetes and slow the progression through the use of ACE inhibitors and/or ARB agents
		Increase AV fistula placement and maturation as part of a timely renal replacement therapy counseling for patients who elect hemodialysis
Care Transitions	(optional theme)	Reduce rehospitalizations

QIO STRUCTURE AND OPERATIONS

QIOs are expected to work *with* health care providers to improve care. Nationally, more than 1 million providers participate in the Medicare program. These range from individual practitioners to large multicity hospitals and health systems (see **Table 15–2**). CMS, which oversees the Medicare program, establishes the requirements for providers to participate in Medicare. These requirements vary by type of provider, but implicit in the acceptance of Medicare payment, and in some settings explicit in the provider agreements, is the expectation that providers will cooperate with Medicare program oversight and quality initiatives, including the work of QIOs.

Requirements of QIOs

CMS contracts with one organization for each U.S. state and territory, although an organization can hold contracts for multiple states. In 2010, there were 38 organizations holding the 53 QIO contracts (http://www .cms.gov/qualityimprovementorgs). Organizations are eligible to be QIOs if they are physician sponsored, can complete case reviews and analyze patterns of care to determine medical necessity and quality of care, and are not a health care organization.

QIOs act as independent contractors to complete their contracts. There are, however, a number of internal and external requirements placed on QIOs by CMS. Internal requirements include the use of a CMS-supplied

TABLE 15–2 Provider Participation in Medicare, by Type

Type of Provider	Number Participating in Medicare
Physicians[a]	667,340
Nonphysician practitioners[a]*	294,499
Hospitals[b]	6,169
Skilled nursing facilities[c]	15,055
Home health agencies[c]	9,407
Hospice providers[c]	3,346

*Includes psychologists, physician assistants, nurse practitioners, dietitians, therapists, clinical social workers, certified nurse midwives, and clinical nurses.
Sources: Centers for Medicare and Medicaid Services, 2009a, 2009b, and 2009c.

standardized computer system to support data management and security, review and verification of data security and confidentiality protocol, and use of a documented internal quality control program. QIOs are tasked with assisting CMS in the event of an emergency and are expected to participate in the state disaster planning process. QIOs are expected to coordinate their work with other stakeholder groups in each state. These stakeholders might include professional associations representing hospitals, nursing homes and home health agencies, state health departments, and voluntary health organizations. External requirements describe how QIOs should interact with other stakeholders. QIOs are expected to conduct education and outreach to beneficiaries and providers and must adhere to CMS requirements when creating and disseminating materials.

Oversight of the QIO program is provided by CMS staff in four regional offices. Each QIO is assigned a project officer who works with the QIO over the life of the contract to ensure that deliverables and contract requirements are met. Project officers hold routine conference calls with their QIOs and make periodic site visits. In addition to their project officers, QIOs can also receive assistance from scientific officers at their assigned regional office.

QIO Staffing

QIO staffing is not dictated by the CMS contract. QIOs are, however, required to have the expertise needed to carry out the contract requirements. QIOs must contract for, or have staff who have, the following areas of expertise: medicine, nursing, health education, coding, quality improvement, epidemiology, statistics, electronic medical records, behavioral sciences including the understanding of human factors, administrative and case review, information technology networking, and database administration, management, and security). In addition, QIOs are expected to have setting-specific expertise, including physician practices, home health, hospital, nursing home, managed care, pharmacy, and prescription drug plans.

Resources Available to QIOs

The QIOs are a national network, linked not only by their similar goals and contractual obligations, but also in a very real sense by shared computer and data systems. A standardized data processing system (SDPS) is required by CMS as part of the QIO contract, which allows all QIOs to have similar data access capabilities and allows CMS to ensure appropriate security standards. The SDPS system allows communication across QIOs from a shared e-mail system and allows access to secure data repositories.

In addition to the shared computer networks, QIOs share expertise through a series of discipline networks (e.g., finance, data, analytic, quality improvement, review, and administrative), which are sponsored by the American Health Quality Association, the professional association that represents QIOs (http://www.ahqa.org). These networks often gather at national meetings to work on common concerns or for shared educational experiences.

Another resource provided to the QIOs is the QIOSCs, or Quality Improvement Organization Support Centers. The QIOSCs are QIOs that have received additional CMS contracts to develop and share content-specific expertise with the QIO network. Beginning in 2005, QIOSCs provided assistance to QIOs for work related to nursing home, home health, hospital, and physician practice. Later QIOSCs were added to provide assistance to QIOs on three clinical topics (patient safety, prevention, care transitions) and two cross-cutting topics (health disparities and communications). The level of assistance provided by the QIOSCs varies, ranging from intensive training (completed through in-person workshops, Webinars, and/or conference calls) to passive resource dissemination (e.g., literature reviews, best-practice examples, sample flow-sheets) through e-mail and Web postings. The QIOSCs also play a role in maintaining the Medicare Quality Improvement Community Web site, a free public resource containing provider settings, and topic-specific quality improvement interventions and associated tools, toolkits, presentations, and links to other applicable Web sites (http://www.cms.gov/qualityimprovementorgs).

Data-Driven CQI

One of the most powerful resources available to QIOs for CQI is access to Medicare data. The national Medicare enrollment database can be accessed by QIO analytic staff to identify appropriate target groups for quality initiatives (e.g., to identify women between 50 and 70 years of age who are eligible for breast cancer screening). Medicare hospital claims data are also available to QIOs. Additionally, files containing claims for services targeted under the contract are available. In most cases, the files are identifiable, making it possible to follow individuals across files and to link persons identified as eligible for a service to the claims files to determine whether they received the service (e.g., to follow the women identified as needing a mammogram to determine whether they received one in a specified time period). In addition to enrollment and claims data, QIOs have access to setting-specific files with quality-measure data collected at the individual level. Files containing hospital, home health, and nursing home quality-measure data can be analyzed at the provider level and used to develop provider feedback reports and to target and evaluate interventions. The easy access to data and the data-driven focus of CQI were natural fits for QIOs.

THE QIO'S ROLE IN CONTINUOUS QUALITY IMPROVEMENT IN MEDICARE

CQI Tools and Strategies Used by QIOs

QIOs are expected to improve both health care processes and health outcomes. For instance, they may be expected to improve flu and pneumonia immunization rates in physician offices or to reduce physical restraint use among nursing homes. Since QIOs do not provide care, they work with volunteer health care practitioners and providers to improve care. QIOs can also intervene at the consumer level to influence consumer behavior. QIOs typically use multiple interventions to impact Medicare beneficiary and health care practitioner and provider behavior to reach the QIO contract goals.

Although QIOs currently work on common clinical conditions, there is variability in how QIOs accomplish the goals established by the contract. The approaches used by QIOs can be grouped into four categories based on the target audience of the CQI activity (**Table 15–3**). Audiences targeted by QIOs include individual consumers, individual providers, groups of providers, and communities. Within each of the four categories, different strategies can be used to influence health behavior, health care processes, and/or health outcomes. More than one approach can be used, and more than one strategy within each approach can be used.

In the individual consumer-level approach, QIOs can directly mail health care reminders to Medicare consumers. Since direct-mail patient reminders, such as those for flu or pneumonia immunization or cancer screening, are more effective when personalized and sent by patients'

TABLE 15–3 CQI Approaches Used by QIOs to Improve Quality of Care in the Medicare Population

Target of Intervention	CQI Approaches Used
Individual Consumers	Direct marketing through mailings directed at consumers and/or information dissemination via Web site
	Case management through direct contact with consumers by health care provider
Individual Providers	Provide educational materials and/or quality improvement toolkits
	Audit and feedback by collecting medical record and/or health care claims data by QIO or external source, with analyses to calculate provider-specific quality measure rates
	Self assessment/data collection by health care provider
	Continuing medical education
	Individual consultation through one-on-one QIO consultation with provider
Groups of Providers	Group education sessions in which providers receive information, either in person or through teleconferences or Webinars; no obligation for participants to act alone or together
	Group improvement with sharing through a modified version of the Institute for Healthcare Improvement (IHI) collaborative method. Participants receive information and support to implement specific activities with defined expectations for participation.
	Collaboratives through the IHI method where QIO offers training and support of quality improvement activities. Participants are expected to submit reports, collect data, attend learning sessions, and share information about their experience.
Communities	Coalition/partnerships, whereby stakeholder participants work together to share resources and jointly address access and quality of care concerns
	Community campaign (mass media) to promote awareness and changes in norms and behaviors

own providers, QIOs often work with providers to prepare and distribute these types of reminders (Stone et al., 2002).

When targeting individual providers, QIOs can use several strategies appropriate for providers and practitioners, including:

- One-on-one consultation to review their established policies
- Procedures and work processes to identify opportunities to improve how care is provided

- Use of provider-specific data feedback comparing their care to established scientific evidence or expert consensus recommendations.

Group approaches include CQI strategies that are described throughout this text. These range from group education sessions, where practitioners/providers are the passive recipients of information, to the intense Institute for Healthcare Improvement's (IHI) Breakthrough Series Collaborative, where practitioners/providers are actively involved in quality improvement projects (IHI, 2003). The value and success of quality improvement collaboratives are also discussed in Chapter 1. The IHI uses its Breakthrough Series Collaborative as a learning method to help hospitals and outpatient settings improve care. Provider participants learn from topic experts and each other over a 6- to 15-month period. Working in teams from their organizations, providers agree to conduct small-scale tests of change, using the Plan, Do, Study, Act (PDSA) cycle (introduced in Chapter 1). In 2002, CMS contracted with IHI to provide training to the QIOs on the Breakthrough Series Collaborative approach, and since that time, QIOs have applied this method and modifications of the method to help various providers improve care.

In 2002, CMS sponsored the national Surgical Infection Prevention (SIP) Collaborative. Fifty-six hospitals volunteered to work with their QIO on a 1-year project to improve quality measures for a predetermined group of surgical procedures. Hospitals agreed to improve the use and timing of antibiotics and other processes of care associated with reductions in surgical site infections. The hospitals also agreed to report monthly clinical process measure data to monitor their improvement. The SIP Collaborative demonstrated a successful QIO-led health care quality improvement project. Hospitals showed improvement in recommended measures related to appropriate surgical care and reduced the rate of surgical site infection (Dellinger et al., 2005).

Within the individual provider and group approaches, QIOs provide training for health care providers on the use of a number of CQI tools and techniques: lean methodology to reduce unnecessary waste (Womack and Jones, 2005); Crew Resource Management (http://www.psnet.ahrq .gov/primer.aspx?primerID=8), an aviation industry technique to improve teamwork and communications; TeamSTEPPS (http://teamstepps.ahrq .gov/), a training program designed by the AHRQ and the U.S. Department of Defense to improve teamwork and communication among health care

workers; and the AHRQ's Patient Safety Culture surveys (http://www
.ahrq.gov/qual/patientsafetyculture/), designed to measure health care
organizational culture to support quality and patient safety.

In most cases, QIO-led CQI approaches are paired with provider-
specific quality measure feedback, trended over time, with benchmark
or comparison data. A frequently used benchmarking approach uses the
ABCs, which stands for *achievable benchmarks of care* (Kiefe et al., 1998).
Under the ABCs approach, quality measure rates are calculated for each
provider, and providers are then rank ordered by performance, from
better to worse performing. Data to be included in the benchmark are
determined by beginning with the top-performing provider and continuing down the ranked list of providers until 10% of the total population is
represented. The benchmark is calculated among the top performers and
represents a level of care attained by providers and experienced by 10% of
the population. This benchmark is, obviously, a higher level of care than
the mean or median and has been demonstrated to result in greater levels
of improvement than provider feedback using the mean performance of
other participating providers (Kiefe et al., 2001). If the initiative is one
for which the QIO has data on all providers in the state, calculated at the
provider level, feedback reports may show graphs ranking all providers in
the state, masking the identity of all providers except the one receiving
the report. In addition, the QIO may provide trended state-level rates or
national rates for comparison.

CQI Across the Continuum of Care

QIOs are unique in that they work with providers across the health
care continuum to improve care (**Figure 15–3**). QIOs have worked
with hospitals, physician offices, home health agencies, skilled nursing
facilities, prescription drug plans, and Medicare Part C plans to improve
health care processes and health outcomes. QIOs are involved in primary
prevention through their activities to increase immunizations to prevent
the development of influenza and pneumonia. QIOs conduct secondary
prevention by working with individuals, providers, and communities to
increase early detection of breast and colorectal cancers and to improve
care for persons with diabetes. QIOs also work in the realm of tertiary
prevention, collaborating with hospitals, home health agencies, and
skilled nursing homes to improve treatments and limit the negative consequences of diseases.

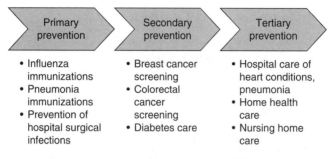

FIGURE 15-3 The Continuum of Care Targeted by QIOs

CQI Example: Clemson Nursing Home

An example of how QIOs work with providers can be seen in the case of Clemson's nursing home. This 95-bed, family-owned nursing home, located in the foothills of North Carolina, was attempting to reduce restraint use in its facility. Clemson received an invitation from the state QIO to participate in a restraint reduction quality improvement initiative. Using data from all nursing homes in the state, the QIO provided Clemson with graphs illustrating that its restraint use was higher than the state and national averages, ranking them as having the fourth highest restraint use rate among nursing homes in the initiative. Working with the QIO, Clemson conducted a root-cause analysis (see Chapter 3 and http://process.nasa.gov/documents/RootCauseAnalysis.pdf) and identified several opportunities for reducing restraints. Testing new processes using PDSA cycles over a period of several weeks, Clemson was able to reduce restraint use from 10% to 6% and ultimately achieved its goal of 3% by the end of the initiative. (See Case 3 of the companion casebook [McLaughlin et al., 2012].)

EVALUATING THE WORK OF THE QIOS

The work of the QIOs can be evaluated from several perspectives. From an organizational perspective, QIO success is judged by the organization's ability to achieve the performance standards set by the CMS contract. Success of a QIO can also be evaluated on a setting- or project-specific initiative. From an oversight perspective, it is important to look at the QIO program on the national level to determine whether the program achieves its goals. The sections that follow address each of these levels of evaluation.

Evaluation Under the CMS Contract

QIOs work on performance-based contracts. State-based QIOs that have acceptably met the performance requirements of the contract are eligible to have their QIO contracts renewed automatically. If a QIO fails the performance requirements, the contract may go out for competition. The evaluation criteria are detailed in the contract and published in the *Federal Register* (http://www.federalregister.gov/articles/2008/07/21/ E8-16757/medicare-program-evaluation-criteria-and-standards-for- quality-improvement-program-contracts-9th). For example, evaluations in the ninth SOW (2008–2011) were conducted in two parts, with measures calculated at 18 months into the contract and again at 28 months. A QIO is considered to have passed the overall contract evaluation if it received a passing score on all themes and components of themes in the contract at both the 18-month and 28-month evaluation periods. A QIO is considered to have failed its contract if it failed any theme or any component in either evaluation period.

QIO contract evaluation is complex. The thresholds for passing the contract vary by theme and are based on preset targets. Primarily, the early evaluation period focuses on achieving tasks and activities (such as provider recruitment), and the later evaluation period focuses on improvements in quality measures (such as increasing immunization rates). The number, type, and data source for quality measures vary by clinical area. Further details on quality measures used by CMS are available on the CMS Web site (https://www.cms.gov/QualityMeasures/). The complexity of evaluation used for QIO contracts has made it difficult to evaluate the overall impact of the QIO program. In response to an IOM review, CMS has contracted for an external review of the ninth SOW contracts (https://www.cms.gov/QualityImprovementOrgs/ downloads/QIO_Improvement_RTC_fnl.pdf).

Evaluation of Outcomes and CQI Strategies Used by QIOs

There is a growing body of literature describing the results of QIO initiatives. The majority of the literature to date has focused on the hospital setting, examining care for patients hospitalized for heart conditions, stroke, and pneumonia and for patients undergoing selected surgical procedures. QIO interventions have been shown to improve care for patients with acute myocardial infarction in multiple studies

(Burwen et al., 2003; Ellerbeck et al., 2000; Marciniak et al., 1998; Schade et al., 2004; Sueta et al., 2001). These studies focused on a common set of detailed, specified quality measures that assessed the timely receipt of medications (aspirin, beta-blockers, and ACE inhibitors) and smoking cessation counseling. QIO interventions have also been reported to improve care for patients with pneumonia (Chu et al., 2003; Schade et al., 2004); heart failure, stroke, and atrial fibrillation (Schade et al., 2004); and CABG surgical procedures (Holman et al., 2001). Interventions have further been shown to reduce surgical infections (Dellinger et al., 2005). However, the studies contain little information about the specific CQI tools used by QIOs. In most of these projects, the primary approaches used by QIOs included hospital-specific data feedback and education and training for hospitals to develop quality improvement plans to address specific quality measures. However, the use of these approaches differed by state and by clinical topic.

Not all QIO interventions with hospitals have been found effective. Hayes and colleagues (2001), in a randomized trial, found no difference in management of deep vein thrombosis for hospitals provided CQI training, tools, and data feedback compared to hospitals not provided the intervention. Similarly, another randomized trial observed no differences in the treatment of patients with unstable angina for hospitals participating in QIO-led CQI activities and hospitals receiving no intervention (Berner et al., 2003).

Evidence of QIO success in physician office settings has been reported for improving care of diabetes through the use of multimodal intervention including education, flow sheets, and chart reminders (Sutherland et al., 2001), by involving providers in a collaborative (Daniel et al., 2004), through the use of provider feedback (McClellan et al., 2003), and through physician feedback with the addition of benchmarks for quality (Kiefe et al., 2001). The latter study also targeted immunizations and showed improvements. As in hospital settings, however, not all QIO reports have demonstrated improvements in care. Schenck and colleagues (2006) reported small increases but no statistically significant improvement in colorectal cancer screening for physicians provided education and practice-based tool kits.

Fewer reports of individual QIO efforts to improve the care provided by home health agencies and nursing homes have been published. One project targeting pain management in nursing homes demonstrated improvement in some targeted care processes—assessing residents for pain and the use of nonpharmacologic treatments for pain—but not in the use of pain medications (Horner et al., 2005). In a report using data from all states, Rollow and colleagues (2006) showed that care in nursing homes that worked with their QIOs improved more than in nursing homes that did not for five quality measures targeting care for patients in pain, reducing restraint use, and reducing functional declines. Similarly, in the same report, home health agencies that worked with their QIO showed greater improvement in 10 of 11 quality measures than agencies that did not work with their QIO.

QIO Program Effectiveness

The Medicare quality program has undergone extensive external review twice since its creation. The 1990 IOM review of the PRO program recommended that the work of PROs be redirected to focus on quality improvement rather than quality assurance and review (Lohr, 1990). In response to the recommendation, successive PRO contracts placed more emphasis on quality improvement. PROs began implementing local quality improvement initiatives. By the end of the decade, the term for organizations holding the contracts had changed, from PROs to QIOs, to reflect the emphasis on quality improvement. In 2003, Congress requested an evaluation of the Medicare QIO program, which resulted in the IOM report *Medicare's Quality Improvement Organization Program: Maximizing Potential* (IOM, 2006). The committee conducted a comprehensive assessment of the QIO program, which included:

- Reviewing the literature on quality improvement and QIOs
- Analyzing QIO program evaluation data and quality measure rates
- Collecting original data from QIOs
- Performing site visits with selected QIOs
- Interviewing CEOs of 20 randomly selected QIOs
- Forming a focus group with 11 additional CEOs
- Reviewing a number of presentations and data reports.

The committee concluded that the care of Medicare beneficiaries had improved over time, but there was insufficient evidence to conclude that the QIO program was responsible for the improvements. Following the publication of the IOM report, CMS issued a report to Congress describing a series of improvement steps that were being undertaken as a result of both the IOM study and CMS's own internal reviews (Leavitt, 2006).

CMS has published two assessments of the QIO program. In 2003, Jencks and colleagues published state-level rates for 22 quality indicators covering seven clinical topics in the hospital (heart attack, heart failure, stroke, pneumonia) and outpatient (immunizations, breast cancer screening, and diabetes care) settings. Baseline data from 1998 to 1999 were compared with data from 2000 to 2001. State-level rates improved in 20 of the 22 indicators, but the study design (observational data from two points in time) made it impossible to determine if the improvements in care were due to the QIO program or individual QIO efforts (Jencks et al., 2003). In 2006, another assessment of the Medicare QIO program was published, including state-level data on quality of care for Medicare delivered in hospitals, nursing homes, home health agencies, and physician practices (Rollow et al., 2006). In this report, care improved in 34 of 41 quality measures from the baseline period to the evaluation period. This study included analyses of differential improvements based on whether the health care provider worked with the QIO. The authors concluded that their findings were "consistent" with an improvement in health care attributable to QIO assistance. However, as with the earlier study, the study results were open to alternative explanations such as secular trend and selection bias, making it difficult to draw causal interpretations.

Snyder and Anderson (2005) also examined the question of the effectiveness of QIOs by examining quality of care data delivered in the hospital setting using data from five states on 15 quality indicators. The authors assessed QIO impact by analyzing the improvement in the quality measures, from baseline to remeasurement, for hospitals that participated with QIOs compared to those that did not. A statistically significant difference in the level of improvement in hospitals that worked with QIOs compared to those that did not was seen in only 1 of the 15 quality measures. The authors concluded that the improvement seen in hospitals did not differ based on participation in QIO projects. This study was criticized, however, because it only included data from five states and assessed improvement at the halfway point in the QIO contract cycle (Jencks, 2005).

Where does the conflicting evidence leave us in our assessment of the QIO program? To borrow a phrase from CQI literature, clearly there is room for improvement in our ability to evaluate the efforts of the QIOs and, undoubtedly, room to improve the work done by the QIOs. However, this problem is not unique to the QIOs; rather, it is a problem shared by the CQI field due to the difficulty of using randomized controlled trials and traditional research approaches in establishing causal associations in community settings. Nonetheless, as the 2006 IOM report noted, "The QIO program is the only public infrastructure devoted to quality improvement with resources on the ground in every state, as well as with electronic communications systems expertise for transmitting, aggregating, validating, and analyzing quality improvement data."

CONCLUSIONS

As described in Chapter 1, quality improvement has evolved and expanded over the years; the development of QIOs in the United States is a clear example of that trend. Interest in the use of CQI in health care has grown tremendously over the past half century since the Medicare program was launched. When CMS broadened the role of PROs and created QIOs, its goal was clearly to take advantage of the increasing knowledge about the process, philosophy, and applicability of CQI in all areas of health care. As this chapter has shown, this trend has continued and QIOs have kept pace with new tools and approaches while also taking full advantage of technology to access larger and more comprehensive data systems spanning a wide variety of providers throughout the United States. As a result, there has been much success in improving the care received by Medicare patients.

National programs such as the public reporting of quality measures, launched by CMS in 2000, have encouraged many providers to implement CQI, and initiatives like "pay for performance" have resulted in some providers viewing quality as important to their financial well-being. Could that mean there will not be a need for QIOs in the future? Despite the CMS goal of ensuring "the right care for the right patient every time," it is likely the services provided by QIOs will be needed in the foreseeable future for a number of reasons. First, there are many organizations and communities that simply do not have the resources or expertise to address quality of care concerns without external support. In the absence of QIO services, which are offered free of charge to providers, or some other publicly available CQI resource, disparities in care would likely grow worse between the organizations with resources and those without. Second, to date, QIOs have targeted a limited number of conditions and procedures in selected settings. Even if optimal levels of care are reached in some settings targeted by QIOs, there are many additional areas in need of CQI that could use the assistance of QIOs, such as care provided in ambulatory care centers and care provided by hospices. Finally, new technologies and procedures are continually being added in health care at a rapid pace, and with the passage of health care reform, additional preventive services and benefits will soon be added to the Medicare program, creating a "moving target" in terms of the universe of care that could be targeted by QIOs.

Reports on quality improvements associated with public reporting and pay for performance have not suggested a ready replacement for the national QIO network. Jung and colleagues (2010) examined 5 years of quality measure data and information about agency characteristics from agencies in the Home Health Compare public reporting Web site. They demonstrated that rates of most quality measures increased after public reporting. However, not all quality measures improved, and the rate of improvement was influenced by agency characteristics. Pay for performance, or *value-based purchasing* as it is now called, was implemented by CMS in 2009 for hospitals and is expected to be employed in other settings soon. Yet evidence for its effectiveness is mixed (Rosenthal and Frank, 2006).

QIOs have evolved over the years in the way they address quality concerns—moving from quality assurance to continuous quality improvement. They have the potential to advance the field of CQI, helping shape our understanding of what works and what doesn't. The most recent IOM report on QIOs recommended specific changes in the way QIOs conduct their work. Some of the recommendations, such as a shift in the QIO strategies toward the provision of technical assistance to low-performing providers, were incorporated into the ninth SOW. Other recommendations, such as removing the review functions from the QIOs (and having review handled by separate contractors) and improving the timeliness of the data available to QIOs, have not yet been implemented. The report concludes that QIOs provide a potentially "valuable nationwide infrastructure dedicated to promoting quality health care." CMS and QIO professionals will need to work collaboratively to strengthen and improve QIOs before the full potential of QIOs can be realized.

Cross-Reference to the Companion Casebook

(McLaughlin, C. P., Johnson, J. K., and Sollecito, W. A. [Eds.]. 2012.
*Implementing Continuous Quality Improvement in Health Care:
A Global Casebook*. Sudbury, MA: Jones & Bartlett Learning.)

Case Study Number	Case Study Title	Case Study Authors
3	Clemson's Nursing Home: Working with the State Quality Improvement Organization's Restraint Reduction Initiative	*Franziska Rokoske, Jill A. McArdle, and Anna P. Schenck*

REFERENCES

Berner, E. S., Baker, S. C., Funkhouser, E., et al. 2003. Do local opinion leaders augment hospital quality improvement efforts? A randomized trial to promote adherence to unstable angina guidelines. *Med Care*, 41(3): 420–431.

Burwen, D. R., Galusha, D. H., Lewis, J. M., et al. 2003. National and state trends in quality of care for acute myocardial infarction between 1994–1995 and 1998–1999. The Medicare Health Care Quality Improvement Program. *Arch Intern Med*, 163(12): 1430–1439.

Centers for Medicare and Medicaid Services. Data compendium. 2009a. Table VI.13a. Retrieved December 2, 2010, from http://www.cms.gov/DataCompendium/15_2009_Data_Compendium.asp#TopOfPage

Centers for Medicare and Medicaid Services. Data compendium. 2009b. Table VI.2. Retrieved December 2, 2010, from http://www.cms.gov/DataCompendium/15_2009_Data_Compendium.asp#TopOfPage

Centers for Medicare and Medicaid Services. Data compendium. 2009c. Table VI.3. Retrieved December 2, 2010, from http://www.cms.gov/DataCompendium/15_2009_Data_Compendium.asp#TopOfPage

Chu, L. A., Bratzler, D. W., Lewis, R. J., et al. 2003. Improving the quality of care for patients with pneumonia in very small hospitals. *Arch Intern Med*, 163(3): 326–332.

Daniel, D. M., Norman, J., Davis, C., et al. 2004. A state-level application of the chronic illness breakthrough series: Results from two collaborative on diabetes in Washington State. *Jt Comm J Qual Saf*, 30(2): 69–79.

Dellinger, E. P., Hausmann, S. M., Bratzler, D. W., et al. 2005. Hospitals collaborate to decrease surgical site infections. *Am J Surg*, 190(1): 9–15

Ellerbeck, E. F., Kresowik, T. F., Hemann, R. A., et al. 2000. Impact of quality improvement activities on care for acute myocardial infarction. *Int J Quality Health Care*, 12(4): 305–310.

Hayes, R., Bratzler, D., Armour, B., et al. 2001. Comparison of an enhanced versus a written feedback model on the management of Medicare inpatients with venous thrombosis. *Jt Comm J Qual Improv*, 27(3): 155–168.

Holman, W. L., Allman, R. M., Sansom, M., et al. 2001. Alabama coronary artery bypass grafting project: Results of a statewide quality improvement initiatifve. *JAMA*, 283(23): 3003–3010.

Horner, J. K., Hanson, L. C., Wood, D., et al. 2005. Using quality improvement to address pain management practices in nursing homes. *J Pain Symptom Manage*, 30(3): 271–277.

Hsia, D. C. 2003. Medicare quality improvement: Bad apples or bad systems? *JAMA*, 289(20): 2648.

Institute for Healthcare Improvement. 2003. *The Breakthrough Series: IHI's Collaborative Model for Achieving Breakthrough Improvement*. IHI Innovation Series white paper. Boston: Author.

Institute of Medicine. 2006. *Medicare's Quality Improvement Organization Program: Maximizing Potential*. Washington, DC: National Academies Press.

Jencks, S. F. 2005. Quality improvement organizations and hospital care. *JAMA*, 294(16): 2028.

Jencks, S. F., Huff, E. D., and Curedon, T. 2003. Change in the quality of care delivered to Medicare beneficiaries, 1998–1999 to 2000–2001. *JAMA*, 289: 305–312

Jencks, S. F., and Wilensky, G. R. 1992. The health care quality improvement initiative. A new approach to quality assurance in Medicare. *JAMA*, 268(7): 900–903.

Jung, K., Shea, D., and Warner, C. 2010. Agency characteristics and changes in home health quality after home health compare. *J Aging Health*, 22(4): 454–476.

Kiefe, C. I., Allison, J. J., Williams, O. D., et al. 2001. Improving quality improvement using achievable benchmarks for physician feedback: A randomized controlled trial. *JAMA*, 285(22): 2871–2879.

Kiefe, C. I., Weissman, N. W., Allison, J. J., et al. 1998. Identifying achievable benchmarks of care (ABCs): Concepts and methodology. *Int J Qual Health Care*, 10: 443–447.

Klees, B., Wolfe, C. J., and Curtis, C. A. Brief summaries of Medicare and Medicaid Title XVIII and Title XIX of the Social Security Act as of November 1, 2009. Retrieved April 4, 2011, from http://www.cms.hhs.gov/MedicareProgramRatesStats/Downloads/MedicareMedicaidSummaries2009.pdf

Leavitt, M. O. 2006. Report to Congress. Improving the Medicare Quality Improvement Organization Program—Response to the Institute of Medicine Study. Retrieved June 5, 2010, from https://www.cms.gov/QualityImprovementOrgs/downloads/QIO_Improvement_RTC_fnl.pdf

Lohr, K. N. (Ed.). 1990. *Medicare: A Strategy for Quality Assurance* (Vol. 1). Washington, DC: National Academies Press.

Marciniak, T. A., Ellerbeck, E. F., Radford, M. J., et al. 1998. Improving the quality of care for Medicare patients with acute myocardial infarction: Results from the Cooperative Cardiovascular Project. *JAMA*, 279(17): 1351–1357.

McLaughlin, C. P., Johnson, J. K., and Sollecito, W. A. (Eds.). 2012. *Implementing Continuous Quality Improvement in Health Care: A Global Casebook*. Sudbury, MA: Jones & Bartlett Learning.

McClellan, W. M., Millman, L., Presley, R., et al. 2003. Improved diabetes care by primary care physicians: Results of a group-randomized evaluation of the Medicare Health Care Quality Improvement Program (HCQIP). *J Clin Epidemiol*, 56(12): 1210–1217.

Rollow, W., Lied, T. R., McGann, P., et al. 2006. Assessment of the Medicare Quality Improvement Organization Program. *Ann Intern Med*, 145: 342–353.

Rosenthal, M. B., and Frank, R. G. 2006. What is the empirical basis for paying for quality in health care? *Med Care Res Rev*, 63(2): 135–157.

Schade, C., Cochran, B., and Stephens, M. 2004. Using statewide audit and feedback to improve hospital care in West Virginia. *Jt Comm J Qual Saf*, 30(3): 143–151.

Schenck, A. P., Peacock, S., Pignone, M., et al. 2006. Increasing colorectal cancer testing: Translating physician interventions into population-based practice. *Health Care Financ Rev*, 27(3): 1–11.

Snyder, C., and Anderson, G. 2005. Do Quality Improvement Organizations improve the quality of hospital care for Medicare beneficiaries? *JAMA*, 293: 2900–2907.

Stone, E. G., Morton, S. C., Hulscher, M. E., et al. 2002. Interventions that increase use of adult immunization and cancer screening services: A meta-analysis. *Ann Intern Med*, 136(9): 641–651.

Sueta, C. A., Schenck, A., Hall, R., et al. 2001. Hospital interventions improve care of North Carolina Medicare patients with myocardial infarction. *N C Med J*, 62(2): 69–73.

Sutherland, J. E., Hoehns, J. D., O'Donnell, B., et al. 2001. Diabetes management quality improvement in a family practice residency program. *J Am Board Fam Pract*, 14(4): 243–251.

Womack, J. P., and Jones, D. T. 2005. *Lean Solutions—How Companies and Customers Can Create Value and Wealth Together*. New York: Free Press.

15–A

Overview of the U.S. Medicare Program

Medicare is a far-reaching, complex program. A brief overview of the beneficiary and provider populations and the services covered under Medicare provides a context for the CQI activities conducted by QIOs.

THE MEDICARE POPULATION

In 2009, the Medicare program had nearly 46 million beneficiaries, making it the largest government insurance program in the United States (http://www.cms.hhs.gov/DataCompendium/15_2009_Data_Compendium.asp#TopOfPage). Approximately 95% of persons 65 years of age and older are enrolled in Medicare (Klees et al., 2009). For individuals in this age group, Medicare data are population based. Yet, although it is considered representative of the older population, it is important to note that Medicare eligibility requirements result in the exclusion of some populations. For example, Medicare eligibility requires that the beneficiary be a citizen or permanent resident of the United States and have contributed to the Medicare system by working for at least 10 years in Medicare-covered employment. Persons who are eligible for railroad retirement benefits or Social Security benefits are automatically eligible for

Medicare Part A. If either the person or his or her spouse has 10 years of Medicare employment, both are considered eligible for Medicare (http://www.medicare.gov/MedicareEligibility/Home.asp?dest=NAV/Home/GeneralEnrollment#TabTop). Persons who have worked as day laborers for employers who do not file appropriate government reports may not accrue enough work time to be eligible.

Although it is typically thought of as an insurance program for older Americans, a substantial portion, 16%, of the Medicare population is younger than 65 years of age and eligible due to a disabling condition; a small portion (less than 1%) of enrollees are eligible due to end-stage renal disease (http://www.cms.hhs.gov/DataCompendium/15_2009_Data_Compendium.asp#TopOfPage). For a person to be eligible for Medicare due to a disabling condition, he or she must have been out of work for 24 months (http://www.medicare.gov/MedicareEligibility/Home.asp?dest=NAV/Home/GeneralEnrollment#TabTop). The demographic and geographic characteristics of the population Medicare recipients younger than 65 years old *are not* representative of the general population.

SERVICES COVERED UNDER MEDICARE

Medicare is not a single program but rather a collection of programs covering different types of care. Medicare Part A is provided to eligible beneficiaries with no monthly payments required. Medicare Part A, sometimes called hospital insurance, covers care provided in a hospital or skilled nursing facility and care provided by home health and hospice providers (http://www.medicare.gov/Publications/Pubs/pdf/10050.pdf). Medicare Part B, sometimes called Medicare Insurance, covers physician office visits and does require the beneficiary to pay a monthly fee. In 2010, the Medicare Part B monthly premium was $110.50 (http://www.medicare.gov/MedicareEligibility/Home.asp?dest=NAV/Home/GeneralEnrollment#TabTop). Medicare Part C, also known as Medicare Advantage and Medicare + Choice, was added in 1997 to offer Medicare coverage under a capitated or managed care system. Medicare Part D, enacted in 2006, provides a prescription benefit.

Most beneficiaries have both Parts A and B through fee-for-service (FFS) Medicare. Nationally, only 17% are enrolled in managed care (Medicare Part C), although that varies dramatically by geographic region, with Oregon having the highest penetration (40%) and Alaska having the lowest (1%) (http://www.cms.hhs.gov/MedicareMedicaidStatSupp/ LT/itemdetail.asp?filterType=none&filterByDID=0&sortByDID=2&s ortOrder=descending&itemID=CMS1212431&intNumPerPage=10). Of enrollees, 58% have Medicare Part D (http://www.cms.hhs.gov/ DataCompendium/15_2009_Data_Compendium.asp#TopOfPage).

Medicare covers most services related to diagnosis, treatment, and rehabilitation. The nursing facility benefit is limited to skilled care, such as might be needed following a hospitalization for a stroke or hip replacement. It does not cover long-term care. Similarly, the home health benefit covers nursing and therapy services when the patient can be expected to gain functional status following a hospitalization. Selected preventive services are also covered, including screening for cancer, heart disease, diabetes, osteoporosis, and HIV, as well as immunizations and other services (http://www.medicare.gov/Publications/Pubs/pdf/10050.pdf).

15–B

Description of Commonly Used Abbreviations in Chapter 15

AHQA—American Health Quality Association The professional association that represents QIOs. The AHQA Web site (http://www .ahqa.org) includes a summary of the QIO mission.

CMS—The Centers for Medicare and Medicaid Services The U.S. federal agency responsible for the Medicare and Medicaid programs. CMS is located administratively in the U.S. Department of Health and Human Services.

DRG—Diagnosis-Related Group A classification system used to group diagnoses of hospital cases into categories based on the expectation that the cases will require similar resources to manage.

HCQIP—Health Care Quality Improvement Program Initially called the health care quality improvement initiative (HCQII), this program was started in Medicare in 1992. The goal of the program was to shift the way in which quality was monitored, from using local criteria and looking at individual cases to using nationally established standards of care and examining patterns of care for the population of patients on Medicare.

PPS—Prospective Payment System   A Medicare payment system for reimbursing providers a predetermined amount to provide patient care. The payment amount is determined differently depending on the setting of care, but it generally involves the patient diagnoses and other conditions.

PRO—Peer Review Organization   Physician-sponsored organizations, established in the 1980s, to review medical care of Medicare beneficiaries. Each state and territory had a PRO responsible for care oversight. PROs were replaced by QIOs in 2002.

PSRO—Professional Service Review Organization   Physician-sponsored organizations, established in the 1970s to review medical care of Medicare beneficiaries. Multiple PSROs were operated within each state. Care was judged as appropriate or not by comparing it to local standards of care and practice patterns. PSROs were replaced by PROs in the 1980s.

QIO—Quality Improvement Organization   Private organizations hired by CMS to help improve the care provided to Medicare beneficiaries. There are 53 separate contracts for QIOs—one for each state and one each for the Virgin Islands, Puerto Rico, and the District of Columbia. Organizations can hold multiple QIO contracts.

QIO Program—Quality Improvement Program   The collective efforts of CMS and its contracts with QIOs to "improve the effectiveness, efficiency, economy, and quality of services delivered to Medicare beneficiaries" (http://www.cms.gov/QualityImprovementOrgs/01_ Overview.asp#TopOfPage).

SOW—Scope of Work   The name given to the contracts between CMS and QIOs, which detail the tasks and performance expectations for QIOs. SOWs are usually 3 years in length and are numbered chronologically.

CHAPTER 16

Continuous Quality Improvement in U.S. Public Health Organizations: Moving Beyond Quality Assurance

Cheryll D. Lesneski, Sara E. Massie, and Greg D. Randolph

"As demands on the U.S. public health system continue to increase, QI strategies may play a vital role in supporting the system and improving outcomes."

—Panel discussion brief: AcademyHealth's 2009
Annual Research Meeting

Public health is "what we, as a society, do collectively to assure the conditions in which people can be healthy" (IOM, 1988, p.1). International health statistics demonstrate that the United States trails other developed nations in many public health indicators. For example, a study of 19 industrialized nations showed that between 1997–1998 and 2002–2003, rates of amenable mortality (i.e., deaths before 75 years of age from certain causes that are potentially preventable with timely and effective prevention strategies) fell by an average of 16% in all countries except the United States, which showed only a 4% decline (Nolte and McKee, 2008). In 2006, the United States ranked 39th for infant mortality, 43rd for adult female mortality, 42nd for adult male mortality, and 36th for life expectancy, despite being first in health care spending per capita (Murray and Frenk, 2010; World Health Organization, 2009). With rankings such as these, it is evident that we need to improve the quality of public health services in the United States.

Over the past two decades, U.S. public health organizations have increasingly undertaken a variety of efforts to ensure and improve the quality of their services. In recent years, accreditation has become part of a national focus to advance the quality and performance of public health. At the same time, public health agencies have begun to implement quality improvement projects using tools and proven methodologies such as Plan, Do, Study, Act (PDSA) cycles (Deming, 2000; Langley et al., 2009). Efforts such as these indicate that public health is poised to move beyond a series of projects and tools toward adopting continuous quality improvement (CQI) as a means of achieving a public health system that is effective and efficient, one that is in step with other industrialized nations around the world.

In this chapter, we provide an overview of CQI in U.S. public health organizations. We begin by clarifying key terms used in this discussion. We then describe the history of quality improvement in public health and current efforts related to CQI. Next, we explore the opportunities and challenges public health organizations face in the adoption of CQI. Finally, we conclude with practical examples of how state, local, and nonprofit public health agencies have applied quality improvement methods and tools.

CLARIFYING KEY TERMS

The *public health system* refers to all public, private, and voluntary entities that contribute to the delivery of public health services within a given area. These systems are a network of entities with differing roles, relationships, and interactions that contribute to the health and well-being of the community or state (CDC, 2007). The term *public health organization* (a subset of the public health system) includes both local and state agencies plus other nonprofit entities whose mission includes the provision of public health services or the development and advocacy of public health policy. *Local public health agencies* (also called local public health departments) are entities providing public health services at the community level. Most local public health agencies are operated by county, multicounty, city, or town government and are governed by either local boards of health or state (or a combination of state and county) government. A *state public health agency* is a unit of state government responsible for identifying health needs and promoting the health of state residents (Turnock, 2009).

A range of public health organizations and agencies undertake efforts to improve quality. In contrast to quality in health care, in public health, *quality* has been defined as "the degree to which policies, programs, services, and research for the population increase the desired health outcomes and conditions in which the population can be healthy" (U.S. DHHS, 2008, p. 2). *Quality assurance* is the systematic monitoring and evaluation of the performance of an organization or its programs to ensure that standards (usually set by public health experts) of quality are being met. *Quality improvement* involves designing and redesigning systems to meet customers' needs by testing and implementing ideas from evidence-based strategies, frontline staff, and customers. In public health, quality improvement has been described as a "distinct management process and set of tools and techniques that are coordinated to ensure that departments [local public health agencies] consistently meet their communities' health needs and strive to improve the health status of their populations" (Riley et al., 2010, p. 5).

Continuous quality improvement in public health organizations is a structured organizational process for involving staff in planning and executing a continuous flow of improvements to provide quality that meets or exceeds the expectations of communities. It focuses on systems change and generally includes these characteristics: a link to the organization's strategic plan, a quality council made up of the organization's top leadership, quality improvement training programs for staff, a mechanism for prioritizing quality improvement projects and launching quality improvement teams, and staff support and motivation for quality improvement activities (McLaughlin and Kaluzny, 2006). An organization that is committed to CQI may have both quality improvement and quality assurance processes, but the predominant focus is on quality improvement.

HISTORY OF ACTIONS TO IMPROVE PUBLIC HEALTH QUALITY

The foundation for CQI in public health rests largely on attempts to identify the core functions and essential services of public health agencies in the last century, initially emphasizing quality assurance approaches to measure performance of these services and standards. During the past 20 years, the public health sector has been clarifying its mission, vision, and core functions. In 1988, an Institute of Medicine (IOM) report declared that the United States "has lost sight of its public health goals and has allowed the system of public health to fall into disarray" (p. 1). The report, *The Future of Public Health*, drew attention to the lack of investment in the public health system and proposed ways to ensure the efficiency and effectiveness of public health service programs. The report identified three core functions of public health: assessment, policy development, and assurance. Operationalizing these core functions and using them to assess local public health system performance was viewed as an important step in changing public health practice (IOM, 1988).

Following the 1988 IOM report, public health experts and analysts promoted a variety of methods and frameworks for changing the public health system and improving performance. By the mid-1990s, the IOM, the Centers for Disease Control and Prevention (CDC), the American Public Health Association, and the National Association of County and City Health Officials (NACCHO) adopted a framework that describes the public health activities that should be undertaken in all communities. The framework, known as the 10 essential public health services (see **Table 16–1**), encompasses all of the activities for identifying and evaluating public health performance that were used in earlier frameworks, including the three core functions of public health.

Using the 10 essential services framework, the National Public Health Performance Standards Program (NPHPSP), a collaborative of seven major public health organizations, developed national performance standards for the public health system. The three NPHPSP assessment instruments are the State Public Health System Assessment Instrument, the Local Public Health System Assessment Instrument, and the Local Public Health Governance Assessment Instrument. With these instruments, organizations can identify gaps in achieving optimal performance and inform quality improvement efforts.

TABLE 16–1 10 Essential Public Health Services

---

1. Monitor health status to identify community health problems.
2. Diagnose and investigate health problems and health hazards in the community.
3. Inform, educate, and empower people about health issues.
4. Mobilize community partnerships to identify and solve health problems.
5. Develop policies and plans that support individual and community health efforts.
6. Enforce laws and regulations that protect health and ensure safety.
7. Link people to needed personal health services and ensure the provision of health care when otherwise unavailable.
8. Ensure a competent public health and personal health care workforce.
9. Evaluate effectiveness, accessibility, and quality of personal and population-based health services.
10. Research for new insights and innovative solutions to health problems.

Source: Public Health Functions Steering Committee, 1995.

The first version of the three instruments was released in 2002, and the second version was released in fall 2007. As of August 2007, more than 30 states had used at least one of the instruments, with fewer states reporting use of the local-level and governance instruments than the state-level instrument (CDC, 2008). One reason for the limited use of the first version of the local-level instrument may be that it is difficult to apply the 10 essential services framework to the actual work of local public health agencies. The work of local public health agencies is not defined, nor is it funded, according to the framework. Instead, local public health agencies receive funding and deliver services in specific programs or content areas, such as family planning or immunization. Often, *Healthy People 2010* (U.S. DHHS, 2000) goals are the focus for many of these programs. The 10 essential services framework was developed to address the variation in program services found across local public health agencies, but alignment of funding, requisite program data collection, and job requirements with the 10 essential services framework did not occur at any level of government. As a result, the NPHPSP is not explicitly linked to the goals of Healthy People, nor does it match the definition of public health activities as defined by many local public health agencies.

In an attempt to address these issues, NACCHO worked collaboratively with public health experts, leaders, and practitioners nationwide to create the *Operational Definition of a Functional Local Health Department* (NACCHO, 2005). This definition was designed to create a shared understanding of what any community member might expect from a local public health agency and to foster a climate of accountability (Lenihan et al., 2007). The operational definition is linked to the 10 essential services and includes 45 standards to help local public health agencies concretely define themselves and demonstrate what they do to improve community health (NACCHO, 2005). Further research is needed to determine the use and value of these standards for local public health agencies.

During this time of standards development, the Turning Point initiative, funded by the Robert Wood Johnson Foundation (RWJF) and the W. K. Kellogg Foundation and directed by NACCHO, sought to transform U.S. public health systems into more community-based and collaborative organizations working to achieve the goals of preventing disease and injury, protecting the public from threats to their health, and promoting healthy behaviors (Turning Point, 2006). Knowledge and tools related to performance management concepts were assembled as part of the initiative and made available in a variety of formats to public health organizations seeking to increase accountability, efficiency, and effectiveness. Performance management is the "practice of actively using performance data to improve the public's health" (Turning Point, 2006). Turning Point promoted an improvement model that emphasized the use of performance standards in conjunction with measurement and reporting of progress and the institution of quality improvement methods to manage change and achieve quality.

ONGOING EFFORTS TO IMPROVE PUBLIC HEALTH QUALITY

Over time, public health organizations have become increasingly interested in standardizing and ensuring quality public health services. This has led to a focus on national public health accreditation through the formation of the Multi-State Learning Collaborative and the Public Health Accreditation Board, the development of a uniform definition of quality in public health, and the use of quality improvement methods and tools in public health agencies.

The Multi-State Learning Collaborative

In late 2004, the RWJF convened a national group of stakeholders to review two background reports on accreditation and determine whether to proceed with public health agency accreditation. A result of the meeting was the establishment of a committee of stakeholders—the Exploring Accreditation Steering Committee—to develop recommendations for implementing a voluntary national accreditation program (Russo, 2007).

In 2005, RWJF launched the Multi-State Learning Collaborative (MLC), an initiative to explore the feasibility of voluntary national public health agency accreditation and provide the Exploring Accreditation Steering Committee with data on existing accreditation practices (Beitsch et al., 2006; Russo, 2007). Five states with mature accreditation or assessment programs received 1-year grants to enhance their existing performance assessment and share information with the Steering Committee and one another. In winter 2006–2007, the Steering Committee published *Exploring Accreditation: Final Recommendation for a Voluntary Accreditation Program for State and Local Public Health Departments*, recommending a national model for accreditation, which was subsequently endorsed by NACCHO and the Association of State and Territorial Health Organizations (ASTHO), among others.

Building on the success of the first year, the MLC later grew to include a second phase in 2007 and a third phase in 2008. In the second phase, 10 states received 1-year grants to focus on quality improvement in the context of accreditation and assessment. During this phase, states explored ways to improve their own accreditation and assessment programs, shared their tools and resources, conducted training in quality improvement, initiated quality improvement practices, and informed the planning for the national public health accreditation program (Gillen et al., 2010).

The third and final phase of the MLC began in 2008. During this phase, 16 states received 3-year grants to prepare for national voluntary accreditation, support the Public Health Accreditation Board in the development of the national voluntary accreditation program, and bolster use of quality improvement methods in local and state health departments through mini-collaboratives in each state (Joly et al., 2010). The mini-collaboratives—teams of local and state health department representatives and other partners—implemented quality improvement projects targeting public health processes (e.g., developing a community health profile) and outcomes in specific topic areas (e.g., tobacco, immunizations) (Gillen et al., 2010; Joly et al., 2010).

The Public Health Accreditation Board

The Public Health Accreditation Board (PHAB) was established to manage and promote a national voluntary accreditation program for state, local, territorial, and tribal public health departments. Using the recommendations in the *Exploring Accreditation* report, the PHAB proposed local standards and measures for accreditation (PHAB, 2009a). Following an alpha test of the standards with two state agencies and six local health departments, a beta version of the standards for state and local public health departments was launched in 30 public health departments in 2009. The beta version of the accreditation standards for state and local use includes two major sections for review and performance assessment. Part A includes standards for the administration and governance of public health agencies. Part B is built around the 10 essential services, the operational definition of a functional local public health agency, and standards of state-based accreditation and assessment programs. PHAB site teams review public health agencies applying for accreditation to assess their operational infrastructure, financial management systems, and engagement of the governing entity, as well as their ability to perform Part B standards.

PHAB's efforts to promote accreditation are reinforced by other groups such as the ASTHO, which has developed an accreditation and performance improvement guide to assist state health agencies with preparing for accreditation and improving the quality of their services (ASTHO, 2009). Resources such as these will help states to prepare and participate in the national public health accreditation program that was launched in 2011.

Consensus Statement on Quality in the Public Health System

In 2008, the U.S. Department of Health and Human Services (DHHS) released the *Consensus Statement on Quality in the Public Health System*, which, for the first time, framed a clear, uniform definition of quality for the public health system: "the degree to which policies, programs, services, and research for the population increase the desired health outcomes and conditions in which the population can be healthy" (p. 2). The statement identifies the optimization of population health as the ultimate goal of quality improvement in public health organizations, consistent with the mission of public health put forward by the IOM in 1988. *Population-based public health services* refers to "interventions aimed at disease prevention and health promotion that affect an entire population and extend beyond medical treatment by targeting risks, such as tobacco, drug, and alcohol use; diet and sedentary lifestyles; and environmental factors" (Turnock, 2009, p. 515).

The *Consensus Statement* includes a set of nine quality aims for the public health system, which are similar to health care's quality aims of providing care that is safe, timely, equitable, effective, efficient, and patient-centered (IOM, 2001). The public health quality aims are *population-centered, equitable, proactive, health promoting, risk reducing, vigilant, transparent, effective,* and *efficient.* All or only some of the aims may apply to a given public health service or function (Honoré et al., 2011; U.S. DHHS, 2008). **Table 16–2** presents an example of how the nine aims may apply to improving an existing public health program whose mission is to deliver targeted, effective, and sustained evidence-based prevention interventions to populations at high risk of HIV infection. For example, improving the frequency and reliability of implementation of evidence-based HIV/AIDS prevention interventions would increase the effectiveness of the office.

Providing a national quality framework through the *Consensus Statement* was deemed necessary to facilitate consistent implementation of quality improvement in the daily routine of public health practitioners and their organizations. Another purpose of the *Consensus Statement* was to demonstrate a national commitment to quality improvement application throughout all parts of the public health system, including finance, programs, management, governance, and education (Honoré, 2009; Honoré et al., 2011). The next steps for the *Consensus Statement* workgroup are developing economic and financial indicators of quality and identifying priority areas for quality improvement in public health, including establishing a core set of quality indicators and measures related to the nine quality aims. These indicators may be useful to public health organizations as they move toward adopting CQI. Case 11 in the companion casebook (McLaughlin et al., 2012) provides further exploration of financial indicators as they relate to CQI in public health organizations.

TABLE 16-2 Application of National Quality Aims for Public Health in a State Office of HIV/AIDS

National Aims for Improvement of Quality in Public Health	Examples of Public Health Practices with Quality Aims in a State Office of HIV/AIDS
Population-centered	• Routine epidemiological studies
Equitable	• Stratification of data by race, gender, and age, and programs built accordingly
Proactive	• Implementation of the Health Education and Risk Reduction program
	• Disease Investigation Specialist program
Health promoting	• Implementation of the "ABC" program (Abstain, Be faithful, use Condoms)
Risk reducing	• Implementation of the Health Education and Risk Reduction program
	• Offering of partner services (notifications, testing, suspect interviews, etc.)
Vigilant	• Statewide surveillance systems
Transparent	• Reporting of data to funders
Effective	• Implementation of national evidence-based programs
Efficient	• Documentation and justification of costs to identify new cases of disease

Source: Adapted from Honoré, 2009, with permission.

Quality Improvement in Local Health Agencies

Across the nation, an increasing number of local public health agencies are applying quality improvement methods and tools. To find out just how widespread such efforts are, NACCHO included a quality improvement module for a representative sample of 545 local health departments in its 2008 National Profile of Local Health Departments survey. Of the 448 local health departments that responded to the module, 55% reported having conducted formal quality improvement efforts during the previous 2 years, and 44% used a specific quality improvement framework such as Balanced Scorecard, Baldrige, or the Turning Point initiative. Of those involved in quality improvement, 68% used at least one of the following methods or tools over the previous year: PDSA cycles, process map, fishbone diagram, and control chart (Beitsch et al., 2010). The quality improvement module requested information on only formal quality improvement activities; however, these results indicate that respondents may have included *informal* quality improvement activities (i.e., with little or no written documentation) as well, given the high response level (NACCHO, 2009). In addition to or in contrast to formal processes, these may be considered as part of a CQI "philosophy," as described in Chapter 1. Later in this chapter, we provide examples of quality improvement efforts, such as these in local public health agencies, as well as efforts in state agencies and nonprofit organizations.

LOOKING AHEAD: THE ADOPTION AND INSTITUTIONALIZATION OF CQI IN PUBLIC HEALTH

Public health is quite early in the process of institutionalizing CQI compared to many industries. The more long-standing experiences of adopting CQI in other industries can provide valuable lessons for public health organizations to consider as they progress along the adoption curve to full institutionalization. Although public health organizations (which are often governmental and nonprofit entities) differ from health care organizations (which are often private, for-profit entities), a review of health care's CQI adoption process, such as that presented in Chapter 1, provides an opportunity to anticipate what is in store as public health organizations adopt CQI. Multiple organizations and multiple strategies were required for health care to begin making progress in adopting CQI. In particular, the steps that led to the national standards, reimbursement strategies, competency development, and incorporation of quality improvement in medical and nursing education provide a good model for how change should be implemented in the U.S. public health system.

Several governmental and nonprofit organizations are already providing substantial leadership in promotion of CQI in public health, just as the IOM and Institute for Healthcare Improvement (IHI) do for health care. We have already mentioned some of the most influential: ASTHO, CDC, DHHS, NACCHO, PHAB, and RWJF. Other influential groups include the National Network of Public Health Institutes (http://www.nnphi.org) and the Public Health Foundation (http://www.phf.org).

All of these organizations are well respected and have the visibility and influence to advance CQI in public health. In addition, these organizations and others have the ability to promote transparency in public health, advocate for the importance of quality improvement (including moving beyond relying primarily on quality assurance), and support resources and models for how CQI can be implemented effectively in public health organizations. In this section, we describe these and other areas within public health that merit significant attention in the future.

Promotion of Transparency

The *Consensus Statement* (U.S. DHHS, 2008) includes transparency as one of the nine aims that characterize quality improvement in the public health system. Transparency in public health refers to "ensuring openness in the delivery of services and practices with particular emphasis on valid, reliable, accessible, timely, and meaningful data that is readily available to stakeholders, including the public" (U.S. DHHS, 2008, p. 5). Two current efforts to promote transparency in public health are the Community Health Status Indicators (CHSI) project and the Mobilizing Action Toward Community Health (MATCH) initiative. CHSI is a DHHS report that provides an overview of key health indicators for local communities in order to encourage dialogue about actions that can be taken to improve a community's health. In 2006, CHSI began providing updated county health status profiles on more than 200 measures for each of the 3,141 counties in the United States (U.S. DHHS, n.d.). MATCH is a 3-year RWJF-funded project at the University of Wisconsin Population Health Institute that is designed to stimulate community-level improvement in health across the United States (Population Health Institute, n.d.). In 2010, the Institute began reporting on a more focused set of health outcomes and major health determinants in comparative county health rankings for each state.

Efforts such as CHSI and MATCH can be powerful change motivators as the public, communities, and states analyze and use data that present sobering evidence of the need to improve community health in many areas. Public health leaders will need to ensure that such data are accurate and properly framed as a stimulus for community health improvement and not used for "shame and blame" of community and state stakeholders. Ultimately, promoting transparency about quality gaps in the health of communities, states, and the nation can help mobilize improvement efforts.

Accreditation as a Tool to Promote CQI

Accreditation, whether in public health, in other areas of health care, or in related industries, has traditionally been primarily a quality assurance strategy focused on meeting standards set by experts. Chapter 18 provides an in-depth discussion of accreditation in health care globally. Accreditation in public health has been described as "the periodic issuance of credentials or endorsement to organizations that meet a specified set of performance standards" (Novick and Mays, 2001, p. 765). In some industries, such efforts have not been particularly successful or popular; of note, they are often unpopular with workers because of the focus on human error, rather than systems, as the source of most problems.

Bender and Halverson (2010) describe accreditation in public health as follows:

> Unlike some health-related agencies and services that are accredited or otherwise regulated, the PHAB board of directors has set the public health accreditation work solidly on the cornerstone of CQI. In other words, accreditation is a means to an end, not an end unto itself. (p. 80)

PHAB envisions accreditation as an accountability approach; it ensures that agencies are organizationally accountable to a set of standards. The goal of PHAB's accreditation program is to "improve and protect the health of every community by advancing the quality and performance of public health departments" (2009b). Implementation of quality improvement is a specific standard in the PHAB beta testing phase (PHAB, 2009c). Case 15 in the companion casebook (McLaughlin et al., 2012) provides a further exploration and an example of public health accreditation in local public health agencies in North Carolina, the first state to pilot test and mandate accreditation of local public health agencies.

The recent establishment of the PHAB, with its systems/organizational approach and its primary aim of promoting CQI, bodes well for public health as the field moves toward adopting CQI. However, fundamentally, improvement requires three things: will, ideas, and execution. Accreditation alone can only provide will and some ideas for where improvement is needed in public health organizations. Ultimately, the success of PHAB in achieving its purpose will depend on public health organizations having the ability to *execute* improvement efforts. Public health must develop and invest in new ways to assist organizations in building the infrastructure for CQI.

Evidence-Based Strategies and Programs

Risk reduction, health promotion, and effectiveness are among the national quality aims for public health. To improve public health, we must generate and apply evidence-based strategies and programs, and we must not invest in public health services that are shown to have uncertain benefit or no effect. The evidence base for public health interventions is lacking in some areas, and additional funding for research on developing new approaches and documenting the effectiveness of current public health interventions is necessary (U.S. DHHS, 2009). However, many evidence-based strategies and programs for improving health and preventing disease in communities are available and catalogued in free online resources. One such resource is the CDC's *Guide to Community Preventive Services* (http://www.thecommunityguide.org/index.html). Another useful resource is the University of Massachusetts Medical School's *Evidence-Based Practice for Public Health* (http://library.umassmed.edu/ebpph/).

Public health organizations can use quality improvement methods to apply and reliably deliver what we already know works and to assess the effectiveness of novel approaches where little or no evidence exists. Many local public health agencies in MLC states are already using quality improvement tools such as flowcharts, trend charts, and fishbone diagrams, among others (Joly et al., 2010). **Table 16–3** illustrates the applicability of such tools within a public health framework known as the 10 organizational practices. Additional information about these and other tools that are applicable in public health settings can be found in Chapter 3, which includes links to online resources, and in the Public Health Foundation's recent publication *The Public Health Quality Improvement Handbook* (Bialek et al., 2009).

Although many evidence-based strategies and programs are catalogued, to be effective these strategies and programs must be *readily* available and in a user-friendly and comprehensively described format for public health organizations and practitioners involved in improvement efforts at the community level. More research and development is needed to increase the availability and usability of evidence-based approaches; likewise, more educational and training opportunities are needed to ensure the effective application of these approaches.

TABLE 16–3 Suggestions for Use of Quality Improvement Tools in the 10 Organizational Practices

Core Function	Organizational Practice	Quality Improvement Tool
Assessment	Assess the health needs of the community	Histogram, run chart
	Investigate the occurrence of health effects and health hazards in the community	Pareto diagram, trend, or run chart
	Analyze the determinants of identified health needs	Fishbone diagram
Policy development	Advocate for public health, build constituencies, and identify resources in the community	Dashboard, stakeholder analysis
	Set priorities among health needs	Prioritization matrix, Pareto diagram
	Develop plans and policies to address priority health needs	Force field analysis, affinity diagram
Assurance	Manage resources and develop organizational structure	Balanced scorecard
	Implement programs	Flowchart, PDSA cycles
	Evaluate programs and provide quality assurance	Process or value stream maps, statistical process control charts
	Inform and educate the public	PDSA cycles

Innovative Partnerships to Increase the Capacity of Local Public Health Agencies

Local and state public health agencies alone cannot address many important public health problems, such as the increasing burden of chronic diseases. There is growing recognition that often a coalition of partners from disparate organizations is necessary (Bonnie L. Zell, MD, MPH, personal communication, July 29, 2009). Private–public partnerships will likely become increasingly important, especially when resources for public health contract. Local partnerships can be an excellent way to leverage public health resources; for example, a partnership between a local public health agency and a nonprofit hospital, which is responsible for providing programs that benefit communities, can be an effective way to expand the capacity and services of a local public health agency.

In Putnam County, Florida, the health department and St. Vincent Health System have collaborated for almost a decade to increase their community's public health services resources. The partnership began when St. Vincent was interested in improving the health of migrant farm workers while the health department was, at the same time, trying to control the spread of tuberculosis among farm workers. The hospital entered into a long-term contract with Putnam County to pay for staff to provide core public health services to their vulnerable population of farm workers. This strategic partnership expanded public health services in the region and increased the agency's capacity to provide services and its ability to continuously improve health. The tuberculosis case rate dropped in the migrant farm worker population, and the tuberculosis infection rate declined (RWJF, 2007). In addition, joint efforts to monitor finances, services, and outcomes revealed opportunities for ongoing quality improvement work.

Financing of Public Health Organizations

A growing body of evidence reveals great variation in the availability and quality of public health services in the United States (Mays et al., 2009). From a funding perspective, even in the best of times, the resources to address the nation's major public health challenges are tight. The financing of public health services is likely a major contributor to this variation, as it primarily focuses on funding services and programs, thereby limiting general funding for infrastructure.

Over time, the absence of flexible, adequate funding streams has resulted in many local public health agencies relying on reimbursable primary care services as a way to generate income. In Florida, Brooks et al. (2009) found that most resources within local public health agencies were used for individual health care services, even as demand for improved population-focused services increased. In Georgia, a public health practice assessment revealed that the core business of public health in the state did not align with the 10 essential services, stating that "the primary drivers or determinants of public health practice are finance related rather than based in need or strategy" (Smith et al., 2007, p. 169). Public health services that treat disease in the short term at the individual level rather than prevent the conditions that cause disease at the population level do not meet the quality aim of population-centeredness.

One way to maximally improve the population's health is to provide new and innovative approaches to financing local and state public health agencies. Financial incentives for improving the most important determinants of population health using evidence-based strategies are needed. For instance, public health could benefit from adapting and testing innovative financial approaches that have been successful in other areas of health care, such as pay-for-performance strategies.

CQI relates to these financial challenges in at least two ways. First, implementing CQI should help reduce overall costs while increasing quality, just as it has in many other industries and organizations (Spear and Bowen, 1999). Reducing costs and inefficiencies can help increase capacity and allow for a greater focus on population-centered services. Second, if the financing of public health services remains focused on funding specific services and programs rather than infrastructure, then public health agencies will likely have great difficulty investing in the infrastructure needed for CQI. Case 11 in the companion casebook (McLaughlin et al., 2012) provides further exploration of financial indicators as they relate to CQI in public health organizations.

Public Health Education and the Public Health Professionals' Paradigm

CQI is focused on making system improvements, which is a familiar paradigm to public health professionals who are trained to think at the system and population levels. This paradigm of system-level thinking provides a tremendous advantage to public health organizations' adoption of CQI, and it helps ensure that public health organizations achieve the quality aim of population-centeredness. To build and reinforce the adoption of CQI in public health organizations, schools of public health and other institutions that educate the public health workforce will need to broaden their curricula to include a greater emphasis on evidence-based practice, systems thinking, and the philosophies, methods, and tools of CQI. In addition, they will need to incorporate experienced practitioners to supplement traditional faculty and provide additional resources needed to teach CQI. Provision of certificates and continuing education in CQI for public health professionals is another untapped opportunity in this regard. The continuing use and expansion of executive and distance education formats to do all of the above will also be critical to ensure the most efficient training of the existing public health workforce.

PUBLIC HEALTH QUALITY IMPROVEMENT IN PRACTICE

Although public health still has far to go in the adoption and institutionalization of CQI, a rapidly growing number of public health organizations have embraced quality improvement, and some are making substantial progress toward creating an organizational infrastructure for CQI. The approaches being used and the problems being addressed vary greatly (Davis, 2008). This section provides practical examples of quality improvement in local public health agencies, state agencies, and nonprofit organizations.

Quality Improvement in Local Public Health Agencies

In recent years, an increasing number of local public health agencies have been doing quality improvement work (Beitsch et al., 2010). We describe three quality improvement efforts that are illustrative of the variety of approaches taken in local agencies. The first is an example of an agency beginning with a quality improvement project using lean methodology to begin its quality improvement efforts and move toward creating an infrastructure for CQI. The second example involves a local agency's effort to integrate CQI throughout the organization while simultaneously conducting projects. The final example shows how an agency began its journey with a focus on developing a CQI infrastructure first.

Beaufort County Health Department

In 2008, the Beaufort County Health Department in Washington, North Carolina, invited local experts from North Carolina State University to propose a quality improvement project to help reduce the 3-hour waiting times in its Family Planning Clinic by at least 50%. The experts suggested using lean, a quality improvement method that focuses specifically on identifying and eliminating non-value-added or wasteful activities (for more information about lean, see http://www.ies .ncsu.edu/leanhealthcare/).

At the beginning of the project, six frontline staff from the Family Planning Clinic formed a project team and served as local experts on the family planning process. The team and members of the agency leadership attended a half-day training session on lean methods and spent three and a half days in an on-site rapid improvement event facilitated by two lean experts. During the rapid improvement event, the team did the following:

- Observed the clinic process from the client's perspective to carefully document the current process and make observations for potential improvements
- Used a "value stream mapping" process to identify which steps provided actual value for their clients and which did not
- Used a five-part, standardized process known as "5S" (Sorting, Straightening, Shining, Standardizing, and Sustaining) to organize the workplace and improve workflow
- Eliminated wasteful or non-value-added steps from the process, such as duplicative and unnecessary forms
- Tested and implemented ideas from frontline staff to improve efficiency (for example, the team revised a Notice of Privacy Practices form, changing it from an 8-page, stapled document to a double-sided, foldable brochure, reducing paper consumption, time spent making copies, and the need for storage space and making it less intimidating for clients)

The pilot project resulted in a 50% reduction in wait times, meeting the agency's ambitious goals. The program was so successful that the leadership at Beaufort collaborated with its 10 regional local public health agency partners to conduct a second round of lean projects in all 10 local agencies. The second wave of projects had similar results in clinical settings and home health programs.

Beaufort County's successful experience with its first quality improvement project, which was proactive and focused on efficiency—two of the nine national quality aims—has spurred its leadership team to commit to developing a culture and infrastructure for CQI. The ability of frontline staff to redesign their processes, thereby making their jobs easier and services better for their clients, was especially important to Beaufort County's leadership. The agency has since trained several staff members to be quality improvement coaches, provided quality improvement training for its managers, and launched additional quality improvement projects. Agency leaders and frontline staff have also served as leaders and teachers of quality improvement for other local agencies across North Carolina.

Tacoma-Pierce County Health Department

In 2006, Washington State's Tacoma-Pierce County Health Department began a multiyear effort to develop an organizational infrastructure for CQI. The primary impetus was the influence of the MLC. Several staff, including the health director, deputy director, and several division directors and managers attended quality improvement training sponsored by the Washington Department of Health, which was engaged in the first phase of MLC. The workshop soon led to the agency deciding to do its first improvement project.

After reviewing the experiences of successful organizations in other industries, leaders at Tacoma-Pierce decided to work on developing the infrastructure for CQI at the same time it initiated several quality improvement projects. The agency formed a quality council, chaired by the Health Director, consisting of top directors and managers. Based on *Healthy People 2010* (U.S. DHHS, 2000) health indicators, the quality council created a performance measures dashboard (including metrics such as the county's immunization rate, tobacco use, and incidence of 10 priority communicable diseases) to assess the agency's performance. The quality council now prioritizes and guides quality improvement efforts through an annual quality improvement plan, which includes selecting major activities, assigning a leader responsible for each activity, and setting timelines. Ideas for improvement are derived from gaps in the performance dashboard and suggestions from other public health agencies. The quality council also is responsible for plans to provide quality improvement training for staff and for staff recognition.

The Tacoma-Pierce County Health Department initially hired a quality improvement consultant to assist in training staff and guiding its CQI infrastructure development efforts but is now relying less on outside consultation and more on dedicated staff in its agency. The agency has one and a half full-time quality improvement staff and uses some of its program staff to assist in facilitating quality improvement activities.

Since beginning its quality improvement efforts in Tacoma-Pierce County, the agency has seen improvements in a number of its dashboard indicators, including increased use of household hazardous waste collection sites/facilities, increased number of children enrolled in public health insurance programs, increased percentage of water systems meeting drinking water standards, and decreased chlamydia positivity rates. For example, chlamydia positivity rates decreased by 20% between 2006 and 2008 after an improvement project was started to reduce the escalating chlamydia rates in the county.

Tacoma-Pierce County Health Department's efforts demonstrate all of the key components of a robust CQI infrastructure, including links to the organization's strategic plan, support and guidance from the organization's top leadership, quality improvement training programs for staff, a mechanism for prioritizing quality improvement projects and launching quality improvement teams, and staff support and motivation for quality improvement activities.

Miami-Dade County Health Department

In 1997, the Miami-Dade County Health Department (MDCHD), which serves the eighth largest county in the United States, began a multiyear effort aimed at developing an organizational infrastructure for CQI. The leadership decided that a drastic organizational culture change was needed due to a combination of budget shortfalls, low staff morale and satisfaction, ongoing difficulties in addressing community needs proactively, and other challenges.

In the first year of this organizational change effort, the MDCHD conducted an organizational self-assessment, using a tool from the Florida Sterling Council, which allowed MDCHD to better understand the organization's overall performance. Furthermore, the MDCHD established a quality unit with quality coaches and mentors, adopted an agency-wide approach to quality improvement using available literature to determine the right approach, and focused on top leadership commitment to quality improvement. The agency found the organizational assessment to be particularly useful, as it identified areas for improvement, helped the organization focus on some common goals, and helped leaders align resources with strategic objectives through targeted quality improvement projects.

Over the ensuing 4 years, MDCHD focused on improving strategic planning around quality improvement (including prioritizing quality improvement projects and activities) and greater involvement and recognition of frontline employees in CQI through quality improvement training, listening sessions, and communications. Senior leadership, midlevel leaders, and frontline staff were trained to use quality improvement tools and methods, such as cause-and-effect/fishbone diagrams and process mapping. Training was initially provided by consulting services; however, MDCHD later moved to a train-the-trainer approach using its own staff.

In addition, MDCHD leadership decided to prepare for the Sterling Quality Achievement Recognition for Focus on Creating Value. In 2002, the department won the prestigious award for its focus on creating value, and in 2006, it won a second Sterling Council Award and served as a pilot site for the national Malcolm Baldrige Award for nonprofits.

Most recently, MDCHD has identified and focused on its key processes related to CQI—workforce development (including leadership development and public health and quality improvement competencies), customer service and satisfaction, organizational self-assessments (such as the Sterling and Baldrige self-assessment tools), employee involvement in CQI activities and systematic recognition, strategic planning, and process and business management results, including benchmarking comparisons to similar state and national organizations.

In return for its investment in quality, the MDCHD has seen impressive measurable improvements. Employee satisfaction has increased from around 40% to 70% or higher, and the department consistently ranks among the top three state health departments in employee satisfaction. In addition, external customer satisfaction has improved. Improvements in community health outcomes have included reductions in teen births, unintended pregnancies, infant mortality, and vaccine preventable diseases, which were reduced by 40% over the past 5 years. Tuberculosis therapy completion rates have increased, as has the percentage of infants in the Women, Infants, and Children program who are breast-fed.

The MDCHD demonstrates all of the key components of a robust CQI infrastructure, including links to the organization's strategic plan, support and guidance from the organization's top leadership, quality improvement training programs for staff, a mechanism for prioritizing quality improvement projects and launching quality improvement teams, and staff support and motivation for quality improvement activities. MDCHD's results are an excellent illustration of the potential impact of CQI in a public health organization.

New undertakings of the MDCHD include becoming an accredited public health department and voluntarily participating as a beta site for the National Public Health Accreditation Program. In addition, the MDCHD plans to pursue a third Sterling Award in 2012.

Quality Improvement in State Agencies

Several state agencies, driven in large part by the MLC, are beginning to explore ways to incorporate CQI into their culture and organizational structure. A few states illustrate the potential, such as Washington and North Carolina, which were among the first states in the MLC. In this section, we describe a state-led quality improvement project in Washington's and North Carolina's attempts to promote and spread CQI implementation at the state and local levels.

Washington Department of Health

The State of Washington Department of Health first became involved in quality improvement initiatives in 1999. At the time, data revealed that the quality of care for diabetes patients in outpatient settings was surprisingly poor and differed substantially from evidence-based practice. In response, the Department of Health funded staff from several clinics to attend an IHI chronic care model collaborative. After the success of these clinics, the Department of Health sent several of its own staff to receive extensive quality improvement training from IHI to continue and expand improvement efforts in the state. The department has since conducted numerous collaborative improvement projects at the local level.

In 2006, the National Immunization Survey showed that Washington State's immunization rate was 71%, and only 36% of children living in Washington had up-to-date immunization records in the state's immunization registry. These concerning statistics prompted the Department of Health to bring together three local agencies—the Spokane Regional Health District, the Snohomish Health District, and CHILD Profile Immunization Registry—to collaborate on a quality improvement project: the Immunization Reminder-Recall Project (2008).

The collaborating organizations completed a brainstorming exercise using a fishbone (cause-and-effect) diagram to explore the reasons for the low rates and potential targets for change and improvement. They decided on three goals: (1) increase the proportion of 19- to 35-month-old children who are fully immunized in provider settings, (2) increase the amount of data in the immunization registry, and (3) increase providers' use of the registry.

During the 15-week project, data were collected from two pediatric practices and one family medicine practice. Results from the 15-week project were promising: the project increased the proportion of 19- to 35-month-old children who were fully immunized, and it improved current data in, and use of, the registry. This project is an example of the national quality aims of being population-centered, proactive, and risk reducing.

North Carolina Center for Public Health Quality

North Carolina was the first state to pilot test state accreditation (Reed et al., 2009), and it was the first state to statutorily mandate statewide accreditation for local public health agencies. Case 15 in the companion casebook (McLaughlin et al., 2012) provides a further exploration and an example of public health accreditation in local public health agencies in North Carolina.

Following the state accreditation pilot test, the North Carolina Division of Public Health (NCDPH) identified numerous areas of improvement. To address these shortcomings, the NCDPH Director of Performance Improvement and Accountability chartered six improvement teams centered on improving internal business operations such as communication and integration between the NCDPH business office and programs. At the same time, the director, in collaboration with five NCDPH nurse consultants, was charged with assisting all 85 of North Carolina's local health agencies with their quality improvement efforts as they went through the statewide accreditation process. In general, the NCDPH and local public health agencies were unable to launch and implement quality improvement activities at the state and local levels without significant support, and it quickly became apparent that additional resources and infrastructure would be needed to serve both the state and local agencies in North Carolina (Denise Pavletic, RD, MPH, personal communication, January 8, 2010).

In 2008, NCDPH began working with several partners—the North Carolina Association of Local Health Directors, the North Carolina Institute for Public Health, the North Carolina Area Health Education Centers, the North Carolina Hospital Association, and three foundations, The Duke Endowment, the Kate B. Reynolds Charitable Trust, and the

BlueCross BlueShield of North Carolina Foundation—to launch the North Carolina Center for Public Health Quality (NCCPHQ). The mission of the NCCPHQ is to create an infrastructure to foster and support CQI and learning among *all* public health professionals in North Carolina.

NCCPHQ's goals for the first 3 years are to provide quality improvement training for more than 50 local health department teams and more than 5 NCDPH teams; provide ongoing technical assistance for quality improvement teams; create a robust interactive Web site for state and local staff with improvement modules, tools, and evidence-based practices; create an NCDPH and statewide local health agency dashboard of quality measures; create and engage state and local quality councils; and celebrate successful improvement teams and efforts.

The NCCPHQ trains public health agency teams experientially through a 6-month training program, *Public Health QI 101*. The program teaches teams lean improvement methods and the Model for Improvement, which is a quality improvement method that focuses on three simple steps: setting measurable improvement goals, testing and implementing changes in series of rapid cycle tests (PDSA cycles), and measuring the impact of the changes on the processes and outcomes related to the improvement goals (Courtlandt et al., 2009; Randolph et al., 2009). Teams also implement a quality improvement project as part of the course. NCCPHQ also provides quality improvement training for agency leaders in conjunction with each team's experiential training in the Public Health QI 101 course to facilitate leadership support for projects and lay the foundation for a commitment to CQI.

In its first year, NCCPHQ trained 12 local agencies and 2 NCDPH teams, facilitated 15 new public health quality improvement projects, and provided CQI training for approximately 100 public health practitioners and 60 public health leaders. In partnership with the MLC and the North Carolina Institute for Public Health, the NCCPHQ also supported one statewide initiative to improve the job satisfaction and retention of public health nurses. This project used the Model for Improvement (Langley et al., 2009) to adapt and implement an evidence-based nurse mentoring program developed by the Georgia Department of Community Health. In addition, NCCPHQ developed a Web site (http://www .ncpublichealthquality.org) for state and local staff with improvement tools and evidence-based practices. NCCPHQ also created both a local and a state quality council for strategic alignment of improvement efforts.

The NCCPHQ is an example of the resources and partnerships needed to build a CQI infrastructure at the state level. Like the Miami-Dade and Tacoma-Pierce county health departments, the NCCPHQ illustrates the key components of a CQI infrastructure, including links to the organization's strategic plan, support and guidance from the organization's top leadership, quality improvement training programs for staff, a mechanism for prioritizing quality improvement projects and launching quality improvement teams, and staff support and motivation for quality improvement activities.

Quality Improvement in Nonprofit Public Health Organizations

As stated earlier, public health organizations include nonprofit entities that focus on the provision of public health services or the development and advocacy of public health policy. An example of CQI in a nonprofit public health organization is the North American Quitline Consortium (NAQC), a membership-based organization formed in 2006 to maximize the use and effectiveness of tobacco quitlines. Quitlines (telephone support) and patient education materials to support tobacco use cessation are part of an evidence-based intervention that is effective in both clinical and community settings (NAQC, n.d.).

The goals of the NAQC are to increase the use, capacity, quality, and cultural appropriateness of quitlines. Each goal is further defined by measurable objectives. For instance, the objective for goal 1 requires that "by 2015, each quitline should achieve a reach of at least 6% of its total tobacco users" (NAQC, n.d., p. 1). NAQC members use a standardized data set for evaluating progress toward shared goals, which fosters the sharing of similar data across organizations.

To assist its members with improving quality, the NAQC supports a strategic framework for improving tobacco quitline quality in North America. The framework is derived from Avedis Donabedian's three quality components: structure, process, and outcome (Donabedian, 1980). Quitline funders and service providers throughout North America apply the NAQC's quality framework to improve the structural areas of funding, contract relationship, and provider capacity. The NAQC promotes and monitors the implementation of evidence-based methods; provides technical assistance, guides, case studies, and checklists to support implementation of recommended quality standards; and provides training programs, including educational seminars, annual conferences, publications, and benchmarking activities, all of which are process components. Outcomes, such as reduction in the rate of tobacco use, are monitored and used to make changes as needed across the three quality components.

The NAQC exemplifies four of the DHHS quality aims: It is population-centered, proactive, risk reducing, and effective. The NAQC also demonstrates many of the key elements of the philosophy and processes of CQI: It links improvement activities to the organization's strategic plan, includes quality improvement training programs for staff, and has staff support and motivation for quality improvement activities.

CONCLUSIONS

The need to improve public health in the United States is evident. Despite efforts to define the mission and functions of public health and a heavy focus on quality assurance strategies, substantial quality gaps persist. The increasing attention placed on the adoption of CQI in public health, a more recent phenomenon, is both timely and encouraging. Although there is a long way to go before CQI will be commonplace in local, regional, state, and national public health organizations, there are many opportunities to accelerate its adoption, including using accreditation efforts to promote CQI and learning from health care and other industries about the facilitators and barriers to CQI adoption. Public health organizations can also capitalize on their many strengths, including:

- National organizations' engagement in promoting CQI
- Knowledge of gaps in the performance of public health services
- An increasing evidence base for public health
- The increasing number of efforts to promote transparency
- A system-thinking approach
- The ability to establish innovative partnerships

All of these factors can enhance efforts to build the organizational capacity to continuously improve public health. Just as in other industries, including health care, the adoption and institutionalization of CQI within public health organizations appears to be a much-needed next step to improve the public's health. Public health organizations that adopt CQI to help employees work as a team, address gaps in performance by analyzing and redesigning processes, and encourage innovation to meet the needs of communities hold the promise for a healthier future, both in the United States and throughout the world.

Cross-References to the Companion Casebook

(McLaughlin, C. P., Johnson, J. K., and Sollecito, W. A. [Eds.]. 2012. *Implementing Continuous Quality Improvement in Health Care: A Global Casebook.* Sudbury, MA: Jones & Bartlett Learning.)

Case Study Number	Case Study Title	Case Study Authors
11	Financial Analysis and Quality Management in Patriot County, Ohio	*Cheryll D. Lesneski*
15	North Carolina Local Health Department Accreditation Program	*David Stone and Mary V. Davis*

REFERENCES

Association of State and Territorial Health Officers. 2009. Accreditation and performance: Raising the bar for state public health. Retrieved January 8, 2010, from http://www.astho.org/programs/accreditation-and-performance/

Beitsch, L. M., Leep C., Shah, G., et al. 2010. Quality improvement in local health departments: Results of the NACCHO 2008 survey. *J Public Health Manage Pract*, 16(1): 49–54.

Beitsch, L. M., Thielen, L., Mays G., et al. 2006. The multistate learning collaborative, states as laboratories: Informing the national public health accreditation dialogue. *J Public Health Manage Pract*, 12: 217–231.

Bender, K., and Halverson, P. K. 2010. Quality improvement and accreditation: What might it look like? *J Public Health Manage Pract*, 16(1): 70–82.

Bialek, R., Duffy, G. L., and Moran, J. W. 2009. *The Public Health Quality Improvement Handbook.* Milwaukee, WI: American Society for Quality, Quality Press.

Brooks, R. G., Beitsch, L. M., Street, P., et al. 2009. Aligning public health financing with essential public health service functions and National Public Health Performance Standards. *J Public Health Manage Pract*, (15)4: 299–306.

Centers for Disease Control and Prevention. 2007. National Public Health Performance Standards Program: Acronyms, glossary, and reference terms. Retrieved January 29, 2010, from http://www.cdc.gov/od/ocphp/nphpsp/documents/glossary.pdf

Centers for Disease Control and Prevention. 2008. National Public Health Performance Standards Program overview presentation. Retrieved November 1, 2009, from http://www.cdc.gov/od/ocphp/nphpsp/PresentationLinks.htm

Courtlandt, C. D., Noonan, L., and Feld, L. G. 2009. Model for improvement—Part 1: A framework, for health care quality. *Pediatr Clin North Am*, 56(4): 757–778.

Davis, M. V. 2008. Opportunities to advance quality improvement in public health: A report prepared for the Robert Wood Johnson Foundation. Retrieved January 10, 2010, from http://nciph.sph.unc.edu/mlc/publications/qi_BackgroundPaper.pdf

Deming, W. E. 2000. *The New Economics for Industry, Government, and Education* (2nd ed.). Cambridge, MA: MIT Press.

Donabedian, A. 1980. *The Definition of Quality and Approaches to Its Assessment*. Ann Arbor, MI: Health Administration Press.

Gillen, S. M., McKeever, J., Edwards, K. F., et al. 2010. Promoting quality improvement and achieving measurable change: The lead states initiative. *J Public Health Manage Pract,* 16(1): 55–60.

Honoré, P. 2009. Quality in the public health system. Presentation at the 137th Annual Meeting of the American Public Health Association. Philadelphia.

Honoré, P., Wright, D., Berwick, D. W., et al. 2011. Creating a Framework for Getting Quality into the Public Health System. *Health Aff,* 30(4): 737–745.

Immunization Reminder-Recall Project. 2008. [PowerPoint slides]. Retrieved May 21, 2010, from the National Network of Public Health Institutes Web site: http://nnphi.org/home/section/3/ecatalog

Institute of Medicine. 1988. *The Future of Public Health*. Washington, DC: National Academies Press.

Institute of Medicine. 2001. *Crossing the Quality Chasm: A New Health System for the 21st Century.* Washington, DC: National Academies Press.

Joly, B. M., Shaler, G., Booth, M., et al. 2010. Evaluating the multi-state learning collaborative. *J Public Health Manage Pract,* 16(1): 61–66.

Langley, G. L., Nolan, K. M., Nolan, T. W., et al. 2009. *The Improvement Guide: A Practical Approach to Enhancing Organizational Performance.* San Francisco: Jossey-Bass.

Lenihan, P., Welter, C., Chang, C., et al. 2007. The operational definition of a functional local public health agency: The next strategic step in the quest for identity and relevance. *J Public Health Manage Pract,* 13(4): 357–363.

Mays, G. P., Smith, S. A., Ingram, R. C., et al. 2009. Public health delivery systems: Evidence, uncertainty, and emerging research needs. *Am J PreventMed,* 36(3): 256–265.

McLaughlin, C. P., Johnson, J. K., and Sollecito, W. A. (Eds.). 2012. *Implementing Continuous Quality Improvement in Health Care: A Global Casebook.* Sudbury, MA: Jones & Bartlett Learning.

McLaughlin, C. P., and Kaluzny, A. D. 2006. Defining quality improvement. In McLaughlin, C. P., and Kaluzny, A. D. (Eds.), *Continuous Quality Improvement in Health Care: Theory, Implementations, and Applications* (3rd ed., pp. 3–40). Sudbury, MA: Jones and Bartlett Publishers.

Murray, C. J. L., and Frenk, J. 2010. Ranking 37th—Measuring the performance of the U.S. health care system. *N Engl J Med,* 362: 98–99.

National Association of County and City Health Officials. 2005. Operational definition of a functional local health department. Retrieved November 10, 2009, from http://www.naccho.org/topics/infrastructure/accreditation/OpDef.cfm

National Association of County and City Health Officials. 2009. 2008 National profile of local health departments. Retrieved April 4, 2011, from http://www.naccho.org/topics/infrastructure/profile/resources/2008report/upload/NACCHO_2008_ProfileReport_post-to-website-2.pdf

Nolte, E., and McKee, C. M. 2008. Measuring the health of nations: Updating an earlier analysis *Health Aff,* 27(1): 58–71.

North American Quitline Consortium. n.d. Promoting evidence-based quitline services across diverse communities in North America. Retrieved December 10, 2009, from http://www.naquitline.org/

Novick, L. E., and Mays, G. P. (Eds.). 2001. *Public Health Administration, Principles for Population-Based Management.* Gaithersburg, MD: Aspen Publishers.

Population Health Institute. n.d. Mobilizing Action Toward Community Health (MATCH): Population health metrics, solid partnerships, and real incentives. Retrieved March 20, 2011, from http://www.pophealth .wisc.edu/uwphi/pha/match.htm

Public Health Accreditation Board. 2009a. Proposed local standards and measures. Retrieved March 20, 2011, from http://www.phaboard.org/ assets/documents/PHABLocalJuly2009-finaleditforbeta.pdf

Public Health Accreditation Board. 2009b. Public Health Accreditation Board [homepage]. Retrieved March 20, 2011, from http://www .phaboard.org/

Public Health Accreditation Board. 2009c. Frequently asked questions. Retrieved March 20, 2011, from http://www.phaboard.org/index.php/ about/faq/

Public Health Functions Steering Committee. 1995. Public health in America. Retrieved January 25, 2010, from http://www.health.gov/ phfunctions/public.htm

Randolph, G., Esporas, M., Provost, L., et al. 2009. Model for improvement—Part two: Measurement and feedback for quality improvement efforts. *Pediatr Clin North Am*, 56(4): 779–798.

Reed, J., Pavletic, D., Devlin, L., et al. 2009. Piloting a state health department accreditation model: The North Carolina experience. *J Public Health Manage Pract*, 15(2): 85–95.

Riley, W. J., Moran, J. W., Corso, L. C., et al. 2010. Defining quality improvement in public health. *J Public Health Manage Pract*, 16(1): 5–7.

Robert Wood Johnson Foundation. 2007, March. TB project screens migrant workers in the field and tracks them from state-to-state. Retrieved March 20, 2011, from http://www.rwjf.org/pr/product .jsp?id=17350

Russo, P. 2007. Accreditation of public health agencies: A means, not an end. *J Public Health Manage Pract*, 13(4): 329–331.

Smith, T. A., Parker, C., Tyler, B., et al. 2007. From theory to practice: What drives the core business of public health? *J Public Health Manage Pract*, 13(2), 169–172.

Spear, K., and Bowen, H. K. 1999. Decoding the DNA of the Toyota production system. *Harvard Business Rev*, 77: 96–106.

Turning Point. 2006. *About Turning Point.* Retrieved January 29, 2010, from http://www.turningpointprogram.org/Pages/about.html

Turnock, B. J. 2009. *Public Health: What It Is and How It Works* (4th ed.). Sudbury, MA: Jones and Bartlett Publishers.

U.S. Department of Health and Human Services. 2000, November. *Healthy People 2010: Understanding and Improving Health and Objectives for Improving Health* (2nd ed.). Washington, DC: U.S. Government Printing Office.

U.S. Department of Health and Human Services. 2008, August. Consensus statement on quality in the public health system. Retrieved August 30, 2009, from http://www.dhhs.gov/ophs/programs/initiatives/phqf-consensus-statement.pdf

U.S. Department of Health and Human Services. 2009. Evaluating sources of knowledge for evidence-based actions in public health. Retrieved March, 20, 2011, from http://www.healthedpartners.org/hc2020/090710call/3_1_Evidenced%20Based%20PH_FINAL-1%2007%2009.pdf

U.S. Department of Health and Human Services. n.d. Community health status indicators report. Retrieved March 20, 2011, from http://www.communityhealth.hhs.gov/homepage.aspx?j=1

World Health Organization. 2009. *World Health Statistics 2009.* Retrieved March 20, 2011, from http://www.who.int/whosis/whostat/2009/en/index.html

CHAPTER 17

Quality Improvement in Nursing

Gwen Sherwood and Cheryl B. Jones

"Who better than nursing to move into the forefront of improving care? While quality and safety are not ours alone, they provide us with a platform for being our professional best."

—Marla Salmon (editorial in *Nursing Outlook*, 2007, p. 119)

INTRODUCTION

Mounting evidence over the past decade reveals a critical need for improvement in all sectors of health care delivery. Despite spending more than any other country in the world, the U.S. health care system is marked by significant shortcomings in efficiency, quality, access, safety, and affordability (Davis et al., 2010). Vigilance in improving quality provides the mechanism through which the health care system can be transformed. It is the continuous work of all health professionals in collaboration with patients and their families, researchers, payers, planners, and educators that leads to improvements that offer better patient outcomes (health), better system performance (care), and better professional development (education) (Batalden and Davidoff, 2007). To address quality issues, all health professionals must be able to assess the scientific evidence to determine what constitutes good care, identify the gaps between good care and actual care in their setting, and know the actions necessary to close gaps. The need for quality improvement intersects all areas of health care, from economic issues to the moral basis undergirding quality. This effort builds on the shared values and moral commitment common to all health professions.

Nurses are at the forefront of quality improvement efforts in health care. They serve as a critical member of the health care team and lead quality improvement initiatives because of their key role in our health care system and society. Their constant presence with patients, their advocacy for patients, their clinical knowledge, the critical thinking gained in their educational preparation, and their capacity as change agents make their contributions to care delivery essential. To capture the essential role of nurses in improving our health care system, nursing education standards now include concepts pertaining to quality. These standards rely on structure, process, and outcome measures to identify clinical questions, describe processes of changing current practice, and evaluate the outcomes of improvement efforts. This focus on quality is consistent with nurses' core values for choosing nursing as a career. By applying quality improvement in their nursing practice, nurses enhance their effectiveness as health care team members, thus accelerating changes in their workplace. This chapter will trace the history of quality improvement as part of the nurse's role in quality and safety, discuss the evolving role of nurses in quality improvements efforts, describe a national project to transform nursing curricula to include quality improvement, highlight nurse-led national and international quality improvement initiatives, and envision future opportunities that lie ahead.

HISTORIC PERSPECTIVES ON NURSING'S INVOLVEMENT IN QUALITY IMPROVEMENT

One need look no further than Florence Nightingale to appreciate the breadth and depth of the nurse's commitment to quality and the science of improvement. A frequently cited quote from her book *Notes on Nursing* (1859) captures the importance of quality to nurses and demonstrates her commitment and enduring contributions to the health care system's understanding of quality:

> I am fain to sum up with an urgent appeal for adopting this or some
> uniform system of publishing the statistical records of hospitals. If
> they could be obtained . . . they would show subscribers how their
> money was being spent, what amount of good was really being done
> with it, or whether the money was doing mischief rather than good.

This simple comment, made more than one and a half centuries ago,
reminds us not only of the complexity of achieving quality in health care,
but also the difficulty in doing so: We are just now showing "subscribers"
how their money is spent and the value of their spending.

Since Nightingale, there have been ongoing efforts from within nursing to improve the overall delivery of care. Professional organizations such
as the American Nurses Association (ANA) (2011) and the International
Council of Nurses (2002) have been actively engaged in quality improvement efforts nationally and globally. Also, research and practice have
advanced from "assuring" quality to improving quality (Doran, 2010;
Montalvo and Dunton, 2007; Rantz, 1995), and the quality of nurses'
education has advanced to focus on ensuring the integration of quality
and patient safety in nursing school curricula (American Association of
Colleges of Nursing, 2006; Cronenwett et al., 2007; Cronenwett et al.,
2009; National League for Nursing, 2010).

Efforts to improve the quality of nursing practice have also evolved over
time. The Magnet initiative, first coined in a report commissioned by the
ANA (McClure et al., 1983), described hospitals that were particularly
successful attracting and retaining nurses in a time of a nurse shortage.
In 1990, the Magnet movement became formalized as one way of demonstrating organizational quality in the delivery of nursing care. Today,
the Magnet initiative provides a framework for specifying the organizational and practice environment conditions that support and facilitate
nursing excellence and draws attention to the critical link between the
organization and delivery of nursing care and quality. Continuous quality improvement is embedded in the standards for Magnet designation
and certification, which recognize excellence in nursing (McClure and
Hinshaw, 2002). Lundmark (2008) summarizes evidence on the characteristics of Magnet hospitals and their link to patient, staff, and organizational outcomes.

The National Database of Nursing Quality Indicators (NDNQI) was
established by the ANA in 1998 with 30 participating hospitals (ANA,
2011). The long-running project now has more than 1,000 diverse

facilities that have sustained an improvement in a designated nursing-sensitive indicator. Nurses from these facilities share their NDNQI experiences from the start of their programs, including details about quality measurement, reporting, and project results in a monograph from Montalvo and Dunton (2007). Quality indicators measured by nurses relate to staffing, hospital-acquired pressure ulcers, falls and prevention of injury from falls, staff satisfaction, and specialty data related to pediatrics and psychiatric mental health areas (ANA, 2011).

Quality improvement efforts in nursing have also been shaped by forces outside of nursing. The call for sweeping reform of the American health care system came from the Institute of Medicine (IOM) in its 2001 report *Crossing the Quality Chasm: A New Health System for the 21st Century*, which identified a set of six performance expectations for the 21st-century health care system. Namely, patient care should be safe, effective, patient-centered, timely, efficient, and equitable. These aims are intended as the measures of quality that ultimately will align incentives for payment and accountability based on improvements in quality; yet recent reports indicate many gaps in the quality desired (Balik and Dopkiss, 2010; Leape and Berwick, 2005; Wachter, 2004, 2010), including how we educate health care professionals.

The push to accomplish the original six aims led to a subsequent IOM report (2003), which declared education to be the bridge to quality. Five competencies were identified as essential for all health professionals if we are to accomplish these sweeping changes: delivering patient-centered care, working as part of interdisciplinary teams, practicing evidence-based health care, focusing on quality improvement, and using information technology (IOM, 2003). Educators and organizations responsible for accreditation, licensing, and certification of health professionals are transforming how we prepare students and working professionals so they are proficient in these competencies essential to quality and safety.

Another IOM report, *Keeping Patients Safe: Transforming the Work Environment of Nurses*, has also drawn specific attention to the important link between nurses, their work environment, and patient safety and quality of care. This report represented an interdisciplinary effort to examine the work of nurses in detail and made several important recommendations (Page, 2004):

- Create a satisfying and rewarding work environment for nurses
- Provide adequate nurse staffing

- Focus on patient safety at the level of organizational governing boards
- Incorporate evidence-based management in the management of nursing services
- Build trust between nurses and organizational leaders
- Give nurses a voice in patient care delivery through effective nursing leadership and participation in executive decision making
- Provide organizational support to promote learning for both new and experienced nurses
- Promote interdisciplinary collaboration
- Design work environments that promote patient safety
- Create cultures that strengthen patient safety

This report has been critical in shaping the role of nurses in patient care quality and safety efforts.

Other efforts have also propelled nursing forward in its engagement in and contributions to quality improvement in health care. A collaboration between the Robert Wood Johnson Foundation (RWJF) and the Institute for Healthcare Improvement (IHI), called Transforming Care at the Bedside (or TCAB), was initiated in 2003 to recognize "nursing's critical but commonly overlooked role" in care delivery (Lavizzo-Mourey and Berwick, 2009, p. 3). This initiative took advantage of an opportunity to take high-performing hospitals to the next level of excellence by creating "learning laboratories" for innovations at the point of care. The result of this initiative has been the development and identification of benchmarks that serve as performance improvement targets to guide organizational leaders in achieving efficiencies and lasting changes. This initiative has spread from 3 organizations at its inception to roughly 160 organizations in 2009, including 40 facilities from the Department of Veterans Affairs (Hassmiller and Bolton, 2009). Many other organizations across the United States have taken advantage of the knowledge gained from TCAB because of the extraordinary published reports that point to better clinical outcomes, increased direct care time for nurses, reduced nurse turnover, and lower costs (Lavizzo-Mourey and Berwick, 2009). A step-by-step guide for implementing innovations from TCAB is provided in the TCAB toolkit, available through the RWJF (2008). This initiative has been so successful that an entire supplement of the *American Journal of Nursing* was devoted to publishing important TCAB efforts in November 2009.

Nurses' involvement in quality also stems from regulatory standards that impact nursing practice, such as those from the Centers for Medicare and Medicaid Services (CMS) or The Joint Commission (TJC). For example, the Deficit Reduction Act of 2005 changed the payment structure for health care, and subsequently, CMS-developed programs focused on reducing hospital-acquired conditions (HACs), or those conditions that were not present at the time of a patient's hospital admission (CMS, 2008). In 2008, CMS announced that it would no longer reimburse hospitals for 10 preventable HACs (known as "never events"), many of which pertained to the delivery of nursing care (Hines and Yu, 2009; Kurtzman and Buerhaus, 2008). Other third-party payers and large employers have followed suit by linking performance indicators to reimbursement plans to focus on value-based purchasing. In these pay-for-performance plans, health systems receive additional economic incentives when specific quality targets are met. TJC has also focused on quality in its accreditation of health care institutions, including the institution in 2002 of a set of annually changing patient safety goals that emphasize a systematic process for quality improvement, patient safety, and outcomes.

Efforts to engage nurses in the quality movement have also come from other federal and nonfederal organizations outside of nursing. The Agency for Healthcare Research and Quality (AHRQ) thought nursing was so critical in ensuring patient care quality and safety that it, in conjunction with the RWJF, supported a handbook for nurses on patient safety and quality that could be used in education and practice, titled *Patient Safety and Quality: An Evidence-Based Handbook for Nurses* (Hughes, 2008). With a comprehensive summary of important patient safety and quality improvement concepts, it also examines published evidence for providing patient-centered care, nurses' working conditions and work environment, and how nurses are involved in improving quality and safety. In this book, Farquhar (2008) outlined quality indicators in which nurses have key roles in four key quality areas: prevention in ambulatory care settings, inpatient settings, patient safety across the health care system (including public health), and pediatric care for children younger than 17 years old. Outcomes of these quality indicators provide other areas of data for pay for performance.

Other initiatives such as those brought about by the IHI have shaped nurses' engagement in quality improvement initiatives. The IHI's 100,000 Lives and 5 Million Lives campaigns (http://www.ihi.org/IHI/Programs/Campaign/) and other efforts to encourage collaborations among hospitals serve as a means of engaging nurses by advancing quality improvement, deploying special projects and evidence-based care bundles, and sponsoring educational forums for all health professionals. Thus, whether through professional organizations, regulation, practice standards, or their education and socialization, nurses at all levels and in all settings must be aware of and involved in addressing the myriad issues that impact the quality and safety of care delivered.

THE EVOLVING ROLE OF NURSES IN QUALITY IMPROVEMENT AND HEALTH CARE TEAMS

Much of the daily work of hospital-based nurses hinges on the delivery of quality care. Hughes (2008) uses the phrase "everydayness of errors" to describe the challenge that nurses practicing within complex health care environments face in staying attuned to a variety of issues, including the disease processes of their patients, the clinicians and others who come in contact with their patients, the technologies used, the policies and procedures that guide practice, and the resources available to them.

Nurses have well-established roles in quality improvement as hospitals have started to build a culture of patient safety (Sammer et al., 2010). Safety culture—or the result of individual, unit, and organizational "values, attitudes, perceptions, competencies, and patterns of behavior that determine the commitment to, and the style and proficiency of, an organization's health and safety management" (Health and Safety Commission, 1993)—is being promoted in health care organizations through the use of quality-related activities as important "safety checks." These checks ensure that certain actions and precautions are taken by clinicians to protect patients during care delivery. Thus, the achievement of quality and safety in patient care is the result of caregivers doing the right thing, the right way, the first time. Promoting a culture of patient safety requires nurses to serve as a critical link to the best quality health care that organizations have to offer. Nurses are now called upon to speak out, speak up, and question aspects of care delivery that put patients' safety in jeopardy. They must also serve on interdisciplinary teams to help create new care protocols, design care pathways to set standards of care, use safety reporting systems to identify safety risks, participate in root cause analyses following sentinel events, examine benchmark data for areas of improvement, and help design system changes derived from analysis of data.

While quality and safety are intertwined concepts in the attempt to deliver exemplary patient care (Caramanica et al., 2003), nurses have not always been trained or educated for the new roles they must play in ensuring patient care quality and safety. Today, nurses must apply quality improvement techniques that improve patient safety in an effort to understand, improve, and standardize care processes based on current evidence (Hughes, 2008). Applying evidence-based standards is one way nurses can improve quality and safety; analyzing clinical pathways and/or developing clinical algorithms to standardize nursing care as a means of improving quality of care is yet another.

Nurses' roles in quality improvement have evolved to also include both membership and leadership on health care teams. Regulatory agencies responded to the staggering IOM data with many changes and initiatives to improve outcomes. New standards for improving quality of care gave new roles and responsibilities to health care workers, particularly nurses. Because nurses are often the first line for communication with patients and their families, both as the constant provider with inpatients and the first link for communication in outpatient settings, they have an essential role on health care teams by coordinating, integrating, and facilitating the delivery of care. Thus, while nurses are often one of several members of the health care team, the very nature of their role means that much of what they do in practice is through their leadership on clinical teams.

Nurses also play key roles in quality improvement initiatives by both being a part of and leading quality improvement initiatives in health care organizations. In their role on quality improvement teams, they often gather data for, help develop, and implement protocols required to meet regulatory standards and economic incentives (Bodrock and Mion, 2008). Nurses gather and use data to monitor the outcomes of care processes, design and apply improvement methods to design and test changes, and use outcomes—of patients, providers, and systems—to improve care processes as well as the system overall. Improvement activities of patient care units are often led by nurses in health care organizations, and these activities must be balanced with those put forward by other organizational leaders at the system level.

It has been reported that the continuous focus on quality has become so pervasive that quality initiatives comprise the majority of the work time of chief nurse executives (Arnold et al., 2006). A study by the Center for Studying Health System Change cites the increasing role and influence for nurses in quality initiatives (Draper et al., 2008). These roles vary according to the hospital's organizational culture and investment in a quality culture. Organizations that offer supportive leadership, embrace a philosophy of quality as everyone's responsibility, promote individual accountability, identify physician and nurse champions, and seek effective feedback experience more staff involvement (Draper et al., 2008).

In any improvement effort, the first step is often making staff aware of breakdowns in communication and work flow hampered by work-arounds that have become the norm. Communicating this information often falls to the unit manager, who is responsible for overseeing the delivery of care on a patient care unit. The leadership style of the nurse manager has been linked to certain unit-level outcomes, including staff nurse retention, satisfaction, turnover, and/or global measures of quality (Bratt et al., 2000; Leveck and Jones, 1996). Increasingly, health care organizations may move in the same direction as other industries and base nurse manager performance evaluation on quality-related metrics, such as patient satisfaction (Light, 2010), which would remove some of the subjectivity involved in the performance evaluation process. Thus, nurse managers and leaders at all levels need in-depth knowledge and understanding of the business side of care delivery to create positive work environments for the nurses who provide care to patients, and to make better decisions that impact both patients and the organizations where they receive care (American Organization of Nurse Executives, 2007).

At times, nurses may feel "caught in the middle"—between the point of care delivery and organizational leadership—or their involvement in quality improvement practice may feel like just another task in an already full workload. Nurses on the front lines often feel too stressed, overworked, and understaffed to adequately deliver care to patients and families; nurses in leadership positions may feel like they are constantly responding to the urgency of ensuring safe staffing levels, keeping up with regulatory mandates, and improving quality of care with limited resources. However, Hall, Moore, et al. (2008) describe how the growing focus on providing high-quality care not only benefits patients but also stimulates joy in nurses' work. There are many system issues that influence nurses' job satisfaction, which can be addressed through quality improvement analysis of such issues as patient flow problems, safe management of high census periods, communication problems around complex patients, and improving medication safety (Hall, Moore, et al., 2008). Having the skills to deliver the kind of care they know meets best practice increases satisfaction, contributes to a more positive work environment (Hall, Doran, et al., 2008), and improves patient satisfaction (Lindberg and Kimberlain, 2008).

While nurses at all levels may at times feel challenged to accept the responsibilities for quality improvement, implementing best practices and continuously improving quality in their everyday nursing activities, failing to do so comes at a high price to patients, their families, other nurses, and the health care system at large. Changing the way nurses practice may seem difficult, but the incentives to do so and the opportunities to contribute to systemic changes in our health care system have never been greater.

Applications in Specific Care Settings

Quality improvement as systematic, data-guided activities designed to bring about immediate improvements in the delivery of health care has implications for how it is applied in particular settings. The role of nurses translates across varied health care settings, including acute care, long-term care, and primary care.

Williams and Fallone (2008) discuss the role of nurses in an acute care setting to monitor, evaluate, and creatively improve their working environment to lead to best practice guidelines and standards for their unit. Applying a Plan, Do, Study, Act (PDSA) (see Chapter 1) quality improvement methodology leads to clearer care processes and improved practice in a continuous cycle of asking questions, seeking new knowledge, and applying to care standards. Braaten and Bellhouse (2007) used an adaptive design and the Toyota production system to redesign work systems in their acute care unit to achieve sustainable improvements in productivity, staff and patient satisfaction, and quality outcomes.

Compas et al. (2008) synthesized the literature to examine quality improvement projects in nursing homes with common approaches to include goal statements, multidisciplinary teams, education needed, project champions, and a feedback loop. Bonner et al. (2007) demonstrate how students can participate in quality improvement in long-term care where overworked staff may lack training in improvement methods.

One example of a nursing standard of care linked to a regulatory standard is urinary incontinence in nursing homes. Palmer (2008) discusses urinary incontinence as part of the Nursing Home Quality Initiative from the CMS. Urinary incontinence remains a quality issue in nursing homes despite intense efforts to alleviate it. Palmer describes the key role of nurses in appropriate assessment and treatment protocols for urinary infections, and the quality improvement strategies used, which are sometimes referred to as "excellent management."

Students are valuable resources to help design and implement quality improvement in settings where few resources are available for quality initiatives such as the one described by Teeley et al. (2006) in a community health setting. Based on an identified gap in their undergraduate community health course, these faculty members saw a need to revise the course to build upon their past work and bring more quality improvement experiences into the curriculum. This 2-year project focused on clinic operations, and a redesign of patient care reflected a collaboration between faculty at Simmons College in Boston, its Learning for Action Institute for Community Health Improvement, and the community health sites within which undergraduate students were placed for clinical experiences. Faculty developed course materials (both lecture and online) and incorporated selected readings to teach students about the quality improvement process; they then guided students in the conduct of a focused quality improvement project. The quality improvement process used eight key steps (Knapp and Lowe, 2001): clarifying the project aim; forming the right team; targeting improvement efforts to the project aim; gathering and using data to inform the process; listening to the customer; using improvement tools and methods; conducting improvement and learning cycles; and making improvements. Students worked in teams to conduct projects focused on issues such as reducing the number of patients with abnormal test results lost to follow-up, reducing clinic no-shows, and improving clinic patients' perceptions of quality care. In the end, students and faculty felt they had given something back to the agency, and faculty reported that the students became engaged and invested in the project outcomes, adding to their understanding of the issues in community nursing.

Jones and colleagues (2009) described another educational initiative that focused on the total revamping of a graduate-level nursing course through strong academic–practice partnerships. Faculty and service partners collaboratively developed a preceptor model with a practicum component that was integrated into the course. This shifted the course focus from the faculty member as "authority" and student as passive learner to the faculty as guide and student as active learner. Students applied quality improvement, patient safety, and outcomes knowledge and skills learned in the didactic portion of the class with real-world experiences gained in the health care facilities. Key features of the process included problem identification, working in teams alongside organizational staff to address problems, accessing organizational experts for guidance, gathering and/or evaluating relevant organizational data, designing solutions that were appropriate to the organization, and integrating quality improvement techniques learned in the didactic portion of the course. By taking advantage of both students' expertise and organizational capabilities, problems were addressed in a manner mutually beneficial to students and the facility where the practicum was conducted. Student team projects ranged from designing a process to improve patient handoffs to an evaluation of rapid response teams to an examination of organizational heart failure core measure performance. Students, preceptors, organizational leaders, and faculty highly praised the course revision, but the greatest indicator of success was that, in every case, team project recommendations were implemented by the partnering organization.

The role of nurses in quality improvement in various settings is further illustrated in Cases 2 and 9 of the companion casebook (McLaughlin et al., 2012).

QUALITY IMPROVEMENT IN NURSING EDUCATION

Similar to other health professionals, nurses have largely learned improvement methods on the job, as traditionally these methods were not included in nursing curricula. The gap in skills and expertise to lead quality initiatives meant hospitals developed longer and more costly orientations and staff development programs (Sherwood and Drenkard, 2007) to prepare new graduates to practice in the current health care environment. The significant quality issues in our health care system demand a redesign in what and how we teach the next generation of nurses and other health care professionals so that they understand the factors that help ensure quality care. Nurses must be able to identify and bridge the gaps between what is and what should be. Emerging views of quality and safety and related competencies applied in practice have corresponding implications for the redesign of nursing education programs.

The Quality and Safety Education for Nurses (QSEN) project was developed to bridge the gap increasingly evident between nurses' education and expectations in practice roles and responsibilities (Cronenwett et al., 2007). Funded by the RWJF, the goal is to help nurses gain the knowledge, skills, and attitudes that support roles in continuously improving the health care systems in which they work. The long-range goal of QSEN is to reshape professional identity formation in nursing to include commitment to creating cultures of quality and safety. The project has developed in three phases to address the challenges of preparing future nurses with the knowledge, skills, and attitudes necessary to help change patient care outcomes. Phases I and II, which have been completed, sought to identify the current status of nursing education related to quality and gaps in the curriculum and to establish a pilot learning collaborative to demonstrate both didactic and clinical learning interventions. Phase III, which is under way, provides faculty development.

In Phase I of the project, a national expert panel employed an iterative process to reach consensus on the six competencies adapted from the IOM report on the future of health professions education to improve quality and safety in health care: patient-centered care, teamwork and collaboration, evidence-based practice, quality improvement, safety, and informatics (Cronenwett et al., 2007). Whereas the IOM combined quality and safety into one competency, the QSEN panel recognized the science undergirding each of these as separate competencies. The 17-member panel included two physicians who were also involved in quality improvement education for physicians; thus, the QSEN work was consistent with developments among other health professional education.

Each competency was defined and further expanded with explication of the knowledge, skills, and attitudes for each competency, first for prelicensure nursing education programs (Cronenwett et al., 2007) (see **Table 17–1**) and subsequently for graduate nursing education programs (Cronenwett et al., 2009). The definition remains the same for both prelicensure and graduate nurses, but **Tables 17–2** and **17–3** illustrate the differences in the knowledge, skills, and attitudes for the two levels of nursing. QSEN leaders completed a national survey of baccalaureate

TABLE 17–1 Quality and Safety Competencies Identified by QSEN for Prelicensure Nurses

Quality and Safety Competencies	Definition	Attributes
Patient-centered care	Recognize the patient or designee as the source of control and full partner in providing compassionate and coordinated care based on respect for the patient's preferences, values, and needs	Applies knowledge of patient values and preferences in caring for patient and with others on the care team
Teamwork and collaboration	Function effectively within nursing and interprofessional teams, fostering open communication, mutual respect, and shared decision making to achieve quality patient care	Use personal strengths to foster effective team functioning Integrate quality and safety science in effectively communicating across diverse team members Include patient and family as members of the health care team
Evidence-based practice (EBP)	Integrate best current evidence with clinical expertise and patient/family preferences and values for delivery of optimal health care	Practices from a spirit of inquiry Bases nursing care standards on evidence Applies technology to investigate latest evidence to determine best care approaches and clarify care decisions
Quality improvement	Use data to monitor the outcomes of care processes and use improvement methods to design and test changes to continuously improve the quality and safety of health care systems	Is integrated into nursing role and identity Uses quality tools, evidence, patient preferences, and benchmark data to assess current practice and design continuous quality improvements
Safety	Minimize risk of harm to patients and providers through both system effectiveness and individual performance	Constantly asks: What about my actions poses a risk to the patient? Where is the next error likely to occur? What actions can I take to prevent near misses?
Informatics	Use information and technology to communicate, manage knowledge, mitigate error, and support decision making	Uses technology to improve and manage care

Source: Adapted from Cronenwett et al., 2007.

TABLE 17–2 Definition of Quality Improvement and the Required Knowledge, Skills, and Attitudes for Prelicensure Nurses

Definition: Use data to monitor the outcomes of care processes, and use improvement methods to design and test changes to continuously improve the quality and safety of health care systems.

Knowledge	Skills	Attitudes
Describe strategies for learning about the outcomes of care in the setting in which one is engaged in clinical practice	Seek information about outcomes of care for populations served in care setting Seek information about quality improvement projects in the care setting	Appreciate that continuous quality improvement is an essential part of the daily work of all health professionals
Recognize that nursing and other health professions students are parts of systems of care and care processes that affect outcomes for patients and families Give examples of the tension between professional autonomy and system functioning	Use tools (such as flowcharts, cause-and-effect diagrams) to make processes of care explicit Participate in a root cause analysis of a sentinel event	Value own and others' contributions to outcomes of care in local care settings
Explain the importance of variation and measurement in assessing quality of care	Use quality measures to understand performance Use tools (such as control charts and run charts) that are helpful for understanding variation Identify gaps between local and best practice	Appreciate how unwanted variation affects care Value measurement and its role in good patient care
Describe approaches for changing processes of care	Design a small test of change in daily work (using an experiential learning method such as the PDSA cycle) Practice aligning the aims, measures, and changes involved in improving care Use measures to evaluate the effect of change	Value local change (in individual practice or team practice on a unit) and its role in creating joy in work Appreciate the value of what individuals and teams can do to improve care

Source: Adapted from Cronenwett et al., 2007.

TABLE 17-3 Quality Improvement Competency Defined by QSEN for Graduate-Level Nursing Practice

Definition: Use data to monitor the outcomes of care processes, and use improvement methods to design and test changes to continuously improve the quality and safety of health care systems.

Knowledge	Skills	Attitudes
Describe strategies for *improving* outcomes of care in the setting in which one is engaged in clinical practice	Use a variety of sources of information to review outcomes of care and identify potential areas for improvement	Appreciate that continuous quality improvement is an essential part of the daily work of all health professionals
Analyze the impact of context (such as access, cost, or team functioning) on improvement efforts	*Propose appropriate aims for quality improvement efforts*	
	Assert leadership in shaping the dialogue about and providing leadership for the introduction of best practices	
Analyze ethical issues associated with quality improvement	*Ensure ethical oversight of quality improvement projects*	*Value the need for ethical conduct of quality improvement*
Describe features of quality improvement projects that overlap sufficiently with research, thereby requiring institutional review board oversight	*Maintain confidentiality of any patient information used to determine outcomes of quality improvement efforts*	
Describe the benefits and limitations of quality improvement data sources, and measurement and data analysis strategies	*Design and use databases as sources of information for improving patient care*	*Appreciate the importance of data that allows one to estimate the quality of local care*
	Select and use relevant benchmarks	
Explain common causes of variation in outcomes of care in the practice specialty	Select and use tools (such as control charts and run charts) that are helpful for understanding variation	Appreciate how unwanted variation affects outcomes of care processes
	Identify gaps between local and best practice	

(continued)

TABLE 17-3 Quality Improvement Competency Defined by QSEN for Graduate-Level Nursing Practice (*continued*)

Definition: Use data to monitor the outcomes of care processes, and use improvement methods to design and test changes to continuously improve the quality and safety of health care systems.

Knowledge	Skills	Attitudes
Describe common quality measures in the practice specialty	*Use findings from* root cause analyses to design and implement system improvements	Value measurement and its role in good patient care
	Select and use quality measures to understand performance	
Analyze the differences between microsystem and macrosystem change	*Use principles of change management to implement and evaluate care processes at the microsystem level*	Appreciate the value of what individuals and teams can do to improve care
Understand principles of change management	Design, *implement, and evaluate* tests of change in daily work (using an experiential learning method such as the PDSA cycle)	*Value local systems improvement (in individual practice, team practice on a unit, or in the macrosystem) and its role in professional job satisfaction*
Analyze the strengths and limitations of common quality improvement methods	*Align the aims, measures, and changes involved in improving care*	*Appreciate that all improvement is change, but not all change is improvement*
	Use measures to evaluate the effect of change	

Source: Adapted from Cronenwett et al., 2009.

Note: Bold italic type indicates variation from prelicensure competencies in Table 17-2.

nursing program leaders and a state survey of associate-degree educators to assess beliefs about the extent to which the competencies were already included in curricula, the level of satisfaction with student competency achievement, and the level of faculty expertise in teaching the competencies. Faculty who responded to the survey identified quality improvement as a learning need to achieve the competency (Smith et al., 2007).

The expert panel examined systems thinking and improvement, error reduction, human factors theory, and safety to identify the knowledge, skills, and attitudes defining each competency. Rather than prescribing a curriculum, the panel identified measurable objectives so that faculty and clinical educators had flexibility in how the competencies were applied in their individual settings. Pedagogical experts on the panel helped develop exemplar classroom, clinical, and simulation-based learning strategies that could be applied with interprofessional student groups (Day and Smith, 2007; Durham and Sherwood, 2008; see also http://www.qsen.org).

As the competencies gained wide recognition and acceptance among nurses, faculty development emerged as key to leading the necessary changes. In QSEN Phase II, a pilot learning collaborative funded 15 schools to model integration of the competencies into their curricula (Barton et al., 2009; Cronenwett et al., 2009). Schools demonstrated different strategies for implementing quality improvement into curricula. To help students achieve the competencies detailed in Table 17–2, a common strategy was to work with faculty to incorporate information about quality improvement tools into the curriculum. This helped students master skills in searching and gathering information from databases and Web sites of national quality initiatives, such as those of the IHI, TJC, and the National Quality Forum, and helped them conduct a simple PDSA process using appropriate tools such as run charts and fishbone diagrams (see Chapter 3). Many students were involved in quality improvement initiatives during their clinical learning time and were coached in asking quality-focused questions. Some students had the opportunity to design a small test of change on a topic of interest to them. This helped increase their awareness of opportunities for quality improvement and gave them a chance to search the literature, design a planned change, test implementation, and measure the outcome.

Phase III (2009–2011) promotes innovative ways to teach, test, and certify the competencies across educational levels of nursing. Faculty development includes teaching and coaching faculty about quality improvement methods so that they can design learning strategies in their curricula in partnership with clinical agencies. Phase III also focuses on incorporating the competencies in textbooks, licensing, accreditation, and certification standards to offer students and faculty the needed learning resources to address quality improvement and produce a new generation of nurses for whom quality is a part of their daily work. A Web site (http://www.qsen .org) provides a worldwide resource for teaching strategies, key links, an annotated bibliography, a teaching video, and other resources.

From the outset, QSEN leaders realized the impact of the changes on standards for nursing education, accreditation of nursing programs, and certification in specialty practice. An advisory council with representative membership from physician education, nursing accreditation and credentialing organizations, nursing care delivery settings, interprofessional education projects, exemplar national change projects, and varied educational entry programs worked alongside the expert faculty panel to help lead the changes. This collaboration enabled swift action to integrate the quality and safety competencies in the educational standards for baccalaureate, master's, and the Doctor of Nursing Practice programs and corresponding accreditation requirements for schools of nursing that offer these programs. Both the National Organization of Nurse Practitioner Faculties and the American Nurses Credentialing Center recognize the quality competencies in their work in credentialing advanced practice and specialty nurses. This work in policy implementation ensures that ultimately all nurses will recognize and embrace the role of quality as part of their professional identify.

FUTURE DIRECTIONS

The evolving role of nurses in quality improvement, regulatory standards, education initiatives, and the societal mandate to improve care suggests several directions for the future. These directions pertain to interdisciplinary education, retooling of nursing faculty, goals to improve nursing practice, and engagement of nurses in national quality initiatives.

Education with Other Disciplines

Accreditation standards for most health professions now mandate inclusion of quality improvement (Batalden et al., 2009). The generations of practicing professionals whose education did not include quality improvement lack the necessary knowledge, skills, and attitudes needed to actively participate in systems improvement, placing the education burden on clinical settings. Quality improvement processes require participation across the disciplines, yet health professions students have few interprofessional learning experiences. Achieving Competence Today is an example of a new model for interprofessional education to prepare professionals for quality, safety, and health systems improvement through a four-module active learning course in which learners from different disciplines develop a quality improvement project to address a quality or safety problem in their own practice system (Ladden et al., 2006).

Implications for Nursing Faculty

The IOM (2004) calls for education in all health professions to be infused with the six quality and safety competencies, and new accreditation standards can be accomplished through significant shifts in attention rather than new courses. Strategies that place less burden on already overloaded curricula include questions embedded in case studies, redirected clinical learning experiences, debriefings in postclinical conferences, mentoring through participation in quality improvement initiatives, and application of the competencies in clinical learning laboratories. A shift from student learning development that focused only on the individual patient to mindful inquiry can position the individual patient within the system of care and provide the first step in broadening the scope of one's practice to include quality and safety (Barton et al., 2009; Day and Smith, 2007).

While there are many approaches to teaching quality improvement, descriptions of what content should be included and reports of the approaches' effectiveness have been limited. Critical thinking is an integral foundation of nursing education. It helps nurses develop a spirit of inquiry to become analytical practitioners, which contributes to the art of asking questions, the first stage of a quality improvement process (Edwards, 2007). Quality improvement is often taught through participation in an improvement initiative and sometimes through interprofessional approaches (Hall, Moore, et al., 2008) or high-fidelity patient simulation exercises (Durham and Sherwood, 2008). The Quality Improvement Knowledge Application Tool (Varkey et al., 2006) determined that medical and nursing participants in an interdisciplinary quality improvement initiative significantly improved their capacity to make changes using quality improvement methods. A systematic review of the effectiveness of published quality improvement curricula in medical education by Boonyasai et al. (2007) concluded that learning strategies do demonstrate sound adult learning principles; the data failed to determine which educational methods have meaningful clinical benefits.

Goals for Practice Improvements

Quality improvement has become an intrinsic part of health care delivery operations that involves both providers and patients. The ethical framework undergirding quality improvement extends from the ethical responsibility to provide the best known care to the ethical conduct of the process itself. While quality improvement activities are distinct from human subjects research and therefore do not require review by an institutional review board, quality improvement activities do require professional supervision and oversight as defined by an expert panel convened by the Hastings Center (Lynn et al., 2007).

Nurses' Roles in National Quality Initiatives

There are many organizations focusing on quality of care. The Association of American Medical Colleges launched the Integrating Quality Project to help educators with the dual role of attending to high-quality care and educating medical students by providing resources for teaching quality improvement. The ANA established the National Center for Nursing Quality to showcase nursing care quality projects, provide quality and safety educational resources and tools, and examine the quality of the work environment for nurses.

CONCLUSIONS

The health care marketplace is rapidly changing, along with increasing regulatory pressures to improve the quality of care delivered. Technologies will allow even faster change in the future. One thing is certain, however: The health care purse strings are not likely to be loosened in the future. The costs of care will continue to be a concern as technological advances make the best possible care more and more expensive. Consequently, health care payers and organizations will continue to place emphasis on ensuring patient care quality and safety through qualifications, capabilities, and competencies across disciplines.

Efforts to improve the quality of care are critically important to nursing practice, the overall delivery of health care, and the quality of care delivered to our society. As the single largest group of health care providers in an industry that consumes more than 17% of the gross domestic product of the United States (Truffer et al., 2010), nurses are an integral component of the current and future health care delivery system by virtue of the roles they play in frontline care delivery, on health care teams, and in quality improvement initiatives. To improve the care environment, the essential role of nurses in ensuring quality and the impacts of change efforts on nurses and patients must be considered and better understood (Jones and Lusk, 2002). Nurses are critical in leading and serving as members of quality improvement teams in the future to more fully enhance the value of care delivered.

Cross-References to the Companion Casebook

(McLaughlin, C. P., Johnson, J. K., and Sollecito, W. A. [Eds.]. 2012. *Implementing Continuous Quality Improvement in Health Care: A Global Casebook.* Sudbury, MA: Jones & Bartlett Learning.)

Case Study Number	Case Study Title	Case Study Authors
2	Holtz Children's Hospital: Reducing Central Line Infections	*Gwenn E. McLaughlin*
9	Forthright Medical Center: Social Marketing and the Surgical Checklist	*Carol E. Breland*

REFERENCES

American Association of Colleges of Nursing (AACN). 2006. Hallmarks of quality and safety: Recommended baccalaureate competencies and curricular guidelines to assure high quality and safe patient care. *J Professional Nurs*, 22(6): 329–330.

American Nurses Association. 2011. The National Database of Nursing Quality Indicators. Retrieved April 7, 2011, from http://nursingworld .org/MainMenuCategories/ThePracticeofProfessionalNursing/Patient SafetyQuality/Research-Measurement/The-National-Database.aspx

American Organization of Nurse Executives. 2007. AONE guiding principles for the role of the nurse executive in patient safety. Retrieved June 29, 2010, from http://www.aone.org/aone/resource/PDF/AONE_ GP_Role_Nurse_Exec_Patient_Safety.pdf

Arnold, L., Campbell, A., Dubree, M., et al. 2006. Priorities and challenges of health system chief nursing executives: Insights for nursing educators. *J Prof Nurs*, 22(4): 213–220.

Balik, B., and Dopkiss, F. 2010. 10 years after *To Err Is Human*: Are we listening to patients and families yet? *Focus on Patient Safety: A Newsletter from the National Patient Safety Foundation*. Retrieved June 29, 2010, from http://www.npsf.org/paf/npsfp/fo/pdf/Focus_ vol_13_1_2010.pdf

Barton, A., Armstrong, G., Preheim, G., et al. 2009. A national Delphi to determine developmental progression of quality and safety competencies in nursing education. *Nurs Outlook*, 57(6): 313–322.

Batalden, P. B., and Davidoff, F. 2007. What is "quality improvement" and how can it transform healthcare? *Quality Safety Health Care*, 16(1): 2–3.

Batalden, P. B., Leach, D., and Ogrinc, G. 2009. Knowing is not enough: Executives and educators must act to address challenges and reshape healthcare. *Healthcare Executive*, 24(2): 68–70.

Bodrock, J. A., and Mion, L. C. 2008. Pay for performance in hospitals: Implications for nurses and nursing care. *Quality Manage Health Care*, 17(2): 102–111.

Bonner, A., MacCulloch, P., Gardner, T., et al. 2007. A student-led demonstration project on fall prevention in a long-term care facility. *Geriatric Nurs*, 28(5): 312–318.

Boonyasai, R. T., Windish, D. M., Chakraborti, C., et al. 2007. Effectiveness of teaching quality improvement to clinicians: A systematic review. *JAMA*, 298(9): 1023–1037.

Braaten, J. S., and Bellhouse, D. E. 2007. Improving patient care by making small sustainable changes: A cardiac telemetry unit's experience. *Nurs Economic$*, 25(3): 162–166.

Bratt, M. M., Broome, M., Kelber, S., et al. 2000. Influence of stress and nursing leadership on job satisfaction of pediatric intensive care unit nurses. *Am J Crit Care*, 9(5): 307–317.

Caramanica, L., Cousino, J. A., and Petersen, S. 2003. Four elements of a successful quality program: Alignment, collaboration, evidence-based practice, and excellence. *Nurs Adm Q*, 27(4): 336–343.

Centers for Medicare and Medicaid Services. 2008. Roadmap for implementing value driven healthcare in the traditional Medicare fee-for-service program. Retrieved July 14, 2010, from https://www .cms.gov/QualityInitiativesGenInfo/downloads/VBPRoadmap_OEA_ 1-16_508.pdf

Compas, C., Hopkins, K., and Townsley, E. 2008. Best practices in implementing and sustaining quality of care: A review of the quality of improvement literature. *Res Gerontol Nurs*, 1(3): 209–215.

Cronenwett, L., Sherwood, G., Barnsteiner, J., et al. 2007. Quality and safety education for nurses. *Nurs Outlook*, 55(3): 122–131.

Cronenwett, L., Sherwood, G., and Gelmon, S. 2009. Improving quality and safety education: The QSEN Learning Collaborative. *Nurs Outlook*, 57(6): 304–312.

Davis, K., Schoen, C., and Stremikis, K. 2010. Mirror, mirror on the wall: How the performance of the U.S. health care system compares internationally, 2010 update. Retrieved July 14, 2010, from http:// www.commonwealthfund.org/~/media/Files/Publications/Fund%20 Report/2010/Jun/1400_Davis_Mirror_Mirror_on_the_wall_2010.pdf

Day, L., and Smith, E. L. 2007. Integrating quality and safety content into clinical teaching in the acute care setting. *Nurs Outlook*, 55(3): 138–143.

Doran, D. M. 2010. *Nursing Outcomes: The State of the Science* (2nd ed.). Sudbury, MA: Jones & Bartlett Learning.

Draper, D. A., Felland, L. E., Liebhaber, A., et al. 2008. The role of nurses in hospital quality improvement. Center for Studying Health System Change. Retrieved March 31, 2011, from http://hschange.org/ CONTENT/972/972.pdf

Durham, C., and Sherwood, G. 2008. Education to bridge the quality gap: A case study approach. *J Urolog Nurs*, Special Topic Issue on Quality, 28(6): 431–438.

Edwards, S. L. 2007. Critical thinking: A two-phase framework. *Nurse Educ Pract*, 7(5): 303–314.

Farquhar, M. 2008. AHRQ quality indicators. In Hughes, R. G. (Ed.), *Patient Safety and Quality: An Evidence-Based Handbook for Nurses* (Vol. 8). Rockville, MD: Agency for Healthcare Research and Quality.

Hall, L. M., Doran, D., and Pink, L. 2008. Outcomes of interventions to improve hospital nursing work environments. *J Nurs Adm*, 38(1): 40–46.

Hall, L. W., Moore, S. M., and Barnsteiner, J. H. 2008. Quality and nursing: Moving from a concept to a core competency. *Urolog Nurs Off J Am Urolog Assoc Allied*, 28(6): 417–425.

Hassmiller, S. B., and Bolton, L. B. 2009. The development of TCAB. *Am J Nurs*, 109(11): 4.

Health and Safety Commission. 1993. *Third Report: Organizing for Safety*. ACSNI Study Group on Human Factors. London: HMSO.

Hines, P. A., and Yu, K. M. 2009. The changing reimbursement landscape: Nurses' role in quality and operational excellence. *Nurs Economic$*, 27(1): 345–352.

Hughes, R. G. 2008. Tools and strategies for quality improvement and patient safety. In Hughes, R. G. (Ed.), *Patient safety and quality: An evidence-based handbook for nurses* (Vol. 3). Rockville, MD: Agency for Healthcare Research and Quality.

Hughes, R. G. (Ed.). 2008. *Patient safety and quality: An evidence-based handbook for nurses* (Vol. 8). Rockville, MD: Agency for Healthcare Research and Quality.

Institute of Medicine. 2001. *Crossing the Quality Chasm: A New Health System for the 21st Century*. Washington, DC: National Academies Press.

Institute of Medicine. 2003. *Health Professions Education: A Bridge to Quality*. Washington, DC: National Academies Press.

Institute of Medicine. 2004. *Patient Safety: Achieving a New Standard for Care*. Washington, DC: National Academies Press.

International Council of Nurses. 2002. Position statement on patient safety. Retrieved July 14, 2010, from http://www.icn.ch/images/ stories/documents/publications/position_statements/D05_Patient_ Safety.pdf

Jones, C. B., and Lusk, S. L. 2002. Incorporating health services research into nursing doctoral programs. *Nurs Outlook*, 50(6): 225–231.

Jones, C. B., Mayer, C., and Mandelkehr, L. K. 2009. Innovations at the intersection of academia and practice: Educating graduate nursing students about quality improvement and patient safety. *Quality Manage Health Care*, 18(3): 158–164.

Knapp, M., and Lowe, J. 2001. Community-based health improvement: Lessons from the Learning for Action Institute, Simmons College. *Quality Manage Health Care*, 9(4): 11–23.

Kurtzman, E. T., and Buerhaus, P. I. 2008. New Medicare payment rules: Danger or opportunity for nursing? *Am J Nurs*, 10(6): 30–35.

Ladden, M. D., Bednash, G., Stevens, D. P., et al. 2006. Educating interprofessional learners for quality, safety and systems improvement. *J Interprofessional Care,* 20: 497–505.

Lavizzo-Mourey, R., and Berwick, D. M. 2009. Nurses transforming care. *Am J Nurs,* 109(11): 3.

Leape, L. L., and Berwick, D. M. 2005. Five years after *To Err Is Human*: What have we learned? *JAMA,* 293: 2384–2390.

Leveck, M. L., and Jones, C. B. 1996. The nursing practice environment, staff retention, and quality of care. *Res Nurs Health,* 19(3): 331–343.

Light, J. 2010. Performance reviews by the numbers. *Wall Street J,* June 29, 2010, D4.

Lindberg, L., and Kimberlain, J. 2008. Quality update. Engage employees to improve staff and patient satisfaction. *Hosp Health Networks,* 82(1): 28–29.

Lundmark, V. 2008. Magnet environments for professional nursing practice. In Hughes, R. G. (Ed.), *Patient Safety and Quality: An Evidence-Based Handbook for Nurses* (Vol. 3). Rockville, MD: Agency for Healthcare Research and Quality.

Lynn, J., Baily, M. A., Bottrell, M., et al. 2007. The ethics of using quality improvement methods in health care. *Ann Intern Med,* 146(9): 666–673.

McClure, M., and Hinshaw, A. S. (Eds). 2002. *Magnet Hospitals Revisited: Attraction and Retention of Professional Nurses.* Washington, DC: American Nurses Publishing.

McClure, M., Poulin, M., and Sovie, M. D. 1983. *Magnet Hospitals: Attraction and Retention of Professional Nurses.* Kansas City, MO: American Academy of Nurses.

McLaughlin, C. P., Johnson, J. K., and Sollecito, W. A. (Eds.). 2012. *Implementing Continuous Quality Improvement in Health Care: A Global Casebook.* Sudbury, MA: Jones & Bartlett Learning.

Montalvo, I., and Dunton, N. 2007. *Transforming Nursing Data into Quality Care: Profiles of Quality Improvement in U.S. Healthcare Facilities.* Silver Spring, MD: American Nurses Association.

National League for Nursing. 2010. Master's education in nursing. Retrieved July 14, 2010, from http://www.nln.org/aboutnln/reflection_dialogue/refl_dial_6.htm

Page, A. 2004. *Keeping Patients Safe: Transforming the Work Environment of Nurses.* Committee on the Work Environment for Nurses and

Patient Safety, Board on Health Care Services. Washington, DC: National Academies Press.

Palmer, M. 2008. Urinary incontinence quality improvement in nursing homes: Where have we been? Where are we going? *Urolog Nurs Off J Am Urolog Assoc Allied*, 28(6): 439–444.

Rantz, M. J. 1995. Quality measurement in nursing: Where are we now? *J Nurs Care Quality*, 9(2): 107.

Robert Wood Johnson Foundation. 2008. The Transforming Care at the Bedside (TCAB) Toolkit. Retrieved June 30, 2010, from http://www.rwjf.org/pr/product.jsp?id=30051

Salmon, M. 2007. Care quality and safety: Same old? [Guest editorial]. *Nurs Outlook*, 55(3): 117–119.

Sammer, C. E., Lykens, K., Singh, K. P., et al. 2010. What is patient safety culture? A review of the literature. *J Nurs Scholarship*, 42(2): 156–165.

Sherwood, G., and Drenkard, K. 2007. Quality and safety curricula in nursing education: Matching practice realities. *Nurs Outlook*, 55(3): 151–155.

Smith, E., Cronenwett, L., and Sherwood, G. 2007. Quality and safety education: Prelicensure nursing educator views. *Nurs Outlook*, 55(3): 132–137.

Teeley, K. H., Lowe, J. M., Beal, J., et al. 2006. Incorporating quality improvement concepts and practice into a community health nursing course. *J Nurs Educ*, 45(2): 86–90.

Truffer, C. J., Keehan, S., Smith, S., et al. 2010. Health spending projections through 2019: The recession's impact continues. *Health Aff*, 29(3): 522–529.

Varkey, P., Reller, M. K., Smith, A., et al. 2006. An experiential interdisciplinary quality improvement education initiative. *Am J Med Q*, 21(5): 317–322.

Wachter, R. M. 2004. The end of the beginning: Patient safety five years after *To Err Is Human*. *Health Aff*, W4: 534–545.

Wachter, R. M. 2010. Patient safety at ten: Unmistakable progress, troubling gaps. *Health Aff*, 29(1): 165–73.

Williams, H. F., and Fallone, S. 2008. CQI in the acute care setting: An opportunity to influence acute care practice. *Nephrol Nurs J*, 35(5): 515–522.

CHAPTER 18

Accreditation: A Global Regulatory Mechanism to Promote Quality and Safety

David Greenfield, Marjorie Pawsey, and Jeffrey Braithwaite

"What has eluded us thus far, however, is maintaining consistently high levels of safety and quality over time and across all health care services and settings."

—Chassin and Loeb (2011, p. 562)

The accreditation of health care organizations is a regulatory mechanism used in many countries around the world. Accreditation is an important strategy by which improvements in quality and safety have been advocated and institutionalized. The purpose of this chapter is to provide an overview of accreditation of health organizations. The chapter has five sections. The first section considers the purpose of accreditation, noting that it has become a global phenomenon found in many industries and sectors of health care. The second section discusses the extent of the accreditation of health organizations, the maturing of accreditation program philosophy from quality assurance to quality improvement, and the self-governing system that has been developed. The third section explores the commonalities and differences in accreditation programs, where increasingly a common model of accreditation is enacted but with variation in standards. The evidence base for accreditation is examined in the fourth section. Finally, the fifth section considers the issues and challenges for accreditation stakeholders.

AN OVERVIEW OF ACCREDITATION

What Is Accreditation?

Accreditation is the formal declaration by a designated authority that an organization, service, or individual has demonstrated competency, authority, or credibility to meet a predetermined set of standards. Accreditation is a mechanism that seeks to reassure external stakeholders that quality and safety standards are demonstrated. A secondary and more recent goal in some applications, notably health care, is to provide a basis for quality improvement initiatives (Davis et al., 2009; Gibberd et al., 2004; Williams et al., 2005). The shift to accreditation, notably from the 1970s onward, is representative of a shift in philosophy by governments whereby they have sought to provide a framework for the governance of services rather than to provide those services themselves. Through accreditation and other regulation strategies, governments have sought abatement or control of risks to society by indirect means (Sparrow, 2000).

Accreditation has become a ubiquitous part of our modern world. For example, it can apply to any of the following:

- Industries, including organic food (Gabriel, 2007), tourism (Australian Government, 2010), and telecommunications services (Association of TeleServices International, 2010)
- Institutions, including education (Stimson, 2003) and health (Australian Council on Healthcare Standards [ACHS], 2007a) organizations
- Products, including automobiles (Casper and Hancke, 1999) and software (Jones and Price, 2002)

- Systems, including management systems (Casile and Davis-Blake, 2002) and laboratory processes (Gough and Reynolds, 2000)
- Individuals, including health professionals (Australia's Health Workforce Online, 2008), statisticians (Statistical Society of Australia, 2009), and builders (Green Building Certificate Institute, 2010)

ACCREDITATION IN THE HEALTH CARE INDUSTRY

Accreditation is found extensively in health care industries around the world. Accreditation is an element in a network of activities that seeks to regulate conduct in the health sector. Health organizations, and individual professionals, are networked together, and their behavior is assessed by independent bodies through accreditation programs, standards, and quality indicators. Regulation via this network has been called "nodal governance" (Shearing and Wood, 2003); that is, organizations, services, and professional behavior in health care are shaped by an increasing variety of government and nongovernment bodies related to but independent of each other.

Health care organizations are accredited for the management and provision of their services, including hospitals, general practices, geriatric care facilities, and public health (ACHS, 2007a; The Joint Commission [TJC], 2010; Simone and Epstein, 2009). Within health organizations, specialized health services can be accredited, such as tissue banks (American Association of Tissue Banks, 2009), pharmacies (American College of Health-System Pharmacists, 2006), and aeromedical transportation services (Association of Air Medical Services, 2010). Additionally, individual professionals from medical (American Academy of Neurology, 2010), nursing (American Academy of Nurse Practitioners, 2010), and allied health (American Physical Therapy Association, 2009; Council on Podiatric Medical Education, 2010) fields, and administrators, including medical administrators (American Academy of Medical Administrators, 2010), are increasingly required to be certified. Given the breadth and complexity of the accreditation measures in the health care industry, this chapter takes as its focus the accreditation of health organizations.

The Self-Governing System of Accreditation of Health Organizations

Accreditation in health was first initiated in the United States through the work of the American College of Surgeons, which in 1917 developed the "Minimum Standards for Hospitals." This organization subsequently collaborated with colleges and associations from the United States and Canada to create, in 1951, the Joint Commission on Accreditation of Hospitals (Viswanathan and Salmon, 2000), which is now referred to as The Joint Commission (TJC). From this beginning, accreditation has spread to be practiced across the world. A few figures highlight the global extent and reach of accreditation. Accreditation is now practiced in more than 70 countries. There are 22 national bodies and an international agency, the International Society for Quality in Health Care (ISQua), that are focused on the issue (Greenfield and Braithwaite, 2008). In the United States, TJC accredits more than 4,000 organizations, or 82% of the hospitals in the country (2010). The Haute Autorité de Santé (HAS) accredits all acute health care organizations in France, which total more than 700 hospitals (Touati and Pomey, 2009). Accreditation Canada (2008) and the ACHS (2007a) each accredit more than 1,000 organizations in their respective countries. These, and many other major international health care accreditation agencies, are independent, not-for-profit, nongovernment agencies.

Accreditation agencies assess organizations and services against standards, and develop and supervise peer reviewers to maintain a surveyor workforce. Additionally, some accreditation agencies set and revise their own standards. Accreditation involves assessment against minimum standards and more recently has evolved, as a result of higher quality and safety expectations, to be a developmental process promoting continuous quality improvement (Cudney and Reinbold, 2002; Parsons and Riley, 2009). This current trend is especially notable in public health in the United States (Parsons and Riley, 2009). This model of accreditation is reflective of practice in many countries, including, for example, in the United States (Viswanathan and Salmon, 2000), Australia (Greenfield, Braithwaite, et al., 2008), Canada (Touati and Pomey, 2009), France (Pomey et al., 2004), and Lebanon (El-Jardali et al., 2008).

Accreditation programs in their initial phase typically focused on standards aimed at the structures and processes of organizations. As programs have matured, and new ones have emerged, attention has shifted so that organizations have been increasingly required to demonstrate that in addition to having structures and processes in place they are functioning effectively. That is, there has been a philosophical shift from *quality assurance* to *quality improvement*. The former is regarded as a program that strives to improve quality through defining and measuring it (Silimperi et al., 2002). The latter incorporates both retrospective and prospective assessments and is aimed at developing strategies to make things better and to create systems to prevent errors (McLaughlin and Kaluzny, 2006; Parsons and Riley, 2009). In simple terms, quality improvement involves health professionals constantly asking themselves "Despite having the 'right' things in place to do the 'right' things, what are we doing now that we can do better?" Furthermore, accreditation is about answering the question posed by external assessors: "What systems have you implemented, how do they work, and can you show me how you are planning to do things better?"

The shift can be illustrated by an example concerning patient satisfaction surveys. An accreditation program promoting a quality assurance approach would focus on a patient satisfaction survey and how it is developed and administered. In contrast, an accreditation program with a quality improvement philosophy would focus on the response rate of the surveys, the issues identified by the patients, the organization's actions, and confirmation of improvement in subsequent surveys.

While the continuous quality improvement model is the dominant accreditation model for health care organizations, there is an alternative, more generic model that can be described as an "audit model." In this model, an external reviewer, with or without health care experience, uses a generic set of quality standards to assess the presence or absence of organizational quality activities. This model is endorsed by the International Organization for Standardization, which accredits organizations in many diverse industries, including health (see http://www.iso.org).

There are external and internal motivations that drive health care organizations to seek accreditation (Greenfield and Braithwaite, 2007). External motivation comes from governments, insurers, and consumers requiring that organizations undertake efforts that demonstrate outcomes that advance high-quality and safer health care (Accreditation Canada, 2009; ACHS, 2007b; El-Jardali et al., 2008; HAS, 2008b; TJC, 2010).

The internal impetus comes from staff who make up the health organizations. They report a desire to improve their services and the care they provide (Greenfield and Braithwaite, 2007). Together these two motivations, which are mutually reinforcing, have combined to draw many health care organizations under the umbrella of accreditation.

Accreditation agencies, involving many of their stakeholders, have constructed a self-governing system (Greenfield, Pawsey, Naylor, et al., 2009a). It is a system responsive to the conduct and culture of those being regulated; this approach has been labeled "responsive regulation" (Braithwaite et al., 2005). The system seeks to influence the attitudes and practices of those involved, whether they are in the role of accreditation agency personnel, surveyors, or health staff, in an organization being accredited. Through participation in the development of accreditation programs or the accrediting of health care organizations, a common understanding of standards and shared expectations is constructed. Additionally, participants regulate their own and other colleagues' behaviors to comply with the standards and expectations. The system combines internal assessment, or self-regulation, with self-directed improvement strategies overseen by external peer review. It is a cultural control strategy whose influence is significant on those directly involved (Greenfield, Pawsey, Naylor, et al., 2009a). Those health professionals who participate in their organization's accreditation activities generally report improvements to quality and safety. However, as recent research has shown, the influence of accreditation can wane as participation in the program declines (Paccioni et al., 2008). Health professionals not directly involved in their organization's accreditation activities are known to remain skeptical about the purpose, value, and benefits of the program. They question the bureaucratic and time-consuming activities associated with an accreditation program.

ISQua promotes self-governance through their accrediting of accreditation agencies. That is, ISQua provides guidelines, support, and assessment of accreditation and surveyor training programs (see http://www .isqua.org). Furthermore, the self-governance modality is reinforced through ISQua's encouragement of participation in its organization and the international health quality and safety conferences it convenes. Consequently, the work of ISQua has evoked an international convergence of understanding about, and similarity in the enactment of, health accreditation programs.

COMMONALITIES AND DIFFERENCES IN THE ACCREDITATION MODEL

The Accreditation Model

A common model of accreditation is enacted by many health accreditation agencies (Accreditation Canada, 2009; ACHS, 2007b; TJC, 2010). A breakdown of the process typically involved in this model is as follows. An organization seeking to be accredited develops, implements, and continuously reviews its quality improvement plan and self-assesses progress against the standards of the accreditation program. It concludes this task by providing a written self-assessment report to the accrediting agency. The accrediting agency assesses the organization's report and dispatches an accreditation survey team, comprised of peer reviewers, to visit and assess the organization on site. The visit comprises observations of facilities, interviews with staff, and a review of documentation. The survey team during and at the conclusion of the survey provides verbal feedback to the organization. The accrediting agency receives a written report from the survey team a short time after the visit. The report summarizes the survey team's assessment of the organization's progress in achieving the standards and makes recommendations or commendations as appropriate. Following the correction of any errors of fact by the organization, the report is then considered by the accrediting agency. The agency assesses the report and decides whether to award accreditation status or not. Accreditation is for a defined period, depending on the program, and typically for 3 to 5 years. It is common for accrediting agencies to send survey teams to reassess an organization during the accreditation period. The survey team reviews the organization's continual progress against the updated quality plan and accreditation standards. The surveyors provide verbal feedback, and, after endorsement by the accrediting agency, a written report is provided to the organization. The improvement cycle continues, with the organization using the report to initiate further reflection and examination of its structures, processes, and practices to identify and drive areas for ongoing improvement.

Accreditation Standards

Accrediting agencies are responsible for the development and revision of standards. It is common for agencies to develop standards using representatives drawn from the health industry. For example, in the United States (TJC, 2010), Canada (Accreditation Canada, 2009), France (HAS, 2008a), and Australia (ACHS, 2007b), standards are developed through consultation with a wide range of stakeholders, including combinations of health care experts, researchers, representatives from industry groups, consumers, and governmental agencies. The number and status of standards vary from accreditation program to program. For example, the U.S. Public Health Accreditation Board program has 32 standards (Parsons and Riley, 2009). For the accreditation of hospitals, Accreditation Canada uses 30 standards (Accreditation Canada, 2009), and HAS, the French accreditation agency, has only 13 standards, or "priority practices," as they are called (HAS, 2008a). ACHS, from Australia, has 43 standards in its program, of which 19 are mandatory and 24 are nonmandatory (ACHS, 2007b). In the ACHS program, failure to meet the requirements of a mandatory standard will result in an organization not being accredited. However, an organization may be assessed as meeting mandatory standards but not meeting a nonmandatory standard and still be conferred accreditation status.

Accreditation standards cover infrastructure, organizational, service, and continuum of patient care issues (Greenfield and Braithwaite, 2007; HAS, 2008a). Standards are focused on organizational processes and systems and the availability of appropriate resources for the organization to deliver the defined services. Accrediting agencies are increasingly examining strategies to expand standards to incorporate organizational performance and clinical measures (Accreditation Canada, 2009; ACHS, 2007a; HAS, 2008b; TJC, 2009). Accreditation Canada, with the introduction of its new accreditation program "Qmentum," has introduced performance measures "to strengthen the rigor and objectivity of the accreditation process" (Accreditation Canada, 2009). The measures are used to direct surveyors to examine particular parts of an organization requiring close assessment.

Alternatively, outcome measures are being reported upon separately to accreditation surveys. Accreditation agencies are producing reports of organizational and clinical compliance with expected guidelines to raise awareness across the industry. For example, in the United States, since 2006, the TJC has tracked and reported upon quality of care measures (TJC, 2009). These items are evidence-based, standardized, national measures that allow comparisons across organizations. Currently, TJC is reporting on 31 measures, with data drawn from more than 3,000 accredited hospitals. In particular, the report documents, over the last 7 years, increased quality performance results for heart attack, heart failure, and pneumonia care. Over shorter time periods, there have been improvements on individual surgical care performance measures (last 2 years), individual heart attack (last 3 years), and pneumonia care (last 4 years) measures. Similarly, 1 year of measurement shows very high compliance, more than 99%, on two individual measures of quality relating to inpatient care for childhood asthma. Two measures were identified as problematic for many organizations: Providing fibrinolytic therapy to heart attack patients within 30 minutes of arrival was achieved by just over 50% of hospitals, and only 60% provided antibiotics to intensive care unit pneumonia patients within 24 hours of arrival. Consequently, the report notes that improvement is still needed, and there remains unacceptable variation between organizations.

As these examples demonstrate, the use of quality of care measures in accreditation surveys and the publication of compliance reports are strategies by which accreditation agencies are working with health organizations to assess, measure, and improve their care. Their use forms part of the system of self-governance within and across health organizations.

THE EVIDENCE BASE FOR THE ACCREDITATION OF HEALTH ORGANIZATIONS

While the accreditation of health services has expanded across the world, to the extent that it is now undertaken in more countries and covers more health settings than ever before, the evidence base remains underdeveloped. There is a pressing need for increased research, transparency, and innovation into accreditation (Greenfield and Braithwaite, 2009). This is not a new development, with calls having been made over a number of years for increased research into accreditation (Fernandopulle et al., 2003; Øvretveit and Gustafson, 2003; Shaw, 2001). What is new is that accreditation agencies are reportedly undertaking research studies and programs. For example, in the last few years, substantial research efforts have been commenced by the HAS, TJC, Accreditation Canada, the ACHS, the Italian Society for Quality of Health Care, the Irish

Health Services Accreditation Board, and the Spanish accrediting agency Fundación Avedis Donabedian. What remains unclear is how transparent the accreditation agencies will be with their results (Greenfield and Braithwaite, 2009).

Systematic Review of the Accreditation Research Literature

A systematic review of the accreditation research literature was published in 2008 (Greenfield and Braithwaite, 2008). The review initially identified nearly 34,000 items of literature associated with accreditation and accrediting agencies. By focusing on substantive work, the sample was reduced to just over 3,000, less than 11% of the original search. Subsequent analysis of the abstracts identified that the vast majority were discussion or commentary papers. There were 66 empirical research articles identified for the review. The studies were analyzed and grouped under 10 headings. The assessment of the accumulative findings for each category is presented in **Table 18–1**.

There was an inadequate number of studies to draw conclusions about three issues: consumer views or patient satisfaction, public disclosure, and surveyor issues. There were consistent findings for two items only. Studies showed that accreditation programs promoted change and professional development. Accreditation programs were noted to have improved the organization of facilities, policies and guidelines, decision making, and safety.

TABLE 18–1 Classification and Assessment of Accreditation Research Literature

Literature Category	Assessment of the Cumulative Findings
Consumer views or patient satisfaction	Inadequate studies to assess
Public disclosure	Inadequate studies to assess
Surveyor issues	Inadequate studies to assess
Promotion of change	Consistent
Professional development	Consistent
Professions' attitudes to accreditation	Inconsistent
Organizational impact	Inconsistent
Financial impact	Inconsistent
Quality measures	Inconsistent
Program assessment	Inconsistent

A link between professional development and accreditation was also identified. Accreditation programs were observed to encourage and support professional development, although the effect was considered to be small.

In the remaining five categories, there were inconsistent research findings. Professionals expressed criticism and support for accreditation programs. Concerns related to issues of cost, compliance, standards, surveyor consistency, and what the program was perceived to add to patient care. Conversely, professionals perceived accreditation programs as a strategy for promoting and making transparent quality and collegial decision making; the programs resulted in improved organizational performance. Many health professionals, whether they participate in accreditation activities directly, indirectly, or not at all, seem to hold strong opinions about the value and benefits, or lack thereof. It is an issue that seems to generate polarized views. The organizational impact of accreditation programs was unclear. Accredited and nonaccredited organizations could not be distinguished in one study, but organizational improvements were noted in other research. The financial impact for accreditation was reported as proportionally greater for smaller organizations and considered by some to be high overall. However, the argument has been made that the costs incurred are not additional but part of an organization's required investment in quality.

At present, the relationship between accreditation and quality measures—clinical indicators, quality indicators, or clinical performance measures—is opaque. Accreditation has been shown to generate improvement in some cases but not in others. The question has been raised as to whether we should expect to find a link between accreditation and different quality measures, given they are developed and implemented separately and not linked. Overall, the assessment of accreditation programs has provided mixed evidence. In some cases, programs were deemed credible; in others, their value and results were questioned.

Findings from Further Research

Since the preceding review, completed in 2008, further research has been published. Unfortunately, these studies do not clarify the picture significantly. One research investigation has argued that professionals who fail to participate in accreditation efforts continue to perceive the efforts as external bureaucratic reporting mechanisms (Touati and Pomey, 2009). Other work shows that participating in accreditation has cultivated communication and cooperation among individuals and teams, thereby promoting change in an organization (Paccioni et al., 2008). Accredited hospitals formalize, and at times realize, improvements in quality management practices (Braithwaite et al., 2010; El-Jardali et al., 2008; Paccioni et al., 2008; Touati and Pomey, 2009). Another study found a positive effect from accreditation on patient satisfaction (Al Tehewy et al., 2009).

There continues to be considerable discussion among stakeholders about the relationship between accreditation and quality measures. Concern has been expressed about the lack of a relationship between the two, and the argument persists that this issue needs further investigation (Braithwaite et al., 2010; Chuang and Inder, 2009). One large-scale randomized study that examined accreditation as a predictor of health care performance has been conducted (Braithwaite et al., 2010). The study investigated relationships between accreditation performance and clinical performance, organizational culture, organizational climate, consumer involvement, and leadership. Positive correlations were found between accreditation performance and organizational culture and leadership. A positive trend was noted with clinical performance. Accreditation was unrelated to organizational climate and consumer involvement.

In the period since the 2008 systematic review, there have been a number of studies examining surveyor issues. Reliability in surveying has been investigated. Reliability is noted as being a critical issue in accreditation, and in health care more broadly. Being able to conduct consistent assessments, interpretations, and judgments, individually and collectively, is a challenge for professionals working in many areas of health care (Greenfield, Pawsey, Naylor, et al., 2009a). As such, the challenges of consistency faced by accreditation surveyors are not unique, and surveyors will have encountered them in their normal professional activities. Recent research has highlighted that because accreditation surveying is an activity based on document analysis, observations, and interviews, survey findings need to be credible and verifiable (Greenfield, Braithwaite, et al., 2008; Greenfield, Pawsey, Naylor, et al., 2009a). Survey teams use these three qualitative data collection methods (document analysis, observations, and interviews) to triangulate their assessments (Denzin, 1989; Ely et al., 1991). The results produced through this complex process are not precisely replicable, as human judgments are central to the data collection and analysis process. Nevertheless, striving for rigor in application of standards, individual and team conduct, and transparency in interpretation and decision making is essential. Hence the finding that "Where surveyors and survey teams achieve process consistency and program interpretation from survey to survey, their findings can then be said to be reliable" (Greenfield, Pawsey, Naylor, et al., 2009a). In other words, accreditation agencies, rather than focusing on reliability of outcome, which is by definition unachievable, need to be encouraged to implement strategies to promote and ensure reliability of process and consistent application of standards. This recommendation is supported by the findings of an empirical study examining two survey teams in situ (Greenfield, Pawsey, Naylor, et al., 2009b). While the study did not unfold as planned—the problems encountered highlighted the difficulties of conducting in situ research into organizations—the study confirmed the need for survey teams to ensure reliability of process and consistent application of standards.

Reliability in surveying has been shown to be promoted or undermined by six factors (Greenfield, Pawsey, Naylor, et al., 2009a):

1. The accreditation program, including documentation requirements for organizations and survey teams

2. Member relationship with the accrediting agency and survey team

3. Accreditation agency personnel

4. Surveyor workforce renewal

5. Management of the surveyor workforce

6. Survey dynamics' effect on the reliability of surveys directly and indirectly

It is argued that reliability in the accreditation process is constructed through the interplay of these factors. They construct shared expectations and conduct among stakeholders; together they promote standardized beliefs and action that become accreditation cultural norms (Greenfield, Pawsey, Naylor, et al., 2009a).

It is important to distinguish between intra- and inter-rater reliability. Intra-rater reliability is high when the assessments made by an individual surveyor or survey team are consistent from case to case. Inter-rater reliability is high when assessments made by different surveyors or survey teams are consistent with one another. Reliability in accreditation is a concern for accreditation agencies and organizations that have been or are considering going through the accreditation process. Two studies developed scenario exercises, using real data, for individual surveyors and survey teams to examine the respective issues. Individual surveyors assessed, at two points in time, scenarios of individual standards relating to a large hospital, and their results were compared. The findings revealed that intra-rater reliability is problematic; that is, individuals struggle to consistently make consistent assessments. A 20% variation in surveyors' individual assessments that potentially could have affected accreditation outcomes was noted (Greenfield, Pawsey, Braithwaite, et al., 2009). Similarly, scenarios based on real data and comprising written information and a role-play were developed and presented to survey teams. In contrast to the intra-rater findings, the results showed that the examination of the inter-rater reliability of survey teams demonstrated more consistent agreement (Greenfield, Pawsey, et al., 2008), thus highlighting the mediating effect of teams on individuals.

A unique typology based on surveyor styles has been developed from the empirical research into reliability (Greenfield, Braithwaite, et al., 2008). The typology, using the dimensions of recording (explicit/implicit) and questioning (opportunistic/structured), classifies four accreditation surveyor styles: the discusser, the explorer, the interrogator, and the questioner. The typology is suggested for use by accreditation agencies in their surveyor training programs and offers the opportunity to match teams of surveyors with a blend of approaches.

Research has been conducted to understand the value of surveying to volunteer surveyors and to the institutions in which they are regularly employed (Lancaster et al., 2010). Health professionals who act as volunteer surveyors derive four benefits from the activity: exposure to new methods and innovations in health organizations, opportunity to engage in a unique form of professional development, opportunity to acquire expertise to enhance quality within the institutions in which they are regularly employed, and opportunity to contribute to the process of quality improvement and enhance public health in organizations beyond their regular employment.

ISSUES AND CHALLENGES FOR ACCREDITATION PROGRAMS

Accreditation stakeholders have a number of significant interrelated challenges to address. A list of these issues is presented in **Table 18–2**.

TABLE 18–2 Challenges Facing Accreditation Stakeholders

Voluntary or mandated accreditation programs
Rigidity or flexibility of accreditation programs
Financial costs to address quality and safety issues
Standards: the role of process and quality indicators to foster improvement
Surveyor workforce: sustainability, role, and reliability
Expanding the evidence base for accreditation

Voluntary or Mandated Accreditation Programs

A majority of accreditation programs, with a few notable exceptions such as the French and Italian accreditation agencies, are *voluntary* programs. However, this term is a misleading one. In many cases, health care organizations are required by external stakeholders to demonstrate efforts at improving quality and safety, including through participation in an accreditation program. Governments, insurers, and consumers, via industry groups and voicing community expectations more generally, seek to be reassured that organizations are making efforts to achieve published standards or address quality and safety. The "choice" many organizations have is not whether to participate but with which accrediting agency and program they will be associated. In effect, accreditation, in many countries, has become a requirement in practice but not in name. If accreditation were made mandatory, what impact would this have on accrediting agencies, health organizations, and surveyors? Would this change the practice of accreditation? Would accreditation agencies and health organizations be under more pressure to achieve a favorable accreditation result?

Chapter 16 presents a discussion of voluntary and mandated public health accreditation initiatives in the United States. One example of successful mandated accreditation is found in North Carolina, where a local health department accreditation program has been in place since 2005, with more than 50 of the state's 85 health departments accredited through 2009. A second round of accreditation is under way, after a brief delay caused by state funding shortages. A full evaluation of this program may yield some answers to these questions. See Case 15 in the companion casebook (McLaughlin et al., 2012) for further details.

Rigidity or Flexibility of Accreditation Programs

An issue that is confused with the question of voluntary or mandated programs is the rigidity and flexibility *within* a program. Some accreditation programs have been shown to be rigid and flexible at the same time. Research contrasting two programs, one mandated and the other voluntary, found that both programs incorporated compulsory and flexible elements. There were positive impacts from both the mandated and voluntary programs, and it was noted that there was a convergence of the two approaches (Touati and Pomey, 2009). The program conducted by the ACHS in Australia has firm and flexible aspects to it. As noted, there are standards that are classified as mandatory or nonmandatory (ACHS, 2007b). The rigidity and flexibility of accreditation programs remain largely an unexamined issue. What is an appropriate degree of rigidity and flexibility within an accreditation program? What are the effects of specified levels of rigidity and flexibility in an accreditation program?

Financial Costs to Address Quality and Safety Issues

Addressing quality and safety issues incurs costs, through consuming organizational resources and requiring health professionals' time. Where accreditation is not considered part of an organization's ongoing or routine activities, the challenge is determining the costs vs. benefits. Separating the costs and benefits associated with accreditation and those incurred independently as part of an organization's ongoing quality and safety efforts is a complicated task, and no one has yet constructed a convincing study. This issue is a significant challenge for accreditation stakeholders. Are the costs incurred by participation in an accreditation program to be considered part of the ongoing organizational costs to address quality and safety issues? If not, what is the cost vs. benefit analysis associated with participation in an accreditation program?

Standards: The Role of Process vs. Outcome and Quality Indicators

Accreditation programs are currently focused on assessing the organizing and delivery of care. The standards have been termed "process indicators," as they focus on how care is delivered rather than the outcomes of the activity. Opponents of programs have argued that because they do not reflect the outcomes of care, they are limited in what they can contribute to our understanding of quality and safety. Quality indicators are advocated as being more effective measures. However, the use of such indicators within an accreditation program is an issue that raises continuing debate (Braithwaite et al., 2010; Chuang and Inder, 2009; Øvretveit, 2005; Touati and Pomey, 2009). Concern is voiced that the use of quality indicators is problematic until the relationship between accreditation and quality indicators is clarified (Braithwaite et al., 2010). The issue remains unresolved as to whether they examine similar or different aspects of health care performance and quality.

This issue is an important one with which to come to terms. How do organizations use the results from process and quality indicators and accreditation programs? Are they to be used independently or together? How do we resolve the differences in their findings? A closely related issue is whether accreditation programs foster quality improvement, and if so, how? (See Case 15 in the companion casebook [McLaughlin et al., 2012], which addresses this issue relative to local public health department accreditation in North Carolina.) With each revision of standards, do we keep raising the bar to stimulate efforts to improve, or will this strategy promote adverse behaviors? Knowing how best to stimulate improvements in quality and safety in health systems facing significant cost pressures and increasing demands is a challenge for accreditation agencies.

Surveyor Workforce: Sustainability, Role, and Reliability Issues

Surveyors are an important element of accreditation programs. Accrediting agencies can have surveyor workforces comprised of full-time or part-time (usually volunteer) surveyors. The ongoing support and development of this workforce requires careful management. Surveyor workforce sustainability and the reliability of their surveys are ongoing challenges for accreditation agencies. Accrediting agencies face difficulties in being able to continually recruit appropriately experienced health professionals as surveyors. The demands of their regular employment can be incompatible with the time required to participate as a surveyor. The surveyor role is a demanding one. It can include educator, judge, evaluator, regulator, or a combination of these functions (Greenfield, Braithwaite, et al., 2008; Plebani, 2001). The status of the accreditation program, whether mandatory or voluntary, will shape the focus of the role and how it is perceived by others. A health professional taking on the surveyor role may be comfortable with some part but not others, or with combining the roles. Additionally, potential or perceived conflict of interest issues have been raised when health professionals are surveying colleagues and organizations with which they have ties or with which they may seek to work in the future (Bohigas et al., 1998; Plebani, 2001). Furthermore, when enacting the surveyor role, intra- and inter-rater reliability are issues of note (Greenfield, Pawsey, Braithwaite, et al., 2009; Greenfield, Pawsey, Naylor, et al., 2009a).

Accreditation agencies that use full-time surveyors see this as a strategy that can work toward increasing the mastery of survey techniques and more consistent interpretation of standards. Conversely, part-time surveyors have current knowledge of the health system, management practices, and clinical expectations, but may not be as consistent in surveying as their full-time colleagues. How then is it possible to sustain, develop, and manage a surveyor workforce to increase the reliability of assessment?

Expanding the Evidence Base for Accreditation

The necessity to expand the evidence base for accreditation is noted in the literature (Greenfield and Braithwaite, 2008; Greenfield and Braithwaite, 2009). Securing more empirically derived findings is necessary to provide a firmer foundation for accreditation programs. It is hoped that studies in progress will be published in the peer-reviewed literature. Doing so will work toward resolving inconsistencies and gaps in understanding. Transparency of findings is important for individual program credibility and contributes to the broader knowledge base (Greenfield and Braithwaite, 2009). In particular, it is worth noting the positive contribution made by ISQua in encouraging and assisting the spread of knowledge between practitioners and accreditation agencies in different countries. Consolidating and expanding the evidence base for accreditation is important to secure its ongoing utility and effectiveness. How can the credibility of accreditation be strengthened? What actions can be taken to expand the evidence base and the publication of results?

CONCLUSIONS

Accreditation has been instituted, and has become institutionalized, in health care sectors and jurisdictions around the world. It is a governance strategy that enables health organizations individually and collectively to self-govern their efforts at improving quality and safety. Empirical studies as to the value and contribution of accreditation present an incomplete and somewhat mixed picture for stakeholders. The research evidence demonstrates that accreditation has resulted in improvements and benefits in some areas and is uncertain in other respects. The challenges facing accreditation stakeholders are significant and include the following:

- Deciding whether programs should be voluntary or mandated
- Achieving a balance between flexibility and rigidity within a program
- Managing the financial costs associated with accreditation
- Understanding the role of process and quality indicators within an accreditation program or their relationship to accreditation results
- Creating a reliable and sustainable surveyor workforce
- Expanding the evidence base for accreditation programs

Accreditation agencies and their partners are actively taking steps to better understand the organizational and clinical impacts of accreditation programs. Further work is necessary, as is the sharing of the knowledge generated, to build upon and continue the improvements made. How the challenges are addressed will shape the regulation of health care and, ultimately, the quality and safety of care provided to consumers.

Cross-References to the Companion Casebook

(McLaughlin, C. P., Johnson, J. K., and Sollecito, W. A. [Eds.]. 2012. *Implementing Continuous Quality Improvement in Health Care: A Global Casebook*. Sudbury, MA: Jones & Bartlett Learning.)

Case Study Number	Case Study Title	Case Study Authors
12	Quality in Pediatric Subspecialty Care	William A. Sollecito, Peter A. Margolis, Paul V. Miles, Robert Perelman, and Richard B. Colletti
15	North Carolina Local Health Departments Accreditation Program	David Stone and Mary V. Davis

REFERENCES

Accreditation Canada. 2008. *Annual Report 2008*. Ottawa, Ontario: Author.
Accreditation Canada. 2009. *2009 Canadian Health Accreditation Report: A Focus on Patient Safety*. Ottawa, Ontario: Author.

Al Tehewy, M., Salem, B., Habil, I., et al. 2009. Evaluation of accreditation program in non-governmental organizations' health units in Egypt: Short-term outcomes. *Int J Quality Health Care*, 21: 183–189.

American Academy of Medical Administrators. 2010. AMAA credentials. Retrieved January 22, 2010, from http://www.aameda.org/ProfAdvancement/professionaladv.html

American Academy of Neurology. 2010. Become an AAN member. Retrieved January 22, 2010, from http://www.aan.com/go/membership/join

American Academy of Nurse Practitioners. 2010. Why AANPCP certification? Retrieved April 1, 2011, from http://www.aanpcertification.org/ptistore/control/index

American Association of Tissue Banks. 2009. Accreditation. Retrieved June 27, 2011, from http://www.aatb.org/Accreditation

American College of Health-System Pharmacists. 2006. ASHP regulations on accreditation of pharmacy residencies. Bethesda, MD: Author.

American Physical Therapy Association. 2009. American board of physical therapy specialties. Retrieved June 27, 2011, from http://www.capteonline.org/WhatWeDo/

Association of TeleServices International. 2010. Industry accreditation/certification/standards committee. Retrieved April 1, 2011, from http://www.atsi.org/atsi/Industry_AccreditationCertificationStandards.asp?SnID=2

Australian Council on Healthcare Standards (ACHS). 2007a. *Annual Report 2007–2008*. Sydney: Author.

Australian Council on Healthcare Standards (ACHS). 2007b. *National Report on Health Services Accreditation Performance 2003–2006*. Sydney: Author.

Australian Government, Department of Resources, Energy and Tourism. 2010. Quality tourism: Quality systems. Retrieved June 27, 2011, from http://www.ret.gov.au/tourism/policy/national_tourism_accreditation_framework/Pages/NationalTourismAccreditationFramework.aspx

Australia's Health Workforce Online. 2008. National registration and accreditation scheme. Retrieved September 3, 2010, from http://www.nhwt.gov.au/natreg.asp

Bohigas, L., Brooks, T., Donahue, T., et al. 1998. A comparative analysis of surveyors from six hospital accreditation programmes and a consideration of the related management issues. *Int J Quality Health Care*, 10(1): 7–13.

Braithwaite, J., Greenfield, D., Westbrook, J., et al. 2010. Health service accreditation as a predictor of clinical and organizational performance: A blinded, random, stratified study. *Int J Quality Health Care*, 19: 14–21.

Braithwaite, J., Healy, J., and Dwan, K. 2005. The governance of health and safety and quality. Canberra, Australia: Commonwealth of Australia.

Casile, M., and Davis-Blake, A. 2002. When accreditation standards change: Factors affecting differential responsiveness of public and private organizations. *Acad Manage J,* 45(1): 180–195.

Casper, S., and Hancke, B. 1999. Global quality norms within national production regimes: ISO 9000 standards in French and German car industries. *Organ Studies*, 20(6): 961–986.

Chassin, M., and Loeb, J. 2011. The ongoing quality improvement journey: Next stop, high reliability. *Health Aff,* 30(4): 559–568.

Chuang, S., and Inder, K. 2009. An effectiveness analysis of healthcare systems using a systems theoretic approach. *BMC Health Serv Res*, 9: 195.

The Commission on Accreditation of Medical Transport Systems. Retrieved June 27, 2011, from http://www.camts.org/component/option,com_frontpage/Itemid,1/

Council on Podiatric Medical Education. 2010. Accreditation: The Council on Podiatric Medical Education. Retrieved January 22, 2010, from http://www.apma.org/Members/Education/CPMEAccreditation.aspx

Cudney, A., and Reinbold, O. 2002. JCAHO: Responding to quality and safety imperatives. *J Healthcare Manage*, 47: 216–219.

Davis, P., Elligers, J., and Solomon, J. 2009. Accreditation as a means for quality improvement. In Bialek, R., Duffy, G., and Moran, J. (Eds.), *The Public Health Quality Improvement Handbook* (pp. 113–125). Milwaukee, WI: ASQ Quality Press.

Denzin, N. 1989. *The Research Act: A Theoretical Introduction to Sociological Methods*. Englewood Cliffs, NJ: Prentice Hall.

El-Jardali, F., Jamal, D., Dimassi, H., et al. 2008. The impact of hospital accreditation on quality of care: Perception of Lebanese nurses. *Int J Quality Health Care*, 20(5): 363–371.

Ely, M., Anzul, M., Friedman, T., et al. 1991. *Doing Qualitative Research: Circles Within Circles.* New York: Falmer.

Fernandopulle, R., Ferris, T., Epstein, A., et al. 2003. A research agenda for bridging the "quality chasm." *Health Aff,* 22(2): 178–190.

Gabriel, S. 2007. Council Regulation EC No 834/2007. *Off J Eur Union,* 1–23.

Gibberd, R., Hancock, S., Howley, P., et al. 2004. Using indicators to quantify the potential to improve the quality of health care. *Int J Quality Health Care,* 16(1): i37–i43.

Gough, L. A., and Reynolds, T. A. 2000. Is clinical pathology accreditation worth it? A survey of CPA-accredited laboratories. *Br J Clin Governance,* 5(4): 195.

Green Building Certificate Institute. 2010. *LEED Green Associate Candidate Handbook.* Washington, DC: Author.

Greenfield, D., and Braithwaite, J. 2007. Researching accreditation. *E-Hospital,* 9(5): 18–19.

Greenfield, D., and Braithwaite, J. 2008. Health sector accreditation research: A systematic review. *Int J Quality Health Care,* 20(3): 172–183.

Greenfield, D., and Braithwaite, J. 2009. Developing the evidence base for accreditation of healthcare organisations: A call for transparency and innovation. *Quality Safety Health Care,* 18: 162–163.

Greenfield, D., Braithwaite, J., and Pawsey, M. 2008. Health care accreditation surveyor styles typology. *Int J Health Care Quality Assurance,* 21(5): 435–443.

Greenfield, D., Pawsey, M., Braithwaite, J., et al. 2009. Intra-rater reliability in accreditation surveys: Is there evidence that the practice exists? The 7th Australian Conference on Safety and Quality in Health Care, Sydney, Australia.

Greenfield, D., Pawsey, M., Naylor, J., et al. 2008. Improving the reliability of an accreditation program: Using research to educate and to align practice. Poster in ISQua 2008, Twenty-fifth International Safety and Quality Conference: Healthcare quality and safety: Meeting the next challenges [International Society for Quality in Health Care], Copenhagen, Denmark.

Greenfield, D., Pawsey, M., Naylor, J., et al. 2009a. Are healthcare accreditation surveys reliable? *Int J Health Care Quality Assurance,* 22(2): 105–116.

Greenfield, D., Pawsey, M. Naylor, J., et al. 2009b. Designing quality into healthcare accreditation surveyor performance: Strategies for professional development. ISQua 2009, Twenty-sixth International Safety and Quality Conference: Designing for Quality [International Society for Quality in Health Care], Dublin, Ireland.

Haute Autorité de Santé. 2008a. *Certification Manual for Healthcare Organisations V2010*. Saint-Denis-La-Plaine Cedex, France: Author.

Haute Autorité de Santé. 2008b. *Haute Autorité de Santé Annual Report 2008*. Saint-Denis-La-Plaine Cedex, France: Author.

The Joint Commission. 2009. *Improving America's Hospitals: The Joint Commission's Annual Report on Quality and Safety 2009*. Oakbrook Terrace, IL: Author.

The Joint Commission. 2010. Facts about hospital accreditation. Retrieved June 27, 2011, from http://www.jointcommission.org/assets/1/18/Hospital_Accreditation_1_31_11.pdf

Jones, L., and Price, A. 2002. Changes in computer science accreditation. *Commun ACM*, 45(8): 99–103.

Lancaster, J., Braithwaite, J., and Greenfield, D. 2010. Benefits of participating in accreditation surveying. *Int J Healthcare Quality Assurance*, 23(2): 141–152.

McLaughlin, C. P., Johnson, J. K., and Sollecito, W. A. (Eds.). 2012. *Implementing Continuous Quality Improvement in Health Care: A Global Casebook*. Sudbury, MA: Jones & Bartlett Learning.

McLaughlin, C. P., and Kaluzny, A. D. 2006. Defining quality improvement. In McLaughlin, C. P., and Kaluzny, A. D. (Eds.), *Quality Improvement in Health Care: Theory and Applications* (pp. 3–40). Sudbury, MA: Jones and Bartlett Publishers.

Øvretveit, J. 2005. *Which Interventions Are Effective for Improving Patient Safety? A Review of Research Evidence*. Stockholm: Karolinska Institute, Medical Management Centre.

Øvretveit, J., and Gustafson, D. 2003. Improving the quality of health care: Using research to inform quality programmes. *BMJ*, 326: 759–761.

Paccioni, A., Sicotte, C., and Champagne, F. 2008. Accreditation: A cultural control strategy. *Int J Health Care Quality Assurance*, 21(2): 146–158.

Parsons, H., and Riley, W. 2009. Public health program design and deployment. In Bialek, R., Duffy, G., and Moran, J. (Eds.), *The Public Health Quality Improvement Handbook* (pp. 53–59). Milwaukee, WI: ASQ Quality Press.

Plebani, M. 2001. Role of inspectors in external review mechanisms: Criteria for selection, training and appraisal. *Clinica Chimica Acta*, 309(2): 147–154.

Pomey, M. P., Contandriopoulos, A. P., Francois, P., et al. 2004. Accreditation: A tool for organizational change in hospitals? *Int J Health Care Quality Assurance*, 17(2–3): 113–124.

Shaw, C. 2001. External assessment of health care. *BMJ*, 322: 851–854.

Shearing, C., and Wood, J. 2003. Nodal governance, democracy, and the new denizens: Challenging the Westphalian ideal. *J Law Soc*, 30: 400–419.

Silimperi, D., Miller Franco, L., Veldhuyzen van Zanten, T., et al. 2002. A framework for institutionalizing quality assurance. *Int J Quality Health Care*, 14(suppl 1): 67–73.

Simone, A., and Epstein, P. 2009. Leading and lagging indicators of public health and public health assessment and accreditation. In Bialek, R., Duffy, G., and Moran, J. (Eds.), *The Public Health Quality Improvement Handbook* (pp. 83–90). Milwaukee, WI: ASQ Quality Press.

Sparrow, M. 2000. *The Regulatory Craft Controlling Risks, Solving Problems, and Managing Compliance*. Washington, DC: Brookings Institution Press.

Statistical Society of Australia. 2009. *Statistics: A Job for Professionals*. Canberra, Australia: Author.

Stimson, W. 2003. Better public schools with ISO 9000:2000. *Quality Progress*, 36(9): 38–45.

Touati, N., and Pomey, M. P. 2009. Accreditation at a crossroads: Are we on the right track? *Health Policy*, 90: 156–165.

Viswanathan, H., and Salmon, W. 2000. Accrediting organizations and quality improvement. *Am J Managed Care*, 6(10): 1117–1130.

Williams, S. C., Schmaltz, S. P., Morton, D. J., et al. 2005. Quality of care in U.S. hospitals as reflected by standardized measures, 2002–2004. *N Engl J Med*, 353(3): 255–264.

CHAPTER 19

Quality Improvement in Resource-Poor Countries

Rohit Ramaswamy and Pierre M. Barker

"Every system is perfectly designed to get the results it gets."

—Paul Batalden

THE NEED FOR QUALITY IMPROVEMENT IN RESOURCE-POOR COUNTRIES

The Gap in Global Health Outcomes

A major gap exists in the health outcomes of populations of high-income countries compared to those of low- and middle-income, or resource-poor, countries (terms that will be used interchangeably throughout this chapter). The most obvious indicator of this disparity is the difference in life expectancy in the countries at the extremes of these income settings. Life expectancy ranges from greater than 75 years in the high-income countries to less than 50 years in low-income countries (Central Intelligence Agency [CIA], n.d.). Yet, while there is a moderate correlation between life expectancy and a nation's economic level, this relationship does not always hold true. This fact is illustrated in **Figure 19-1**, which presents the association between current estimates of life expectancy and gross domestic product (GDP), a measure of purchasing power or standard of living, for selected countries. For example, the United States and Chile have about

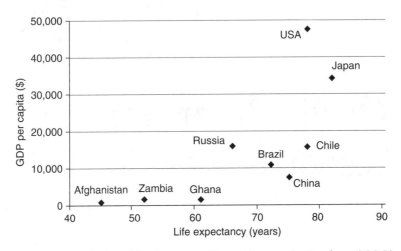

FIGURE 19–1 Relationship Between Gross Domestic Product (GDP) and Life Expectancy in Selected Countries

Source: Data compiled from *The World Factbook 2009*. Washington, DC: Central Intelligence Agency, 2009. https://www.cia.gov/library/publications/the-world-factbook/index.html.

the same life expectancy (78 years), although their populations experience a threefold difference in their average per capita GDP.

A similar general correlation exists between life expectancy and per capita spending on health, which could lead to a misguided conclusion that the principal way to close the gap in outcomes is through introduction of new resources. But major variations in current health outcomes and the rate at which different countries improve those outcomes can be seen in regions with similar resource levels. This observation suggests that other factors such as policy, health system functionality, health program priorities, and burden of different diseases are also major determinants of outcome. Good examples of the variation in rates of improvement in outcomes that are independent of health spending can be found in Asia, where much better infant mortality rates are found in resource-poor countries such as Bangladesh than in countries like Cambodia and central Asian countries that have similar or better resources (CIA, n.d.). We can learn much about how we might improve health systems from analyzing these different countries; factors to analyze should include, at a minimum, the emphasis each country places on primary vs. curative care, how accessible care is to the population, which cadre of health workers are the focus for expansion (i.e., doctors vs. primary care workers), what innovations are introduced, and what approach to improvement in public health is used.

The burden and type of disease are distributed differently between poor and wealthy countries. Low-income countries carry the major burden of infectious diseases. Sub-Saharan Africa, which has 12% of the world's population, accounts for 70% of the world's people living with HIV, 80–90% of the malaria deaths, and 37% of the world's tuberculosis (TB) cases. This region is also grappling with mortality rates among mothers, infants, and children that are 10 to 100 times those seen in the high-income countries (http://www.who.int [CIA, n.d.]). Noncommunicable diseases, chronic diseases, and cancers are major determinants of health outcomes in high-income countries, but because they become more prevalent in the aging population, they have received little attention in low-income countries where they occur at proportionately lower incidence than communicable and maternal and child health problems. There is a growing awareness that these diseases are rapidly increasing in prevalence, particularly in middle-income countries, and can and must be managed as part of the strategy for improving health systems in the developing world. While noncommunicable diseases account for less than half the global deaths, it is estimated that this will rise to 80% by 2020 (Boutayeb and Boutayeb, 2005; World Health Organization [WHO], 2003a, 2003b).

While the level of resources at the disposal of a particular country and the type and burden of disease that each country faces are of great importance, we propose that there is a common approach to improving health systems—optimizing the way in which care is organized and delivered—that can be used in any health setting, wealthy or poor. In fact, countries that face the highest burden of disease and have the least resources at their disposal have the most to benefit from this approach. In this chapter, we will discuss how a quality improvement approach can be used to improve outcomes in low- and middle-income countries. These methods have been used successfully in high-income settings (Ayers et al., 2005) and in some private, for-profit, urban health systems in resource-poor countries (Gupta et al., 2009). However, the effort to introduce these concepts and to train field staff in quality improvement methods and tools has, until recently, been limited in low-resource countries (Berwick, 2004; Smits et al., 2002). In this chapter, we will trace some examples of the evolution of quality improvement to solve health problems in the developing world, and in particular, we will describe some recent successes. We will describe some of the common process improvement paradigms and describe how these could work together to address the enormous challenges to the quality of health systems around the world.

Approaches to Closing the Health Outcome Gap

Millennium Development Goals

The gap in outcomes between low-, middle-, and high-income countries has received significant attention in the new millennium. Possibly the most influential event that galvanized the world's attention was the United Nations' Millennium Declaration in September 2000, when world leaders committed their nations to a new global partnership to reduce extreme poverty and gender inequality, mitigate the effects of climate change, and improve health outcomes by establishing a series of time-bound targets—with a deadline of 2015. These targets have become known as the Millennium Development Goals (MDGs) (United Nations, 2010).

Three of the MDGs were specifically targeted at improving health outcomes: tackling maternal deaths and improving reproductive health, reducing child mortality by two-thirds, and halting the HIV, malaria, and TB epidemics. The MDG initiative was a breakthrough on a number of fronts; it represented a commitment, backed by considerable funding, by a broad range of global leaders who, for the first time, agreed to work together according to a specific agenda to alleviate the major life-shortening problems in low- and middle-income countries. Even more importantly, again for the first time, the leaders quantified the problem and set numerical targets for each of the MDGs and an aggressive timeframe (by 2015) to reach those targets.

Launch of International Health Improvement Programs

Since that time, there has been a massive increase in aid for low- and middle-income countries from a number of multilateral and bilateral organizations, much of it specifically focused on improving health outcomes through direct assistance to governments or through partner organizations. In many instances, this aid has been coupled with specific initiatives such as the World Health Organization (WHO) "3 by 5" initiative to rapidly scale up antiretroviral treatment (2011), the President's Emergency Response for AIDS Relief (PEPFAR) initiatives to increase access to treatment for HIV (USA.gov, n.d.), the Roll Back Malaria Partnership (2011), the Stop TB Partnership (2011), and the Global Initiative for Vaccines and Immunizations (GAVI) initiative to introduce vaccines (GAVI Alliance, 2009). More broad-ranging initiatives, such as the Bangladesh Rural Advancement Committee (BRAC) program in Bangladesh (2011), have been particularly effective in improving child survival through a range of programs using novel ideas including those directed toward effective management of diarrhea (Chowdhury and Cash, 1996).

What Has Been Achieved

The setting of time-bound goals and the significant infusion of new funding has resulted in some successes. Specifically, interventions that have been targeted at improving processes and outcomes for specific diseases, using intense support from donors and outside NGOs (nongovernmental organizations) have been more successful in achieving improvements at a population level. A multilateral effort coordinated by the GAVI (2009) to prevent disease through better access to vaccines has been highly successful in improving vaccine coverage rates and is reported to have averted about 4 million deaths through its program over the past 10 years. The last decade has seen similar major inroads against specific diseases—such as using coordinated campaigns to improve access to antiretrovirals for AIDS (USA.gov, n.d.) and some regional progress in eradicating malaria (Maintaining momentum, 2009)—but at the same time, we have seen setbacks in management of TB with the emergence of extensively resistant TB strains in southern Africa (Singh et al., 2007).

What Is Still Missing

Beyond these types of initiatives, progress in improving health outcomes is still slow and limited. For each of the health-related MDGs, there exists a strong evidence-based body of knowledge that, if implemented through effective programs, could unquestionably result in every country reaching the MDG targets. For example, if every family in sub-Saharan Africa had access to a set of currently recommended, simple, affordable interventions for maternal and child health, 85% of the current maternal and child deaths—representing about 4 million lives—could be prevented each year (U.S. National Academy of Science, 2010). Modest gains have been posted for both child and maternal mortality over the past 10 years, but in most of Africa, the pace of improvement has been slow, with little prospect of reaching MDGs for many countries (see http://www.countdown2015mnch.org/).

Some of the lack of progress has been due to the effects of the HIV epidemic, with some countries in southern Africa experiencing an increase in annual maternal mortality rates over the past 10 years. But the core problem is that we still do not have a delivery system to implement the current body of medical knowledge that could save millions of lives (Barker et al., 2011). This gap between knowing what should be done and what is currently being done is called the "knowing-doing gap" (Pfeffer and Sutton, 2000). For example, a systematic review suggested that the much-vaunted, evidence-based Integrated Management of Childhood Illness program led by the WHO and the United Nations Children's Fund (UNICEF) does not live up to its promise to deliver simple child care interventions that could save millions of lives (Bryce et al., 2003). The study concluded, "We must continue to have clear, consistent, and evidence-based technical guidelines, but we must couple them with expanded capacity to develop, implement, monitor, and assess better combinations of interventions provided through locally-designed delivery strategies" (p. 163).

Similar efforts by UNICEF to introduce a highly targeted "bundle" of child health interventions to health districts in West Africa showed no benefit over the districts that did not receive these interventions (Bryce, 2010). In this study, shortages of drugs, lack of policy support, and weak community participation were stated as reasons for the lack of success. In another report, the effectiveness of one of the principal tools for global health improvement—targeted training of health care workers—was questioned by a report issued in 2010 that showed no effect on neonatal mortality of a program that trained health care workers to resuscitate newborn infants (Waldemar, 2010).

These studies have led to the realization that effective and sustainable improvements in outcomes will require an approach that is directed at strengthening health systems. The most widely adopted model was proposed by the WHO in 2007 based on "six pillars" of the health system, which include health services, information, workforce, commodities, financing, and leadership/governance (WHO, 2007). The importance of "systems thinking" has also been emphasized because health systems are complex, dynamic, and nonlinear systems, the function of which is dependent on the interplay of all of a system's elements (Atun and Menabde, 2008). In other words, in order to improve outcomes, it is not enough to simply increase resources or training. All aspects of the health system—improved delivery of health services, collection of data and availability of information for appropriate decision making, timely availability of the right commodities, adequate financial and human resources, and appropriate leadership and policies—need to be strengthened.

The Promise of Quality Improvement Methods for Health System Strengthening

The WHO has recognized the importance of quality improvement approaches to help countries achieve the MDGs. A recent WHO paper states, "If the majority of barriers to health-related MDGs can be seen as quality-related, quality improvement approaches may be able to tear down some of them" (Spies, 2006). But the paper also lists the following challenges faced by resource-poor countries in implementing quality improvement programs:

- Use of quality improvement approaches that are not aligned with a country's reality
- Lack of an overall vision that prevents scale-up of pilot projects
- Difficulty of building an evidence base for the impact of quality improvement programs because of the need for context-specific approaches

These challenges do not suggest the need for a completely new quality improvement methodology for poor countries. What is needed is the adaptation of models that have been successfully implemented in rich countries to take into consideration the particular contexts, barriers, and constraints of low-income countries. More specifically, the implementation of quality improvement models needs to be done in ways that "respect the rights and abilities of people to exercise constructive control and ownership of processes that affect them" (Spies, 2006). This requires the following key elements to be in place:

- Working in partnership
- Using lessons from the past to ensure a better future

- Balancing short-term and long-term goals
- Local ownership of processes and contents
- Genuine consultation and participation
- A strategic focus rather than ad hoc tactical interventions
- Moving beyond awareness to change in behavior
- Attention to management, support, and continuous evaluation

In summary, as proposed by the WHO, quality improvement methods can successfully bring about much-needed improvements in the health systems of poor countries as long as we pay attention to these critical implementation components.

PRINCIPLES AND MODELS OF QUALITY IMPROVEMENT

Principles of Quality Improvement

The fundamental assumption behind all quality improvement methodologies is that work in any system is conducted through *processes*, and a health system is no exception. Davenport (1993) defines a process as "the structure by which an organization does what is necessary to produce value for its customers." Hammer and Champy (1993) present an almost identical definition of a process as "a collection of activities that takes one or more kinds of input and creates an output that is of value to the customer." There are three aspects to this definition.

- First, a process consists of a series of activities, all of which impact its quality. Quality improvement cannot come about by just fixing one component. As mentioned previously, a systemic view is needed.
- Second, all processes have a customer at their outputs. The word "customer" is broadly defined. In the health system context, depending on the process, it could be a service provider such as a doctor, a nurse or a community health worker, or the recipient of a service such as a patient or a community member. The point is that at the individual or population levels, quality improvement should result in a change that affects outcomes for a person or a community of people. Keeping the focus on the customer is important because it helps to define the goal of a quality improvement effort.

- Third, the goal of a process is to add *value* for the customer. If a process does not add value, it is merely a set of meaningless activities that must be eliminated. A quality improvement effort enhances the value of the process to its customers. Depending on the process, value can be expressed in terms of better outcomes, greater efficiencies, improved consistency, reduced errors, fewer delays, or shorter cycle times. Irrespective of the measure, the principle remains the same.

The Core of Quality Improvement: The PDSA Cycle

As discussed in Chapter 1, quality improvement methods are grounded in operations research and management science, well-established fields that for more than 90 years have combined the disciplines of statistics, psychology, systems engineering, and iterative learning, producing a major impact, across countries and industries, on processes and outcomes. These methods have evolved from industry to health care and from local applications in developed countries to the developing world. The core of many approaches to continuous quality improvement (CQI) is a four-step iterative change cycle known as Plan, Do, Study, Act (PDSA), which was introduced in Chapter 1. This approach was popularized in the 1930s by W. Edwards Deming (1994), who is considered one of the founders of the modern analytical quality movement.

The power of the PDSA cycle is that it is a framework that can be readily adapted to different countries and contexts and that it can be applied by a wide variety of practitioners from different backgrounds and educational levels. This rapid change cycle puts improvement in the hands of those who are most directly responsible for the processes and outcomes to be improved. It encourages local innovation, allowing for local testing, adaptation, and refinement of ideas.

The purpose of the PDSA cycle is to ensure that local ideas for change are tested and evaluated on a small scale before they are spread. This is because it is possible to run into unexpected barriers when trying to implement a new way of doing things, and those barriers are likely to be different and often unpredictable in different settings. The PDSA method is used for action-oriented learning at the front line and is an important departure from top-down strategies where changes are planned by system leaders and the health care workers are then expected to implement them using a manual or some other guide. For each change that is to be introduced to improve the system, the PDSA cycle puts the planning (Plan), testing (Do), evaluating (Study), and decision making (Act) in the hands of front-line health workers and gives them latitude to adapt processes to suit local conditions. In contrast to traditional improvement "deployment," which cycles from management to the facilities and back over months, the PDSA cycle occurs within the facility, in a matter of hours, days, or at most a couple of weeks; furthermore, it empowers frontline workers to "own" the process of change. Importantly, the PDSA cycle places measurement at the heart of the process, encouraging frontline staff to record, collect, and analyze their own data to guide improvement.

After testing a change on a small scale, learning from each test, and refining the change through several PDSA cycles, the team can imple-ment the change on a broader scale. The chances that the changes will be sustained are much greater if the ideas for change originated and were tested by the frontline staff, rather than imposed from "above."

Whether we are talking about changes in local health systems in high-income industrialized countries or in resource-poor countries, the PDSA approach has been shown to be effective for engaging local practitioners in the implementation of CQI. For example, one of the earliest applica-tions of CQI in sub-Saharan Africa was a program, initiated in 1999, to address malaria control in Ghana. The central approach to this coun-trywide improvement initiative was the PDSA change cycle (Agyepong, 2000; Agyepong et al., 2001; Agyepong et al., 2003).

Quality Improvement Models

The PDSA cycle provides a flexible framework within which to imple-ment quality improvement activities, and a variety of quality improve-ment models have been developed over the years for different types of problems. Primarily, these models differ in how improvement activities are planned and conducted and in the analytical tools that are used in the "Do" and "Study" steps. The following models are the ones that have been most commonly used in health care settings.

The Model for Improvement

Under the leadership of the Institute for Healthcare Improvement (IHI), a number of organizations and countries have used a version of the PDSA cycle, called the Model for Improvement, to transform health care in local, regional, and national projects in developed nations like the United States and the United Kingdom (Oldham, 2005), as well as in emerging and developing economies like Russia (Abdallah, 2002), Rwanda (Furth et al., 2005), and South Africa (Barker et al., 2007).

The Model for Improvement, which is shown in **Figure 19–2**, is centered around the application of the PDSA cycle. It helps to structure the thinking and activities that are needed to improve a health care system (Langley et al., 2009). The model has two components: an "inquiry" component and an "activity" component. The inquiry component asks

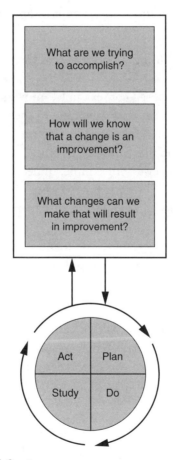

FIGURE 19–2 Model for Improvement

Source: The "Model for Improvement"—A Systematic Approach to Rapid Improvement of Health Processes (Langley et al., 2009).

three questions. The first question establishes the aim of the quality improvement effort, the second identifies the measures that need to be in place to ensure that the system is improving, and the third generates ideas to bring about the required improvements. The activity component uses PDSA cycles to test the ideas generated during the inquiry.

Lean

Relative to medical care, the lean quality improvement paradigm (Liker, 2003) is based on the belief that improving a health care system involves the reduction of *waste* in the system. Waste is defined as all activities that do not add value. The lean approach identifies seven categories of waste:

- Overproduction—using more resources than needed to deliver the service
- Unnecessary transport—for example, moving patients from one clinic to another rather than attending to them at the same location
- Unnecessary motion—for example, doctors or nurses walking long distances to get supplies or medication
- Inventory inefficiency—for example, unnecessary stocking of medicines or supplies until they expire without being used
- Errors—for example, making mistakes in paperwork, diagnostics, procedures, or medication
- Overprocessing—for example, too many steps to process paperwork or to requisition medicines or supplies
- Excessive waiting—for example, long queues to see the doctor, waiting for medicines and supplies to arrive

Improving a health system to make it leaner would require identifying and eliminating one or more of these waste categories. Overall, lean systems improve flow, reduce waits, decrease costs, and eliminate errors. Lean thinking is a powerful way of identifying aims and goals for an improvement effort.

Six Sigma

The focus of the Six Sigma quality improvement paradigm (Trusko et al., 2007) is on *eliminating defects and reducing variability.* A defect is defined as an outcome that does not meet the requirements of its customers.

Long cycle times for access to the health system, delays in immunization or neonatal checkups, and variability in service delivery by facility, district, or region are all examples of defects. A basic principle of Six Sigma thinking is that process variability causes defects, and by reducing process variability, the overall quality of the output will be improved. Systems operating at the Six Sigma level produce only 3.4 defects per million opportunities. Thinking about defect reduction is another way of identifying aims for quality improvement of health systems (Trusko et al., 2007).

Lean and Six Sigma approaches are becoming very popular health care quality efforts in high-income countries. In 2007, more than half the titles or abstract texts of papers in the health care quality improvement literature mentioned these terms (Walshe, 2009). However, the application of these models to date has been limited to resource-poor countries. One potential limiting factor in applying Six Sigma in resource-poor countries is the system capabilities and mathematical skills required of local staff who must apply these procedures. Six Sigma methods have been used in developing countries such as India and South Africa, but so far only in relatively well-resourced public systems or private care settings where the organizational resources exist to train staff and run this type of project (Shukla et al., 2008; Vanker et al., 2010; Wharton School, 2010).

IMPLEMENTING QUALITY IMPROVEMENT: CHALLENGES AND SUCCESS FACTORS

Challenges to Quality Improvements in Resource-Poor Settings

In a recent article, a district health officer in Micronesia underscores the quality improvement needs in low-income countries by stating:

> Narrowly focused, outcome oriented quality improvement initiatives and sporadic accreditation visits fail to address the most pressing need of district health services—to improve manageability. To improve quality at the district level, attention should be directed first toward this need—by building widely focused systems for ongoing, operational monitoring and response. (Durand, 2009, p. 70)

Implementing a quality improvement program in resource-poor countries will necessarily involve change to the organization's processes and ways of doing work. All change will not result in improvement, but any improvement will need to result in change.

Change is hard for all systems, irrespective of whether they exist in wealthy or poor countries. Typical systems are designed to evolve slowly over time, building on many layers of previous activity and norms. This design tends to support the status quo and makes it hard for a system to change, and hard to introduce new ideas successfully or rapidly. The way that change is introduced will have a major bearing on whether its introduction is resisted or embraced.

Common reasons for resistance to change (Phyllida et al., 2004) can include:

- Uncertainty about the need for or adequacy of the new strategy
- Uncertainty about the consequences of the new strategy for the individual's career or the future company size, structure, and employee qualification requirements
- Fear of learning new skills or new ways of doing work
- Unwillingness to accept change ideas from external sources
- Perceived lack of participation in planning the change activities
- Dissatisfaction with communication
- Fear of the magnitude of change or fear of failure, based on previous efforts

While these factors exist in all systems, they are exacerbated in many resource-constrained contexts. In many situations, because the problem is so large, has existed for so long, has proven resistant to multiple previous attempts to change, and has been framed purely in terms of a resource deficit, there is often apathy, indifference, frustration, or despair and a belief that the problem is insoluble.

In addition, the health systems of resource-poor countries face constraints of financial accessibility, physical accessibility, inappropriately skilled staff, poorly motivated staff, weak planning management, and lack of intersectoral action and partnership (Schneider, 2006). These constraints make the barriers to change even more acute and the need to address these factors during quality improvement a critical priority.

An illustration of these constraints is found in the interim evaluation report of the aforementioned Malaria control project in Ghana.

Agyepong et al. (2003) report that demotivation among health care workers was an important factor that had a negative impact on quality of health service delivery. Based on surveys and Pareto chart analyses (see Chapter 3) carried out as part of their rigorous program evaluation, several resource issues were identified that directly affected motivation of health care workers; the issues reported by health care workers as being most important included low salaries, lack of transportation, inadequate staffing, lack of essential equipment and supplies, and issues related to promotions. It was also noted that financial and human resource constraints, including inadequate training, had a direct impact on the ability to carry out the CQI initiative itself.

Factors for Successful Implementation of Quality Improvement Initiatives

In order to be successful, the implementation of a quality improvement initiative has to directly address the barriers and resistance to change. The following factors, assembled from several academic and practitioner sources, are critical for success:

1. Creating clear improvement aims focused on both process and outcomes

2. Encouraging and ensuring active participation of all stakeholders

3. Defining measures that are relevant to the aims of the improvement activity

4. Engaging participants in data collection

5. Generating change ideas collaboratively

6. Creating a learning network for change acceleration and sustainability

These factors are described in greater detail in the following sections.

Factor 1: Creating Clear Improvement Aims

Clear improvement aims are important for rallying all participants in the health system around a common aim, a notion that is directly related to Deming's concept of constancy of purpose (1994). To establish conditions for change, there has to be agreement at all levels of the system that this is everyone's problem to solve. The role of leadership from the outset is to show that the issue being tackled is of great importance, and to show a commitment to engaging and supporting all levels of the system in identifying solutions to the problem. It is especially important to ensure that changes are not "imposed" by leadership through mandate.

The aim of the improvement effort could be to close a gap in performance or to improve an outcome that is important to all participants. In a low- and middle-income country context, the aim could be addressing a major life-threatening issue (e.g., maternal and child health, HIV, TB, malaria) affecting that country, or fixing a major gap in delivery of care (e.g., unsafe hospital care, poor organizational infrastructure). Not all improvement efforts focus on health outcomes alone. If the health system as a whole is working poorly, there may be a number of process and organizational issues that need to be addressed to establish a coherent, sustainable, and effective health system. Poor employee motivation, absenteeism, lack of information systems, waste, and inefficiency in handling materials and supplies are examples of operational problems that could be important aims for quality improvement activities. (Chapter 2 presents further details on the importance and role of leadership at all levels in CQI implementation.)

Factor 2: Encouraging Participation of All Stakeholders

Stakeholders of an improvement activity are not only the staff of clinics and hospitals, but are also members of the community, who are the recipients of health care services. In many cases, these stakeholders may include people who are not motivated or empowered to participate in discussions about what needs to be improved. The *World Bank Participation Sourcebook* (2006) suggests the following approaches to ensure participation of those who may normally be excluded:

- Building the capacity of community members to articulate their interests
- Mandating participation through design
- Organizing separate events for vulnerable groups
- Using explicit power-leveling techniques (e.g., ground rules on speaking) to ensure that all parties get an opportunity to speak
- Using trusted surrogates to represent the poor

- Providing incentives for the poor to participate
- Taking prompt action and demonstrating results
- Understanding societal roles, contexts, and constraints

Health systems in high- and low-income countries alike are poorly designed to include patients or the members of the community in improvement efforts. For many of the poorer countries, where decisions are often made by the government at the state level and handed down to the district level, the gaps are even larger. Engaging local leadership to support staff and community involvement in improvements is an important preparation activity of the Plan step in the PDSA cycle, and extra time and effort taken for this activity can be repaid by the momentum it generates to stimulate larger, systemwide change.

Factor 3: Defining Relevant Measures

Measures should be directly relevant to the aims of the improvement effort; they should be defined in the same language used to define the aims, and proxy measures should be avoided if possible. The importance of doing this is not only to produce the specific analyses required by the project, but also to foster stakeholder participation and engagement. For example, if the aim is to reduce inefficiencies in transport of a primary health care worker who visits pregnant mothers in a community, then one measure might be the average number of bus trips per day or the number of villages visited. If the aim is to reduce the variability in communications between the delivery room and postdelivery patient care, then the measure might be the percentage of deliveries for which written instructions for patient care were not transferred with the patient or the percentage of deliveries for which the instruction forms were not completely filled out. The idea is that, as far as possible, the measure should be expressed in concrete, tangible terms that are directly observable as part of the process that is being improved. Measures such as the number of steps taken, the number of bus trips, or the number of unfilled forms are easier for a stakeholder to connect with than more abstract measures such as time or distance. Sometimes a balance is required between tangibility and accuracy; for example, the average number of bus trips is not as accurate as the average distance traveled, but this trade-off must be considered if it is helpful in gaining community support around the change.

In addition, because reporting requirements to governments or international donors are often primarily focused on health outcome measures, these are often the ones that are regularly collected, or the ones for which resources and training are provided. However, for the community using the health system, process measures might be more important because these measures are often more directly related to a user's experience of the system. Measures such as the percentage of days when free seats are not available in clinic waiting rooms, the number of seats available for men and women, the availability of female clinical staff to examine female patients, the amount of up-front payment required for access to a clinic or medical center, the time taken to receive reimbursement from the government for medical expenditures, or the extent and complexity of paperwork needed to file claims for reimbursement may be equally important to the users of the health system and may be areas where quality improvement, though often ignored, is much needed. When thinking about measures for quality improvement, it is important to think more broadly about the process issues faced by the providers and users of the health system.

Factor 4: Engaging Participants in Data Collection

Collecting the appropriate data for analysis is never easy, but it is a special challenge in countries with educational, economic, technological, cultural, or geographic constraints. Even data that are routinely required to be collected for ongoing health surveillance and monitoring are often incomplete and inaccurate. A study measuring the accuracy and completeness of six key data elements on prevention of mother-to-child transmission of HIV (PMTCT study) routinely collected in three districts in South Africa showed that data elements were reported only 50.8% of the time and were accurate only 12.8% of the time (Mate et al., 2009). While every effort should be made to work within the existing data systems, for many quality improvement efforts that focus on process efficiency or nonclinical issues, data systems may not be available, and data collection processes may need to be developed to meet specific project requirements.

To evaluate the success of a quality improvement effort, it is not enough to collect data just once. At the very least, before and after measurements must be made to assess whether improvement occurred. But successful ongoing monitoring is needed even after the improvements have been achieved to make sure that the system is not sliding back to poor levels of performance. Even as the data collection plan is being designed for the quality improvement project, it is important to think about the methods for regular collection, storage, and analysis. There is often a tension between data collection for a particular project and ongoing data collection. While the former can be designed to be engaging and participatory, using checklists, diaries, pictorial charts, and other practical and concrete tools, the latter is more institutional and requires resources and infrastructure that do not always exist. It is important to ensure that the burden of data collection does not become so tedious that interest in quality improvement is lost. The authors of the PMTCT study (including one of the authors of this chapter) state that "data needs to be perceived by frontline clinic staff as intrinsically valuable in the management of their patients, and in the performance of their delivery of health care." Clearly communicating how the data will be used, developing concrete and tangible instruments, and simplifying recording and tallying tasks will increase data collection compliance and improve data accuracy.

Due to potential limitations on the use of traditional data collection technologies in resource-poor countries, other technologies may need to be considered. For example, the effectiveness of personal digital assistant (PDA) technology to collect and analyze data is being studied (Yu et al., 2009), and pilots using mobile phone technology to collect and transmit data in remote settings are being evaluated (Ramaswamy and Whelan, 2010). While these technological advances are exciting, and hopefully will allow better large-scale data management, at the local quality improvement project level, it remains critical to focus on simplicity, parsimony, and relevance in order to make sure that the best data are available to measure and evaluate improvements on the ground. (Further details on data collection and systems needs and characteristics are presented in Chapter 12, and data analysis is discussed in Chapter 3.)

Factor 5: Generating Change Ideas Collaboratively

Generating ideas involves the analysis of data to identify and prioritize the failure points, defects, or waste to be addressed by the improvement initiative. Simple tools for analyzing performance data have existed for many years. The so-called "seven basic quality tools" (cause-and-effect diagram, check sheet, histogram, Pareto chart, run chart, control chart, and scatter plot) are suitable for frontline workers or community members who can use these tools with limited formal training in statistics. Additional information about these and other tools is presented in Chapter 3 and is widely available through online Web sites.

The challenge in the field is to use the tools appropriately to lead to data-driven solutions, but at the same time ensure that the tools themselves do not become barriers to discussion, engagement, and participation. To engage a broad range of participants in the improvement process, it may be helpful to train as many members of the staff as possible on the data analysis tools and to rotate them in and out of different projects. It is also helpful to make sure that those selected for training are balanced across gender and the organizational hierarchy and culture/ethnicity lines. Finally, as the data analysis is completed and the priorities are presented for change ideas, it is good practice to revisit those opportunities that did not surface as priorities to ensure that the logic for not considering these opportunities was sound. The practical application of analytical tools requires a balance between staying true to objective, data-based decision making and ensuring that this process is executed in a balanced and transparent way that encourages broad participation.

The generation of ideas based on the analysis should also be a participatory process, and there are many tools, such as brainstorming and multivoting, that have been successfully used in quality improvement projects for many years. The practical challenges of running successful idea-generation sessions are similar to those faced with data analysis. Skilled facilitation is needed to make sure the ideas that are generated are based on the results of the data analysis and are not just articulations of perceived solutions based on personal opinions. Facilitation is also needed to ensure that everyone participates and contributes ideas and that idea generation is not dominated by those with power. Once again, it is important to maintain diversity and balance among those selected for training as facilitators.

As a result of idea generation, two categories of change ideas can emerge:

1. Change ideas that can be tested and refined quickly on a small scale. These ideas are often focused on waste reduction, process

simplification, and elimination of failures and errors; they lend themselves to making the healthy system "leaner." Kinds of solutions include better instructions, documentations and job aids, co-location of aligned activities, use of checklists, color coding to identify emergency or fast-track conditions, and a variety of other solutions that can be readily implemented and rapidly tested at a facility, center, or organizational level.

2. Change ideas that require more complicated interventions may include a complete redesign of processes, the hiring of new staff, a large-scale training program, community-level awareness programs, a redesign of internal or external facility spaces, or the introduction of new technology. These and other, more complex solutions may require district-wide coordination, approvals from government officials, or more detailed cost vs. benefit analysis. These ideas focus on making deeper and systemic changes to the health system to improve overall reliability and quality and to enable the system to meet critical quality requirements.

When organizational leaders contemplate quality improvements, there is a temptation to emphasize working on the larger, systemic change ideas because they offer the promise of greater change in a shorter time. However, as we have emphasized several times in this chapter, a top-down approach that does not involve enthusiasm, engagement, and participation of frontline staff is unlikely to be sustainable. An approach that begins with small-scale, local improvements and then expands to larger, systemic changes has a much greater probability of success.

Factor 6: Creating a Learning Network: Accelerating the Pace of Change and Improving the Sustainability of the Changes

It requires considerable investment of resources (time and personnel) to effect major changes in health care performance and outcomes over a large area. IHI (2003) has successfully deployed an approach called the Breakthrough Series (BTS) Collaborative to accelerate change through a structure, executed over a clearly demarcated time frame, that improves the efficiency of this change process and improves likelihood of sustaining the changes. The BTS allows a system to be improved as a whole, rather than trying to improve it one facility at a time.

This BTS design brings together representatives from some or all levels of the health system. In a resource-poor country, these could include various stakeholders within a health district, such as district managers as well as representatives from primary care clinics and hospitals. While many of these networks are conducted virtually in high-income countries, the encounters between participants of low- and middle-income countries are typically face-to-face. The BTS mechanism allows teams to meet to develop common aims and targets for care processes and outcomes relevant to the improvement effort. In addition, participants share successful practices with others and solicit ideas from their peers for overcoming challenges. In this setting, managers are able to communicate policy and remove obstacles identified by the participants. These workshops are held every 3 to 6 months over the span of improvement activities, which typically last 12 to 24 months. To ensure sustainability of the changes and the ability of the health system to continuously improve into the future, the latter part of the BTS process is directed toward teaching participants how to "hardwire" the changes so that the system does not slip back to its former state, and how to integrate the quality improvement activities into daily work at both the facility and management levels. The BTS design has now been applied to successfully improve outcomes in a number of low- and middle-income countries.

SCALING UP: SPREADING IMPROVEMENTS RAPIDLY THROUGH THE HEALTH SYSTEM

While prototyping and facility-based interventions are crucial to demonstrate the viability and applicability of a health system change intervention, the large scale of the health problems facing low- and middle-income countries requires a design that can rapidly spread workable strategies throughout districts, provinces, regions, or nations, while staying true to the philosophy of local ownership of the change process and adaptability to the variable local environment.

Rogers (1995) has described five characteristics of change that make it more likely to spread rapidly:

1. Relative advantage—How well does the innovation appear to address the needs of the larger community that is adopting the change?

2. Compatibility—How closely do the change ideas align with the existing culture and environment?

3. Simplicity—How simple and understandable are the changes?

4. Trialability—Can the changes be adapted and tested in the new environments in which they are being spread?

5. Observability—How transparent are the innovation and its results from the viewpoint of the potential adopter?

Each of these characteristics can help to decrease potential resistance to spreading the changes. (See Chapter 2 for a further discussion of diffusion of innovation and change.)

In high-income countries, these characteristics have been incorporated into fast-moving campaigns. In the United States, the IHI's "100,000 Lives" campaign to reduce unnecessary hospital deaths utilizes relatively simple interventions, supported by a coalition of major stakeholders and a network of trained change agents. Such campaigns have been successful in galvanizing hospitals across the nation to work together toward a common aim, using a common method and common measurement system to dramatically change processes and outcomes on a massive scale (Berwick et al., 2006).

In low- and middle-income countries, a more deliberate design and phased timetable may be needed to support rapid scale-up of change. Low-income countries do not have much experience with quality improvement methods, and change ideas for issues that are relevant to organizations in these countries (e.g., hospital safety and access to care) are less well developed than in some of the successful programs in higher income countries. Therefore the experience and knowledge do not exist for rapid adoption through a campaign-style scale-up approach. The most effective scale-up design in these countries is one that allows maximum learning on a fairly small scale (e.g., in one district) and then moves to an exponential scale-up (using factors of 5–10 times the size of the original project) in successive phases until the whole region is covered. An example of this approach from Ghana is the Project Fives Alive! program, which is shown in **Figure 19–3** and described in greater detail in the next section.

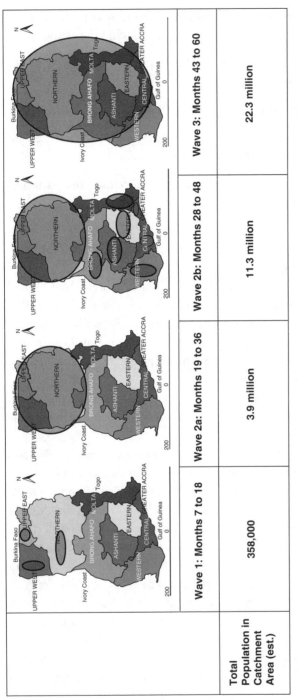

	Wave 1: Months 7 to 18	Wave 2a: Months 19 to 36	Wave 2b: Months 28 to 48	Wave 3: Months 43 to 60
Total Population in Catchment Area (est.)	358,000	3.9 million	11.3 million	22.3 million

FIGURE 19-3 Example of Wave Rapid Scale-Up of Intervention in Ghana to Improve Outcomes for Children Younger Than 5 Years Old

Notes: In wave 1, three northern regions were seeded with prototype collaboratives that tested changes that were then disseminated through the regions in wave 2. In wave 3, a similar set of "innovators" were developed in the southern regions before full-scale spread in wave 4.

Source: http://www.ihi.org/IHI/Topics/DevelopingCountries/FivesAlive.htm.

IMPLEMENTING QUALITY IMPROVEMENT IN RESOURCE-POOR COUNTRIES— SOME EXAMPLES

The following are some examples that show the power of quality improvement methods in improving health processes and outcomes in low- and middle-income countries:

- Despite limitations in documenting consistent intermediate outcomes in their preliminary evaluation report, the malaria control program in Ghana, introduced earlier, has been successful in implementing PDSA techniques and CQI tools at the local level. These tools included survey sampling techniques, Pareto charts, and fishbone diagrams, as well as statistical process control techniques. The program also identified clear indications for further improvements, including the need for greater resource support for staff and providers (internal customers). This program demonstrated the viability of large-scale implementation of CQI in Ghana, and the knowledge gained from this program can now be directed at other health issues in this and other sub-Saharan countries (Agyepong, 2000; Agyepong et al., 2001; Agyepong et al., 2003). For further details, see Case 4 in the companion casebook (McLaughlin et al., 2012).

- There is also a CQI program (Project Fives Alive!) that was launched in 2008 in the northern regions of Ghana by the IHI and the National Catholic Health Service (NCHS) to accelerate the Ghana Health Service efforts to reduce morbidity and mortality in children younger than 5 years of age. This program is pursuing a sequential rapid scale-up approach (see Figure 19-3) to improving systems of care throughout the NCHS and the public health care system, applying systems improvement methods to significantly improve health outcomes for children younger than 5 years while improving the delivery of care (quality, continuity, reliability, safety) and the capacity of the system (leaders and frontline providers) across the nation (IHI.org, n.d).

- In Russia, a team from the University Research Company used improvement teams and redesign efforts to improve processes and outcomes for a broad range of maternal and child health processes and outcomes. Using the model for improvement, a Breakthrough Series Collaborative linked several sites—clinics or hospitals—in a common system of measurement, testing, and learning. Starting with 20 clinics, the project expanded within 18 months to more than 500 clinics, and expanded from 5 hospitals and their associated maternity clinics to all 42 hospitals in the state and every maternity clinic (Berwick, 2004). Significant improvements in systemwide health included:

- Sevenfold increase in patients managed for hypertension at the primary care level
- 70% success rate in controlling blood pressures
- 85% reduction in admissions for hypertension
- 60% reduction in admissions for hypertensive crises
- 64% fewer deaths from respiratory distress syndrome in newborns
- 50% reduction in neonatal mortality

- In South Africa, the Model for Improvement and Breakthrough Series Collaborative were used with a rapid scale-up design to rapidly increase access of whole district populations to antiretroviral treatment for HIV (Barker et al., 2007) and to decrease transmission of HIV from mother to child (Doherty et al., 2009; Youngleson et al., 2010). The methods have now been adopted by the South African government to redesign and rapidly scale up HIV services in the country.

- Max Healthcare, a private, for-profit hospital in India, used Six Sigma methods to reduce the number of catheter-related bloodstream infections by 66% (Gupta et al., 2009).

- At a tertiary hospital in Blantyre, Malawi, redesigning the physical layout and improving the flow of patients by adding an emergency department and outpatient clinic for children younger than 5 years of age reduced the inpatient mortality rate from 10–18% to 6–8% (Molyneux et al., 2006).

DOCUMENTING THE IMPACT OF CQI IN RESOURCE-POOR COUNTRIES

While many examples exist of the use of approaches to improve quality in resource-poor countries, there are fewer published examples of quality improvement being used in resource-constrained settings. This is likely to change as quality improvement methods come increasingly into the mainstream of health systems improvement in high-income countries (Berwick et al., 2006), and the methods are increasingly endorsed by organizations and countries that are influential in driving health systems improvement in resource-poor countries (Berwick, 2004). One reason for the absence of published materials to support the method is the difficulty in associating systemic health system improvements with the quality improvement methods used to achieve those improvements. It is not possible (or it is at least very difficult) to undertake a randomized controlled trial of quality improvement projects, because often we cannot "control" the environment in which the intervention occurs. By definition, quality improvement encourages a constantly changing environment, adapting to changing needs and circumstances. By its nature, quality improvement encourages diffusion of its results, and it is therefore virtually impossible to isolate the intervention from matched control or comparator environments. In addition, there are often multiple factors influencing the environment to change while the study is being undertaken. As a result, even the use of quasi-experimental designs, where entire segments of a population (e.g., regions) are assigned to study and control groups, can be difficult to implement; when implemented, they may suffer from threats to validity due to external influences that cannot be prevented or controlled for at the analysis stage (Shadish et al., 2002).

These design and reporting issues are as likely, or perhaps even more likely, to be a factor in resource-poor settings as they are in high-income countries. For example, Agyepong et al. (2003) faced this problem in their malaria control program in Ghana. Despite implementing a carefully planned quasi-experimental design, which included study and control districts, their ability to measure the direct impact of their CQI intervention was confounded by several external factors, including a national media campaign to increase knowledge about the use of insecticide-treated mosquito nets, which had an impact on both study and control districts.

Nevertheless, since many quality improvement changes result in direct modifications of processes of care delivery, it is possible to evaluate the effect of these changes at the operational level, even in the absence of "gold standard" randomized control studies. For example, in lean implementations, where processes have been eliminated or process steps have been streamlined, it is possible to directly attribute reduced costs to activities that are no longer being performed. It is also possible to demonstrate reduced variability and improved stability of process performance using statistical process control techniques (Shu-Chiung, 2002) to measure reduction in waiting times, increases in capacity of facilities and services, or diminished error rates. These operational-level changes are an important part of the strategy to convince field staff about the need to improve and to demonstrate their ability to directly plan and implement improvements that have an immediate daily effect on their work. These local activities have great value even if their impact on overall or population-wide health outcomes cannot easily be assessed. However, if an organization's quality improvement plan includes large, resource-intensive, strategic projects, a robust evaluation design, such as that described for the malaria control program in Ghana (Agyepong et al., 2003), is definitely needed. Since the implementation of such projects often requires major investments of the organization's time, effort, and money, exposing senior management to the risks associated with failure, it is important to ensure that these projects will indeed bring about the promised improvements in health outcomes.

CONCLUSIONS

In conclusion, major disparities in health outcomes continue to exist between high-income and low- to middle-income countries. The large gap in resources between rich and poor nations will likely continue for the foreseeable future. In this chapter, we have shown that these disparities can, to a certain extent, be overcome by the systematic application of quality improvement methods to improve health system performance within existing resource constraints. The approaches we have described in this chapter, using rapid-cycle improvement methods, accelerated by learning networks and scale-up designs that are sensitive to the local environment and culture, can produce local and population-wide improvements in access to services and quality of care. Many hospitals, public health departments, pharmaceutical companies, health insurers, medical equipment manufacturers, and pharmacies in high-income countries are already using lean methods, Six Sigma, or robust quality improvement programs, such as the Model for Improvement and others based on the PDSA cycle, to improve the quality of their services. The next steps, which are already under way, are to adapt these methods to the local resource and cultural contexts of low- and middle-income countries and to ensure that the capacity for designing and executing quality improvement programs is developed among health care workers, managers, and leaders in government and NGO partners in these countries.

Cross-References to the Companion Casebook

(McLaughlin, C. P., Johnson, J. K., and Sollecito, W. A. [Eds.]. 2012. *Implementing Continuous Quality Improvement in Health Care: A Global Casebook*. Sudbury, MA: Jones & Bartlett Learning.)

Case Study Number	Case Study Title	Case Study Authors
4	CQI for Malaria Control in Ghana	*Irene A. Agyepong, William A. Sollecito, and Curtis P. McLaughlin*
10	**Prince Court Medical Centre: A Private Malaysian Healthcare Institution Prepares for a Pandemic of Influenza A (H1N1)**	*Roswitha M. Wolfram*

REFERENCES

Abdallah, H. 2002. Assessing the economic impact of the new system of care for arterial hypertension in Tula Oblast, Russia. *Operations Res Results*, 2(13). Bethesda, MD.

Agyepong I. A. 2000. *An implementation model for a district management system to achieve continuous quality improvement in malaria control as part of primary health care in Ghana*. Doctoral dissertation, University of North Carolina at Chapel Hill, School of Public Health.

Agyepong, I. A., Anarfi, P., Ansah, E. K., et al. 2003. *Evaluation of the impact of continuous quality improvement on malaria control in Greater Accra region, Ghana*. Unpublished research report. Obtainable from the Ghana Health Service Research Unit, P.O. Box 184, Adabraka, GHANA or from the Dangme West District Health Administration and Research Centre Library, Ghana Health Service, P.O. Box 1, Dodowa, GHANA.

Agyepong, I. A., Sollecito, W. A., Adjei, S., et al. 2001. Continuous quality improvement in public health in Ghana: CQI as a model for primary health care management and delivery. *Quality Manage Health Care*, 9(4): 1–10.

Atun, R., and Menabde, N. 2008. Health systems and systems thinking. In Coker, R., Atun, R., and McKee, M. (Eds.), *Health systems and the challenge of communicable disease*. Berkshire, UK: Open University Press.

Ayers, L. R., Beyea, S. C., Godfrey, M. M., et al. 2005. Quality improvement learning collaboratives. *Qual Manag Health Care*, 14(4): 234–247.

Bangladesh Rural Advancement Committee. 2011. About BRAC. Retrieved April 1, 2011, from http://www.brac.net/index.php

Barker, P. M., McCannon, C. J., Mehta, N., et al. 2007. Strategies for the scale-up of antiretroviral therapy in South Africa through health system optimization. *J Infect Dis*, 196(suppl 3): S457–S463.

Barker, P. M., Mphatswe, W., and Rollins, N. 2011. Antiretroviral drugs in the cupboard are not enough: The impact of health systems' performance on mother-to-child transmission of HIV. *J Acquir Immune Defic Syndr*, 56(2): e45–e48.

Berwick, D. M. 2004. Lessons from developing nations on improving health care. *BMJ*, 328(7448): 1124–1129.

Berwick, D. M., Calkins, D. R., McCannon, C. J., et al. 2006. The 100,000 Lives campaign: Setting a goal and a deadline for improving health care quality. *JAMA,* 295(3): 324–327.

Boutayeb, A., and Boutayeb, S. 2005. The burden of noncommunicable diseases in developing countries. *Int J Equity Health*, 4(1): 2.

Bryce, J. 2010. The Accelerated Child Survival and Development program in West Africa: A retrospective evaluation. *Lancet*, 75(9714): 572–582.

Bryce, J., el Arifeen, S., Pariyo, G., et al. 2003. Reducing child mortality: Can public health deliver? *Lancet*, 362(9378): 159–164.

Central Intelligence Agency. (n.d.). The world factbook. Retrieved April 15, 2011, from https://www.cia.gov/library/publications/the-world-factbook/

Chowdhury, A. M. R., and Cash, R. A. 1996. *A Simple Solution: Teaching Millions to Treat Diarrhoea at Home.* Dhaka: University Press.

Davenport, T. 1993. *Process Innovation: Reengineering Work Through Information Technology*. Cambridge, MA: Harvard Business School Press.

Deming, W. E. 1994. *The New Economics for Industry, Government, Education* (2nd ed.). Cambridge: Massachusetts Institute of Technology Center for Advanced Engineering Study.

Doherty, T., Chopra, M., Nsibande, D., et al. 2009. Improving the coverage of the PMTCT programme through a participatory quality improvement intervention in South Africa. *BMC Public Health*, 9: 406.

Durand, M. A. 2009. Quality improvement and the hierarchy of needs in low resource settings: Perspective of a district health officer. *Int J Quality Health Care*, 22(1): 70–72.

Furth, R., Gass, R., and Kagubare, J. 2005. Quality Assurance Project (QAP). Rwanda human resources assessment for HIV/AIDS scale-up. Phase 1 report: National human resources assessment. operations research results. Retrieved April 20, 2011, from http://pdf.usaid.gov/pdf_docs/PNADH076.pdf

GAVI Alliance. 2009. Saving lives and protecting health: Results and opportunities. Retrieved April 1, 2011, from http://www.gavialliance.org/resources/2009_GAVI_Alliance_Saving_Lives_and_Protecting_Health.pdf

Gupta, A., Verma, A., and Singh, O. 2009. Six Sigma—It's a culture, let's spread it! Retrieved April 1, 2011, from http://www.maxhealthcare.in/services_facilities/our_departments/mer/pdfs/medical_journals/may2009/sixsigma.pdf

Hammer, M., and Champy, J. 1993. *Reengineering the Corporation: A Manifesto for Business Revolution.* New York: HarperBusiness.

IHI.org. n.d. Fives Alive! Initiative in Ghana. Retrieved April 1, 2011, from http://www.ihi.org/IHI/Topics/DevelopingCountries/FivesAlive.htm

Institute for Healthcare Improvement. 2003. *The Breakthrough Series: IHI's Collaborative Model for Achieving Breakthrough Improvement.* IHI Innovation Series. Boston: Institute for Healthcare Improvement.

Langley, G. L., Nolan, K. M., Nolan, T. W., et al. 2009. *The Improvement Guide: A Practical Approach to Enhancing Organizational Performance* (2nd ed.). San Francisco: Jossey-Bass.

Liker, J. 2003. *The Toyota Way.* New York: McGraw-Hill.

Maintaining momentum for malaria elimination. 2009. *Lancet,* 74(9686): 266–266.

Mate, K. S., Bennett, B., Mphatswe, W., et al. 2009. Challenges for routine health system data management in a large public programme to prevent mother-to-child HIV transmission in South Africa. *PLoS One,* 4(5): e5483.

McLaughlin, C. P., Johnson, J. K., and Sollecito, W. A. [Eds.]. 2012. *Implementing Continuous Quality Improvement in Health Care: A Global Casebook.* Sudbury, MA: Jones & Bartlett Learning.

Molyneux, E., Ahmad, S., and Robertson, A. 2006. Improving emergency care for children. *Bull World Health Organization*, 84(4): 314–319.

Oldham, J. 2005. *Sic Evenit Ratio Ut Componitur: The Small Book About Large System Change.* Chichester, UK: Kingsham Press.

Pfeffer, J., and Sutton, R. 2000. *The Knowing-Doing Gap: How Smart Companies Turn Knowledge into Action.* Boston: Harvard Business School Press.

Phyllida, T., Bennett, S., Haines, A., et al. 2004. Overcoming health-systems constraints to achieve the Millennium Development Goals. *Lancet*, 364(9437): 900–906.

Ramaswamy, R., and Whelan, J. 2010. Exploring the use of mobile phone text messaging to supplement discussion forums in a global distance learning program [poster presentation]. American Public Health Association Annual Conference, Denver, CO, November 2010.

Rogers, E. 1995. *Diffusion of Innovations.* New York: Free Press.

Roll Back Malaria. 2011. Retrieved April 1, 2011, from http://www.rollbackmalaria.org/

Schneider, A. 2006. How quality improvement in health care can help to achieve the Millennium Development Goals. *Bull World Health Organ*, 84(4): 259–260.

Shadish, W., Cook, T., and Campbell, D. 2002. *Experimental and Quasi-Experimental Designs for Generalized Causal Inference.* Boston: Houghton Mifflin.

Shu-Chiung, C. 2002. Statistical process control for health care. *Int J Quality Health Care,* 14: 427–428.

Shukla, P. J., Barreto, S. G., Nadkarni, M. S. 2008. Application of Six Sigma towards improving surgical outcomes. *Hepatogastroenterology*, 55(82–83): 311–314.

Singh, J. A., Upshur, R., and Padayatchi, N. 2007. XDR-TB in South Africa: No time for denial or complacency. *PLoS Med*, 4(1): e50.

Smits, H. L., Leatherman, S., and Berwick, D. M. 2002. Quality improvement in the developing world. *Int J Qual Health Care*, 14(6): 439–440.

Spies, C. F. J. 2006. Resolutionary change: The art of awakening dormant faculties in others. Berghof Research Center for Constructive Conflict Management. *Berghof Handbook Dialogue*. Retrieved April 15, 2011, from http://www.berghof-handbook.net/documents/publications/dialogue5_spies_comm.pdf

Stop TB Partnership. 2011. Retrieved April 1, 2011, from http://www.stoptb.org/

Trusko, B. E., Pexton, C., Harrington, J., et al. 2007. *Improving Healthcare Quality and Cost with Six Sigma*. Upper Saddle River, NJ: FT Press.

United Nations. 2010. We can end poverty: 2015 millennium development goals. Retrieved April 1, 2011, from http://www.un.org/millenniumgoals/childhealth.shtml

U.S. National Academy of Science. 2010. African Science Academy Development Initiative. Retrieved April 1, 2011, from http://www.nationalacademies.org/asadi/2008WebSite/ReportsAndPublications.html

USA.gov. n.d. The United States President's Emergency Plan for AIDS relief. Retrieved April 1, 2011, from http://www.pepfar.gov/

Vanker, N., van Wyk, J., Zemlin, A. E., et al. 2010. A Six Sigma approach to the rate and clinical effect of registration errors in a laboratory. *J Clin Pathol*, 63(5): 434–437.

Waldemar, A. C. 2010. Newborn-care training and perinatal mortality in developing countries. *N Engl J Med*, 362: 614–623.

Walshe, K. 2009. Pseudoinnovation: The development and spread of healthcare quality improvement methodologies. *Int J Quality Health Care*, 21(3): 153–159.

Wharton School. 2010. Compassion vs. cost: Improving the prognosis for India's health care sector. Retrieved April 1, 2011, from http://knowledge.wharton.upenn.edu/india/article.cfm?articleid=4447

The World Bank. 2006. *The World Bank Participation Sourcebook*. Washington, DC: Author.

World Health Organization. 2003a. *The world health report: Today's challenges*. Geneva, Switzerland: Author.

World Health Organization. 2003b. *Diet, nutrition and the prevention of chronic diseases*. Technical Report Series 916. Geneva, Switzerland: Author.

World Health Organization. 2007. *Everybody's business: Strengthening health systems to improve health outcomes: WHO's framework for action*. Retrieved April 1, 2011, from http://www.wpro.who.int/sites/hsd/documents/Everybodys+Business.htm

World Health Organization. 2011. *The 3 by 5 initiative*. Retrieved April 1, 2011, from http://www.who.int/3by5/en/

Youngleson, M. S., Nkurunziza, P., Jennings, K., et al. 2010. Improving a mother to child HIV transmission programme through health system redesign: Quality improvement, protocol adjustment and resource addition. *PLoS One*, 5(11): e13891.

Yu, P., de Courten, M., Pan, E., et al. 2009. The development and evaluation of a PDA-based method for public health surveillance data collection in developing countries. *Int J Med Inform*, 78(8): 532–542.

A Call to Action for Transforming Health Care in the Future

Julie K. Johnson and William A. Sollecito

"Everyone in healthcare has two jobs: to do their work and to improve it."

—Batalden and Davidoff (2007)

The future of health care is tied directly to improvements in quality and safety and our ability to meet the challenges of adapting new ideas to everyday practices in health care. In much the same way that continuous quality improvement (CQI) in health care has evolved over the last 60 years, we are now experiencing an acceleration in ideas, technology, and research that affects both health care and CQI. The gap from data to decisions is closing. This trend is further fueled by vast amounts of easily available information that leads to greater awareness of choices and expectations on the part of internal and external customers, including payers, providers, and patients, as well as their families and communities. These trends lay the foundation for the next wave of CQI ideas and initiatives. As the field of quality improvement in health care is rapidly evolving, the organization and delivery of health care are becoming more complex, and health care professionals are continuing to grapple with the best ways to improve quality of care and add value to the patient experience. The aim of this chapter is to create a road map for those who will be leading the transformation of health care.

SETTING THE STAGE FOR CQI

In patient care settings, we operationalize CQI by asking two separate but related questions:

1. How can I improve care for my patients?

2. How can I improve the system of care?

It is generally agreed that the systems we work within are at the root of many of our patient safety and quality problems (Institute of Medicine, 1999). Quality and safety are both properties of systems, and many of our quality and safety initiatives—the specific changes we put into place to make improvements—belong to the system. Many of these initiatives are addressed in the preceding chapters and together, these initiatives create a road map for those who wish to lead the future transformation of health care.

The translation of research into practice requires a certain set of skills; similarly, health care professionals will need to be proficient in specialized skills to be able to translate quality improvement concepts into sustained improvements in patient care processes and health outcomes. A health system can improve by demonstrating excellence in three domains—will, ideas, and execution. Achieving results at the system or organizational level requires *will* at all levels to provide better care and better services; new *ideas* about how work gets done, how relationships are built, how patients participate in their care, and so on; and finally, *execution*, or the implementation of the ideas, including small tests of change (Nolan, 2007). System-level results do not come from a single initiative or even a series of initiatives when these efforts are not aligned. System improvements require a portfolio of projects that are aligned with strategy to produce and sustain results (Nolan, 2007).

As illustrated in **Figure 20–1**, there are three fundamental aims of a health system—better patient outcomes, better system performance, and better professional development. Furthermore, a fourth necessary component is for everyone in the health system to be actively engaged in helping to achieve those fundamental aims (Batalden and Davidoff, 2007; Nelson et al., 2008).

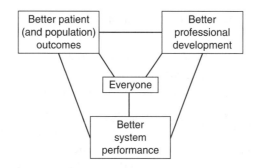

FIGURE 20–1 Fundamental Aims of a Health System
Source: Batalden and Davidoff, 2007.

THE CURRENT STATE OF QUALITY

The state of health care quality has made tremendous progress, but quite frankly, the quality of health care in the 21st century is still lacking. One study estimates that only a little more than half (54.9%) of adults in the United States receive recommended preventive care, and further studies show that the results do not vary significantly in other countries (Hussey et al., 2004; McGlynn et al., 2003). In regard to safety, health care, as an industry, has failed to make as many gains as other industries. Although much of the patient safety debate has focused on the United States, the safety problem is not unique to the United States. Across the world, people seeking care in hospitals are harmed 9.2% of the time, with death occurring in 7.4% of these events. Of significance for CQI efforts, it is estimated that 43.5% of these harm events are preventable (de Vries et al., 2008).

One would think that with the increased efforts to improve safety, outcomes would be improving. Yet a 2010 study—the most rigorous effort to date to collect data about patient safety since the oft-quoted landmark reports from the U.S. Institute of Medicine (IOM) at the beginning of this century (IOM, 1999)—found that harm to patients was common and that the number of incidents did not decrease over time (Landrigan et al., 2010). The study, conducted from 2002 to 2007 in 10 North Carolina hospitals, found that the most common problems were complications from procedures or drugs and hospital-acquired infections. Most disturbingly, many of the problems have solutions, but they had not been implemented in the hospitals that were studied. Reviews of the progress made toward achieving safer systems of care 5 and 10 years following the release of the IOM reports acknowledged that while progress has been made, there are still troubling gaps (Altman et al., 2004; Leape and Berwick, 2005; Wachter, 2004, 2010).

Another indicator of system failure is that in some instances where hospitals have focused on measuring and improving safety, the measurement tools are not adequate for the task. For example, it has been estimated that using standard measurement procedures, such as voluntary reporting and the AHRQ Patient Safety Indicators, adverse events are undercounted in the United States by as much as 90 percent; whereas the use of alternative technologies, such as the Institute for Healthcare Improvement's Global Trigger Tool (see Chapter 3) can rectify this system failure (Classen et al., 2011).

Barriers for achieving potential improvements in quality and safety are reviewed in Chapter 2, with a focus on the role of diffusion theory and identification of organizational factors that should be emphasized to improve the spread of CQI in health care.

ACCELERATING CQI IN THE FUTURE

"Knowing is not enough; we must apply. Willing is not enough; we must do."

—von Goethe

Given the abundance of evidence about best practices in patient care and evidence about how to improve quality and safety using CQI methods and tools, how can we ensure progress in the future? As stated by Denise Grady (2010):

> Process changes, like a new computer system or the use of a checklist, may help a bit, but if they are not embedded in a system in which the providers are engaged in safety efforts, educated about how to identify safety hazards and fix them, and have a culture of strong communication and teamwork, progress may be painfully slow.

This problem highlights the difference between "passive learning," in which lessons, such as what we can learn from the existing evidence about improving quality and safety, are identified but not put into practice, and "active learning," in which lessons are embedded into an organization's culture and practice. Active learning results in the system changes that are needed to sustain CQI as well as the culture that supports the initiatives. As outlined in Chapter 2, the goal of any health care organization wishing to implement ongoing quality improvement is to create a safety culture or a culture of excellence. It is also a direct reflection on the rate of diffusion of innovation, which is slow in health care for several reasons, described throughout this book, including the need to protect patients from unproven therapies and the need to prove that a change is truly an improvement, which are important considerations. But the most important reason for the slow rate of change and diffusion in health care is the complexity of health care systems, with many layers of decision makers coming into play when new ideas are proposed. Furthermore, change needs to be embraced by all the frontline practitioners who are responsible for implementation—not only physicians, but nurses and others who interact directly with patients and communities (e.g., public health practitioners).

Health care has been described as a complex adaptive system (Rouse, 2008; Swensen et al., 2010) and, as such, supports the need for active learning in developing solutions. Much has been written about the "system" and solutions that target various levels of the system, so it is not a lack of evidence about system solutions that is holding us back. As Avedis Donabedian, one of the most well-recognized forefathers of quality, wrote:

> Systems awareness and systems design are important for health professionals, but they are not enough. They are enabling mechanisms only. It is the ethical dimensions of individuals that are essential to a system's success. Ultimately, the secret of quality is love. You have to love your patient, you have to love your profession, you have to love your God. If you have love, you can then work backward to monitor and improve the system. (Best and Neuhauser, 2004, p. 472)

This sentiment addresses the "will" that may be at the heart of those wishing to improve the systems they work within, but what about the "ideas" and "execution"?

FRAMEWORKS FOR IMPROVING CARE

To close the quality chasm, it is time to move from a reactive measurement phase to a more proactive design phase (Battles, 2006). A three-level conceptual framework design would use the six IOM quality aims (safety, timeliness, equity, efficiency, effectiveness, and patient-centered care) (Battles, 2006; IOM, 2001). As illustrated in **Figure 20–2**, the first

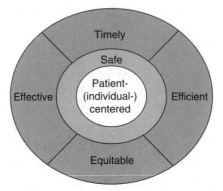

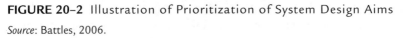

FIGURE 20-2 Illustration of Prioritization of System Design Aims
Source: Battles, 2006.

level of the framework would be designing for patient- (individual-) centered care, the second level would be designing for safety, and the third level would be designing for the remaining aims of efficiency, effectiveness, timeliness, and equity.

The significance of placing the individual at the center of the framework is that doing so shapes all other considerations in systems design. This focus on the individual person is an important reminder for those who wish to lead the future improvement of health care and is highlighted by Don Berwick in "A User's Manual for the IOM's *Quality Chasm* Report," in which he suggests that there are four levels of interest (which are addressed in chapters throughout this book):

- Level A—the experience of patients (individuals)
- Level B—the functioning of small units of care delivery (or microsystems)
- Level C—the functioning of the organizations that house or otherwise support microsystems
- Level D—the environment of policy, payment, regulation, accreditation, and other such factors that shape the behavior, interests, and opportunities of the organizations at Level C

"True north," Berwick writes, "lies at Level A: patients [individuals] and their experiences" (Berwick, 2002). More recently, Berwick et al. identified a "triple aim" to improving health care: "improving the experience of care, improving the health of populations, and reducing per capita costs of health care" (Berwick et al., 2008, p. 759). The primary drivers that will make it possible to simultaneously optimize all three aims in the United States are:

1. Measurement that is transparent

2. Public health interventions

3. Design and coordination of care at the patient level

4. Universal access to care

5. A financial management system

Note that the triple aim (improving the experience of care, improving the health of populations, and reducing per capita costs of health care) is slightly different from the fundamental aims shown in Figure 20–1 (better patient outcomes, better system performance, and better professional development). While these aims are not in conflict, better professional development is a key difference in the two models. We believe that this aim is necessary in achieving the other aims, and a more detailed discussion about educating professionals to lead quality improvement is presented later in this chapter. Education is also discussed in Chapters 13 and 17, which can serve as models for large-scale changes in the education of other health professions.

For CQI to add value, have impact, and realize its potential, it will need to be managed at multiple levels. An ecological perspective provides a potential framework for thinking about CQI, because it acknowledges many levels of contextual layers, such as the environment, organization, health care provider, family, and individual patient characteristics, which directly or indirectly influence a range of patient care outcomes. It also provides a model for breaking down the complexity into manageable components and identifying linkages and interdependencies that must be considered when making changes. **Figure 20–3** illustrates the ecological perspective in public health; it encompasses the vision that is the critical step in developing constancy of purpose (Deming, 1986) and ultimately developing a culture that embraces improvement (see Chapter 2).

The model shown in Figure 20–3 was developed by the public health profession, which has made great strides in quality improvement, spanning education and practice, in recent years and provides another model for accelerating CQI in health care. Much of that progress was initiated

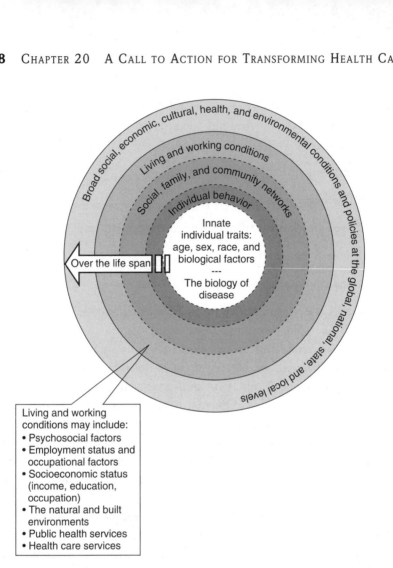

FIGURE 20-3 Ecological Model of Public Health

Gebbie, K., Rosenstock, L., and Hernandez, L. (Eds.). *Committee on Educating Public Health Professionals for the 21st Century.* IOM: Board on Health Promotion and Disease Prevention. The Future of the Public's Health in the 21st Century. 2003. Reprinted with permission from the National Academies Press, Copyright 2003, National Academy of Sciences.

with the release of a 2003 IOM report that "reviews the nation's public health capabilities and presents a comprehensive framework for how the government public health agencies, working with multiple partners from the public and private sectors as an intersectoral public health system, can better assure the health of communities" (IOM, 2003). Great progress has been made in public health, as discussed in Chapter 16, as well as in Cases 4 and 15 in the companion casebook (McLaughlin et al., 2012).

The extension of this model to other sectors of health requires a conversion of terms, but not concepts; it is another example of cross-disciplinary thinking and interprofessional sharing of ideas.

ROAD MAP FOR THE FUTURE

What does the future hold for the further development of CQI? How do we motivate health professionals to engage in improvement activities? Who are the future leaders, where do we find them, and how can we support their development? While to a large extent the future is uncertain, certain trends are currently under way that we believe will be important themes for the future of CQI. These themes, which are discussed in the following paragraphs, include education, research and publication, collaboration, information management and health information technology, leadership, teamwork, and value-added care.

Education

Education is the first, and perhaps the most important, step toward accelerating CQI in health care. During the past decade, we have seen an increased focus on educating health professions students to improve the systems they are training to work within by teaching quality improvement skills. This has been seen across the continuum of medical education, from students in medical schools to postgraduate residency training programs to initial board certification and maintenance of certification programs. (See also Case 12 in the companion casebook; McLaughlin et al., 2012.) However, further formal efforts are needed—learning from and building upon successful models. Dartmouth Medical School has documented its success in incorporating quality improvement, using an experiential approach, into its education and provides a good model for others to study, including emphasis on the importance of careful evaluation to ensure successful curricular reform (Ogrinc et al., 2011).

While medical education has been criticized because it has not traditionally prepared physicians to work as part of teams, we have seen more efforts to train health professionals to work as part of a team or "microsystem" (see Chapter 13). We have also witnessed an increased focus on quality improvement in nursing education. The Quality and Safety Education for Nurses (QSEN) approach serves as a model for consensus building and, spanning 15 nursing schools, is also an example of how to implement broad levels of change on a national scale. It provides for education of students and faculty on the skills needed to practice CQI (see Chapter 17). (Additional information is available at http://www.qsen.org.)

One criticism of educational approaches for CQI in medical care is that clinicians, especially physicians, were brought along later, or not at all—sometimes because they were thought to be too busy with the work of caring for patients. Not only did this lead to slow diffusion of CQI in health care, but it sometimes led to frustration or even a sense of failure from frontline clinicians (Ofri, 2010) that could perpetuate a resistance to CQI initiatives (Balestracci, 2009). It is clear now that physicians should be included early on, with their ideas and concerns addressed as part of the education process (Berwick and Nolan, 1998). As noted by Solberg and colleagues (2006, p. 298):

> The net result of all of these changes has been to focus attention and pressure on clinicians, especially those in primary care. They are feeling both stressed and unappreciated, as they have to run faster to keep up while being constantly told that what they do isn't good enough. At the same time, it is becoming clearer that if we are to address the cost and quality conundrums we face, clinicians must not only be involved, they must take the lead in making change happen.

In addition to CQI, there is a need to focus educational efforts on leadership and teamwork. They are critical competencies associated with quality improvement and are part of the critical "non-technical skills" (Flin et al., 2008) that will better prepare health care practitioners to shape the quality and safety of health care in the future. As depicted in **Figure 20–4**, leadership, teamwork, and CQI skills are the overlapping, complementary foundations of an educational process needed to develop future health care quality improvement leaders. Within those disciplines are specific skill sets that are beneficial to health care in general and CQI specifically.

For everyone to be actively engaged in doing their work and improving their work, there is a basic assumption that everyone will develop a basic understanding of the standards of their own work, as well as the quality improvement skills they need to test changes in that work (Batalden and Davidoff, 2007). As we develop educational programs, an additional consideration for education is that there is a concurrent need to ensure that faculties are both knowledgeable and experienced in the techniques required to implement CQI broadly. It is critical that practitioners learn what to

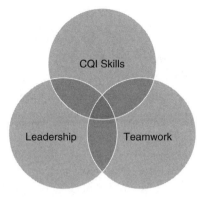

FIGURE 20–4 Educational Components for Future Health Care Leaders

do to improve quality and also become experienced in how it can be done most effectively. This is explained in management science as overcoming the knowing–doing gap (Pfeffer and Sutton, 2000). It is a gap that has stalled some very well-intentioned CQI initiatives. For example, in a CQI program to control malaria in Ghana, increases in knowledge about the proper use of insecticide-treated bed nets was not followed by actual increases in use. (See Case 4 in the companion casebook; McLaughlin et al., 2012.)

An example of how to build "doing skills" into the educational process is illustrated by the Dartmouth Medical School experiential learning approach (Ogrinc et al., 2011), introduced earlier, which serves as model to be considered, not only for other medical schools, but for other health professions and other areas of health care as well.

One key to process improvement, which also illustrates overcoming the knowing–doing gap, is statistical thinking. Training in the quantitative sciences is necessary, but not sufficient; statistical thinking must be woven into the culture for all to understand; to drive decision making—especially decision making about changes and improvements. In an organization or culture that is dedicated to CQI, "statistical thinking means looking at everything the organization does as a series of processes that have the goal of consistently providing the results your customer desires" (Balestracci, 2009, p. 85). The basics of statistical thinking start with measurement and the ability to learn from the data we have collected; we must then take the time to understand what the data tell us, particularly about causes of variation (Deming, 1986), before taking action to make changes. This is a central principle of the application of the Plan, Do, Study, Act (PDSA) cycle.

Research and Publication

In health care, and especially medical care, evidence-based practice is defined by rigorous research methods. At times, quality improvement research has been criticized because it does not always require the rigor that is expected of more traditional biomedical studies. As a consequence, the results of important CQI initiatives may not be disseminated in the literature because they do not meet publication standards regarding clarity of the study population, interventions, outcome measurements, and procedures for data collection (Pronovost and Wachter, 2006). In addition, in some sectors, such as public health, the evidence base is insufficient to address the wide range of issues that practitioners face. As CQI continues to evolve—and there is an increased focus on benefits, costs, and the value of health care—there will be increased demand for rigorous CQI studies, which will lead to better education of health professions students as well as better education in research methods for individuals working in the field. Furthermore, there will be more widespread adoption of guidelines for publishing quality improvement initiatives. In this discussion, it is important to clarify that rigor does not always require large-scale randomized, controlled clinical trials (RCTs). In fact, RCT designs can sometimes be at cross-purposes with quality improvement studies (Balestracci, 2009). Instead, rigorous studies should emphasize careful design, careful selection of representative patients for study, and analyses appropriate for the design chosen and the decision to be made; that is, in some cases a descriptive analysis may be most appropriate. Most important, rigor implies the use of the scientific method and appropriate attention to patient rights and privacy.

Research methods play an important role but should not serve as an impediment to application of CQI innovations; rather, our research perspective should be broadened to use a wider array of methods to achieve our ultimate goal, which is to make the correct decisions about the application of new CQI ideas. In many cases, the most cost-effective approach is best; to reach the correct decision, we may be better served by implementing a number of repetitive small-scale trials by which we learn and adapt from each stage.

Many decisions can be made by simple analyses of properly collected data, perhaps substituting control charts for complex p-values. In some cases, the use of complex design and analysis strategies has produced strong evidence in favor of change, and the widespread adoption of a new approach or CQI tool has met resistance for reasons other than scientific conclusions (see Chapter 2). Value considerations also enter into this discussion, as the use of RCTs may be unduly expensive and may not always be required.

Where more complex methods are required to make decisions, a broader array of research tools that have been proven to be effective should be considered, spanning both traditional experimental designs and observational studies using quasi-experimental designs (Shadish et al., 2002). (See Cases 4 and 19 of the companion casebook; McLaughlin et al., 2012.) Likewise, consideration should be given to qualitative research methods, as they offer unique tools and perhaps more in-depth probing to help understand the needs of patients, providers, and administrators while complementing and providing context to traditional quantitative methods. Qualitative research has an important role in that it can provide insights into both the quality and safety of care. More importantly, it can provide insight into what may be required to improve care because improvement work requires contextual data about health care settings—specifically the people, processes, and patterns that make up the daily work of providing health care.

In 2005, draft guidelines were published for reporting studies of quality improvement interventions. This was the initial step in a consensus process for developing a more definitive version of the guidelines, which the authors refer to as SQUIRE (Standards for QUality Improvement Reporting Excellence) (Davidoff et al., 2008). The SQUIRE guidelines help authors write peer-reviewed, usable articles about quality improvement in health care so that findings may be easily discovered and widely disseminated. The SQUIRE guidelines for quality improvement reporting are the result of an effort to improve the evidentiary base of quality improvement. The premise is that the structure of quality improvement publications will drive the structure (and rigor) of the quality improvement initiatives. The SQUIRE statement consists of a checklist of 19 items that authors need to consider when writing articles that describe formal studies of quality improvement. Most of the items in the checklist are common to all scientific reporting, but virtually all of them have been modified to reflect the unique nature of health care quality improvement (Ogrinc et al., 2008).

Finally, one important limitation related to research considerations in CQI is a lack of funding to pursue appropriate research and, in turn, to further build the evidence base. This issue has been highlighted as an important limitation in regard to CQI applications in public health (Chapter 16) as well as applications in resource-poor countries (Chapter 19). Efforts may be needed to build the funding base before the issues described above can be fully addressed.

Collaboration

Collaboration (working across institutions to improve quality and safety) is a clear direction for the future and an important leadership and team-work skill. Improving value can be accomplished through effective collaborations, including acceptance of shared goals among all stakeholders, measurement of process and outcomes, and sharing of best practices. Indeed, outcome improvements and meaningful cost reductions are unachievable without active cooperation among providers committed to functioning as synergistic units.

For example, in 2010, six leading health care organizations in the United States (Cleveland Clinic, Dartmouth-Hitchcock, Denver Health, Geisinger Health System, Intermountain Healthcare, and Mayo Clinic) announced a collaborative effort to improve care and lower costs (Adams, 2010). The collaboration includes sharing data on outcomes, quality, and costs on eight conditions and treatments: knee replacement, diabetes, heart failure, asthma, weight-loss surgery, labor and delivery, spine surgery, and depression. The group will determine best practices for delivery of care for these conditions and then rapidly disseminate the best practices to other health systems. This form of alliance has been well established in business and in health care as a successful way to share knowledge and create synergy. It has also been a long-standing research model (e.g., multicenter clinical trials) that has led to acceleration of treatment break-throughs, both locally and globally.

There are many examples of successful collaborations in CQI (de Vries et al., 2010; Haynes et al., 2009), but the broad scope of this initiative makes it stand out as a model for the future; it is similar to a "virtual organization" structure (Byrne, 1993), which has been used successfully to join complementary organizations in the pursuit of a common goal in industry and health care. This collaboration is also similar to formal collaborative networks such as the National Cancer Institute's Community Clinical Oncology Program (Minasian et al., 2010) and the National Community Cancer Centers Program (Clauser et al., 2009; Johnson et al., 2011) developed to provide access to state-of-the-art cancer care in community settings.

Information Management and Health Information Technology

Information is the connector between ideas and decisions about improvement; technology is especially valuable in more effective sharing of information. However, the gaps in health care technology infrastructure need to be overcome. One large step in this direction for the future is described in Chapter 12; the Health Information Technology for Economic and Clinical Health (HITECH) Act portion of the American Recovery and Reinvestment Act of 2009 (ARRA) provided about $30 billion to support electronic health records (EHRs) and other related functions. As noted in Chapter 12, this type of infrastructure will benefit CQI initiatives now and in the future by supporting and promoting data availability, reliability, and access (including interoperability and transparency) and statistical analysis (including data mining) and presentation. This will support CQI at many levels, including the individual (provider and patient), organizational, community, and international levels.

Advances in information technology are a source of both opportunities and challenges. First and most important are opportunities to ensure education to support and further develop this infrastructure and to make the most efficient use of it. The use of telemedicine and the implementation of EHRs can offer major benefits to quality improvement, especially in measurement, through ensuring consistency and transportability of data. However, challenges need to be overcome as well. For example, we currently face the dilemma of EHR systems that cannot communicate with each other; it is by recognizing this issue and the benefits of fluency that this challenge is being addressed.

The availability of large-scale databases, accessible through data-mining techniques, has been successfully used by Quality Improvement Organizations in the United States for improving quality among Medicare and Medicaid patients (see Chapter 15). Large databases can be studied in a number of ways and may provide sufficient rigor equivalent to the use of complex designs applied to smaller databases; access to very large databases involving relevant data from much of the population can ultimately serve many of the same quality improvement purposes at much lower costs. Data mining, with the goal of defining evidence-based practices and process improvement, is a very broad area for future research, and with proper investment, long-term benefits will result.

The availability of the Internet and social media to engage patients and their families more directly in their own care has already served as a bridge to mass personalization by providing greater understanding of choices. This phenomenon relates to the concept of disintermediation in the economics literature; like many other information technology innovations described here, it is a double-edged sword that we have been facing for several years. McLaughlin and Kaluzny (2006) describe the challenges posed by these new sources of information:

> Patients come in with a set of printouts or notes from direct-to-consumer drug advertising and may be perceived as demanding a prescription for that product. A less visible example is the patient who checks a Web site and decides that a doctor visit is not warranted. Increasingly patients are receiving advice directly from their insurers through personalized Web pages and from drug companies, pharmacy chains, advocacy groups, government agencies, and a host of other would-be providers. The quality impacts of this information are mixed. The educated patient may make better choices or may be stressed and confused by the information which may or may not be valid. (p. 430)

Further complicating this picture is that the information available on the Internet may be too broad and is often at a level that a lay audience cannot understand. Sometimes the information is simply inaccurate. Nonetheless, as noted earlier in this text, the trends toward mass personalization are increasing and are expected to produce a higher level of quality and patient satisfaction in the long run.

Advances in technology will continue to accelerate at an exponential rate at the system level and at the individual level of the patient and the provider. Education will provide the bridge from challenges to opportunities, leading inevitably to higher levels of quality safety and greater patient satisfaction.

Leadership

As noted previously, any educational initiative must incorporate leadership as part of understanding CQI. The role of leadership is recognized as fundamental to improving quality and safety because leaders enable connections between the aims (see Figure 20–1 and the preceding discussion of Berwick et al.'s triple aim) and the design and testing of those improvements. Chapter 2 addresses many important aspects of leadership. Leadership has a critical role in setting a vision for change, or constancy of purpose (Deming, 1986) and shaping a culture that embraces quality and safety. Leadership is the first of seven Health Care Criteria for Performance Excellence for the Malcolm Baldrige National Quality Award. According to the Baldrige National Quality Program:

> An organization's senior leaders (administrative and health care provider leaders) should set directions and create a patient focus, clear and visible values, and high expectations. . . . Leaders should ensure the creation of strategies, systems, and methods for achieving excellence in health care, stimulating innovation, and building knowledge and capabilities. (Baldrige National Quality Program, 2011, p. 49)

Leading an organization that is committed to improving quality and adding value requires creating a "learning organization" that learns from within and formally seeks new ideas from outside as well, which are keys to the diffusion of CQI in health care (Berwick, 2003). (See Chapter 10.)

Leadership is not about applying a collection of tools and techniques to those being led; it involves integrating the learning disciplines throughout the organization—vision, values, and purpose; systems thinking; and mental models (Senge, 1990). Successful leaders share their own personal vision and demonstrate their commitment to achieving it. They "inspire" the vision throughout the organization. When defining leadership in the terms of creating a learning organization, the role of the leader is to take responsibility for learning, as a designer of the learning process, a steward of the vision, and a teacher by fostering the learning throughout the organization (Senge, 1990). In so doing, leaders ensure the development of an organizational culture that embraces change and improvement.

Leadership includes not only defining the vision but living that vision and leading by example. Also important to note is that leadership must occur at all levels within an organization, including scientific leaders, opinion leaders, and those who champion change ideas. These individuals may or may not have administrative leadership roles. As discussed earlier, education and training are the critical factors to ensure leadership in the future—and not merely for those at the top levels of an organization. If we want to establish leaders at all levels, then we need leadership training at all levels. Public health provides a good model by emphasizing the need for adding leadership to the list of competencies that are taught in schools of public health. As a result, this has been accomplished on a national scale (IOM, 1988). The literature suggests that leadership training should take into account the multiple roles, disciplines, and systems that shape professional behaviors and clinical interactions with patients (Millenson, 2002). Educational programs should address the predisposing, enabling, and reinforcing factors that lead to higher quality, safer health care, including:

- Management—organizational dynamics and diffusion of innovation
- Human factors engineering—systems and devices
- Quality and safety—philosophy and culture
- Measurement and data systems
- Education and socialization of health care professions—theory, practice, and simulation
- Improvement methods—rapid cycle, design system engineering, flowcharts, Pareto charts, and so on
- Systems theory—complexity, root cause analysis, failure mode analysis
- Crisis management, risk communication, and risk management
- Culture—elements that promote a safety culture
- Team training

Many of the elements listed are addressed in this book as well as in the companion casebook (McLaughlin et al., 2012).

Teamwork

Closely associated with the role of leadership is the need for teamwork (described in greater detail in Chapters 2 and 4). Teamwork, especially in modern health care, is no longer an option but a requirement. Characterized by distribution of responsibilities and leadership at all levels, the use of teams adds value, and improves efficiency, by driving decisions to their lowest competent level. Also important in ensuring the development of a culture that is devoted to safety and quality is empowerment of team members and high levels of individual motivation as a result (Grove, 1995). The role of teams in CQI has long been recognized (Deming, 1986); coupled with technology to communicate most effectively, teams are even more important and easier to implement than in earlier years. However, like many other factors associated with health care CQI, there is an important need to teach practitioners how to be effective members of health care teams, especially CQI teams.

A Focus on Value-Added Health Care

Clearly a trend that we think will continue is the focus on adding value. "The value of health care is a function of three elements: its design (the right treatment for the right patient at the right time), its execution (reliably doing it right every time to achieve the best outcomes), and its cost over time" (Swensen et al., 2010). More simply, value can be defined as "health outcome achieved per dollar spent" (Porter, 2010). This definition implies that value is created around the patient, for the patient (Porter, 2010). If value improves, patients, payers, providers, and suppliers all benefit since the economic sustainability of the health care system increases. This is critical for all health care systems, including those in resource-poor countries since they are dealing with limited resources for access and services as well as for CQI initiatives.

Value, as a framework for efficiently improving outcomes, is a concept that all stakeholders—patients, providers, payers, and policy makers—can embrace (Lee, 2010). But how is it achieved? The first step is measurement; however, this step is hampered by our ability to collect data on outcomes and costs for a patient over meaningful episodes of care. Teamwork will be essential, because data will need to be captured across different parts of the health care setting. Furthermore, everyone will have to share accountability for patient outcomes instead of perpetuating a focus on the individual silos of the current organizational structures, which make it challenging to measure (and deliver) value (Lee, 2010; Porter, 2010).

There is a need for the quality movement to shift. Instead of "trying to fill gaps in knowledge about the epidemiology of quality, the focus should be on developing an epidemiology of value, which contains both measurement of cost and quality, and is applicable to both the developed and developing world" (Brook, 2010). It will be necessary to distinguish between a level of quality that is a good value and a level that is the best available care when enormous costs and small incremental improvements are involved (Brook, 2010). While measures of cost and quality are generally at the population level, Ofri (2010) challenges the value of top-down standards and reinforces the need to have practitioner involvement in setting standards about how to use data in a way that does not leave frontline providers feeling victimized.

The conversation about value needs to address value to the internal customers as well as the overall population. Individual physicians are not necessarily compelled to change when faced with data on their own patients; data must be given with the context of an organizational culture that is dedicated to quality and safety, as illustrated by the Intermountain Health Care example (Case 5 in the companion casebook; McLaughlin et al., 2012) and as demonstrated as a factor in the success of quality improvement collaboratives.

Developing a business case for quality to demonstrate value highlights the fundamental importance of data collection, storage, protection, analysis, and use. Whatever the setting or population, the dual value imperatives of cost control and quality improvement can be met only by analyzing processes of care and their impacts on outcomes. Although value has reemerged as a key concept for the future, its roots go back many years to Philip Crosby and others. Crosby does not talk about the business case for quality, but his idea that "quality is free" is at the heart of this concept, in that the cost of poor quality is the expense of not doing things correctly the first time, which directly relates to the value proposition; the costs of a quality program are more than offset by the value produced, and avoidance of costs of rework and the loss of customers as well (Crosby, 1980).

CONCLUSIONS

Our vision for this edition of *Continuous Quality Improvement in Health Care* was to provide a foundation for those interested in learning about CQI—the history of the field as well as some of the most relevant topics in improving quality and safety. While we started this text with the concept of the evolution of CQI from industry to health care, what we have described in these chapters is actually a revolution in the way health care has embraced CQI and surpassed the industries from which it evolved. This is quite natural given the high-stakes scenarios that are played out each day in health care systems around the world. At the same time, we have offered a sobering note regarding what must be done to bring value to the patient experience as we continue our improvement work.

A key issue that has been demonstrated is the robustness of CQI as it has evolved across multiple dimensions, not only from industry to health care but from wealthy manufacturing economies to resource-poor countries. Because of the sparse data on applications in resource-poor counties, we have illustrated what has been accomplished thus far. Only through further applications will we be able to fully understand which factors will be most successful in adapting the CQI processes of the developed world to other nations. The need is there, and those who have worked in addressing these needs are the new pioneers who will lead the way. The commonalities are greater than the differences, and this will lead to mutual learning through shared research and practice.

The other important growth trend has been within health care. The interprofessional learning and adaption from medicine to nursing to public health is illustrative of the growth that has occurred. The goal in health care should be to treat not one condition at a time but the total patient—as the patient progresses through the many phases of care, across diverse care settings, with different teams of providers caring for the patient's multiple overlapping conditions. The future will surely bring linkages aided by technology for collaboration across health care sectors and will lead to a new, broader goal for CQI to break out of our silos. In turn, we may add a new acronym to our lexicon: THCQI—total health care quality improvement.

Finally, we recognize the challenges of ongoing CQI growth, including the need for the greatest rigor in CQI research and the need to emphasize value—not only in the large health care systems of the industrialized world but perhaps especially in resource-poor countries where health challenges are enormous and funding is in short supply.

With these challenges in mind and with the future growth of CQI not an option but a necessity, we close this discussion with a strong emphasis on education to meet the challenges of the future. This education must be more than just training; it must span CQI, leadership, and teamwork and must apply both to current practitioners and, most importantly, to new health care professionals in schools of medicine, public health, and other health professions, especially nursing, which has taken a lead in developing a model that can be applied broadly.

We have explored many issues and often raised new questions. One further question remains, "Who are the future leaders in health care, and where are they from?" The answer is easy: They will come from us, our students, and our children.

Cross-References to the Companion Casebook*

(McLaughlin, C. P., Johnson, J. K., and Sollecito, W. A. [Eds.]. 2012. *Implementing Continuous Quality Improvement in Health Care: A Global Casebook*. Sudbury, MA: Jones & Bartlett Learning.)

Case Study Number	Case Study Title	Case Study Authors
4	CQI for Malaria Control in Ghana	*Irene A. Agyepong, William A. Sollecito, and Curtis P. McLaughlin*
5	The Intermountain Way to Positively Impact Costs and Quality	*Lucy A. Savitz*
12	Quality in Pediatric Subspecialty Care	*William A. Sollecito, Peter A. Margolis, Paul V. Miles, Robert Perelman, and Richard B. Colletti*
15	North Carolina Local Health Department Accreditation Program	*David Stone and Mary V. Davis*
19	Cal Mason, COO, Metro Children's Hospital: Planned Experimentation in CQI	*Lloyd P. Provost*

*Although there are other case studies that apply to this summary chapter, these are the cases with the most direct relevance to concepts presented in Chapter 20.

REFERENCES

Adams, R. 2010. Leading health care organizations announce collaborative effort to improve care, lower costs. Retrieved April 2, 2011, from http://www.dhmc.org/webpage.cfm?site_id=1&org_id=2&morg_id=0&sec_id=2&gsec_id=58387&item_id=58387

Altman, D. E., Clancy, C., Blendon, R. J., et al. 2004. Improving patient safety—five years after the IOM report. *N Engl J Med*, 351(20): 2041–2043.

Baldrige National Quality Program. 2011. *2011–2012 Health Care Criteria for Performance Excellence*. Gaithersburg, MD: National Institute of Standards and Technology.

Balestracci, D. 2009. *Data Sanity: A Quantum Leap to Unprecedented Results*. Englewood, CO: Medical Group Management Association.

Batalden, P. B., and Davidoff, F. 2007. What is "quality improvement" and how can it transform healthcare? *Quality Safety Health Care*, 16(1): 2–3.

Battles, J. B. 2006. Quality and safety by design. *Quality Safety Health Care*, 15(suppl 1): i1–i3.

Berwick, D. 2002. A user's manual for the IOM's *Quality Chasm* report. *Health Affairs*, 21(3): 80–90.

Berwick, D. M. 2003. Disseminating innovations in health care. *JAMA*, 289: 1969–1975.

Berwick, D., and Nolan, T. 1998. Physicians as leaders in improving health care. *Ann Int Med*, 128: 289–292.

Berwick, D. M., Nolan, T. W., and Whittington, J. 2008. The triple aim: Care, health, and cost. *Health Aff (Millwood)*, 27(3): 759–769.

Best, M., and Neuhauser, D. 2004. Avedis Donabedian: Father of quality assurance and poet. *Quality Safety Health Care*, 13(6): 472–473.

Brook, R. H. 2010. The end of the quality improvement movement: Long live improving value. *JAMA*, 304(16): 1831–1832.

Byrne, J. A. 1993. The virtual corporation. *Business Week*, February 8, pp. 98–103.

Classen, D. C., Resar, R., Friffen, F., et al. 2011. "Global Trigger Tool" shows that adverse events in hospitals may be ten times greater than previously measured. *Health Aff (Millwood)*, 30: 581–589. doi:10.1377/hlthaff.2011.0190

Clauser, S. M., Johnson, D., O'Brien, J., et al. 2009. A new approach to improving clinical research and cancer care delivery in community settings: Evaluating the NCI Community Cancer Centers Program. *Implementation Sci*, 4: 63. doi:10.1186/1748-5908-4-63

Crosby, P. 1980. *Quality Is Free: The Art of Making Quality Certain*. New York: Penguin Group.

Davidoff, F., Batalden, P., Stevens, D., et al. 2008. Publication guidelines for quality improvement in health care: Evolution of the SQUIRE project. *Quality Safety Health Care*, 17(suppl 1): i3–i9.

Deming, W. 1986. *Out of Crises*. Cambridge, MA: Massachusetts Institute of Technology Center for Advanced Engineering Study.

de Vries, E., Ramrattan, M., Smorenburg, S. M., et al. 2008. The incidence and nature of in-hospital adverse events: A systematic review. *Quality Safety Health Care*, 17: 216–223.

de Vries, E. N., Prins, H. A., Crolla, R. M., et al. 2010. Effect of a comprehensive surgical safety system on patient outcomes. *N Engl J Med*, 363(20): 1928–1937.

Flin, R., O'Connor, P., and Crichton, M. 2008. *Safety at the Sharp End: A Guide to Non-Technical Skills*. Aldershot, UK: Ashgate.

Grady, D. 2010. Study finds no progress in safety at hospitals. *New York Times*. November 10, 2010.

Grove, A. 1995. *High Output Management*. New York: Random House.

Haynes, A. B., Weiser, T. G., Berry, W. R., et al. 2009. A surgical safety checklist to reduce morbidity and mortality in a global population. *N Engl J Med*, 360: 491–499.

Hussey, P. S., Anderson, G. F., Osborn, R., et al. 2004. How does the quality of care compare in five countries? *J Health Aff*, 23(3): 89–99.

Institute of Medicine. 1988. *The Future of Public Health*. Washington, DC: National Academies Press.

Institute of Medicine. 1999. *To Err Is Human: Building a Safer Health System*. Washington, DC: National Academies Press.

Institute of Medicine. 2001. *Crossing the Quality Chasm: A New Health System for the 21st Century*. Washington, DC: National Academies Press.

Institute of Medicine. 2003. *The Future of the Public's Health in the 21st Century*. Washington, DC: National Academies Press. Retrieved April 2, 2011, from http://www.iom.edu/Reports/2002/The-Future-of-the-Publics-Health-in-the-21st-Century.aspx

Johnson, M., Clauser, S., O'Brien, D., et al. 2011. Improving community cancer care and expanding research in community hospitals. *Oncol Issues*, January/February: 26–28.

Landrigan, C. P., Parry, G. J., Bones, C. B., et al. 2010. Temporal trends in rates of patient harm resulting from medical care. *N Engl J Med*, 363(22): 2124–2134.

Leape, L., and Berwick, D. 2005. Five years after *To Err Is Human*: What have we learned? *JAMA*, 293(19): 2384–2390.

Lee, T. H. 2010. Putting the value framework to work. *N Engl J Med*, 363(26): 2481–2483.

McGlynn, E. A., Asch, S. M., Adams, J., et al. 2003. The quality of health care delivered to adults in the United States. *N Engl J Med*, 348(26): 2635–2645.

McLaughlin, C. P., Johnson, J. K., and Sollecito, W. A. (Eds.). 2012. *Implementing Continuous Quality Improvement in Health Care: A Global Casebook*. Sudbury, MA: Jones & Bartlett Learning.

McLaughlin, C. P., and Kaluzny, A. D. (Eds.). 2006. *Continuous Quality Improvement in Health Care: Theory, Implementations, and Applications* (3rd ed.). Sudbury, MA: Jones and Bartlett Publishers.

Millenson, M. 2002. Pushing the profession: How the news media turned patient safety into a priority. *Qual Saf Health Care*, 11: 57–63.

Minasian, L. M., Carpenter, W., Weiner, B., et al. 2010. Translating research into practice: The National Cancer Institute's Community Clinical Oncology Program. *Cancer*, 116(19): 4440–4449.

Nelson, E., Godfrey, M., Batalden, P. B., et al. 2008. Clinical microsystems, part 1. The building blocks of health systems. *Joint Commission J Quality Patient Safety*, 34(7): 367–378.

Nolan, T. 2007. *Execution of strategic improvement initiatives to produce system-level results*. [IHI Innovation Series white paper]. Cambridge, MA: Institute for Healthcare Improvement.

Ofri, D. 2010. Quality measures and the individual physician. *N Engl J Med*, 363(7): 606–607.

Ogrinc, G., Mooney, S. E., Estrada, C., et al. 2008. The SQUIRE (Standards for QUality Improvement Reporting Excellence) guidelines for quality improvement reporting: Explanation and elaboration. *Quality Safety Health Care*, 17(suppl 1): i13–i32.

Ogrinc, G., Nierenberg, D. W., and Batalden, P. B. 2011. Building experiential learning about quality improvement into a medical school curriculum: The Dartmouth Experience. *Health Aff (Millwood)*, 30: 716–722. doi:10.1377/hlthaff.2011.0072

Pfeffer, J., and Sutton, R. 2000. *The Knowing–Doing Gap: How Smart Companies Turn Knowledge into Action*. Boston: Harvard Business School Press.

Porter, M. E. 2010. What is value in health care? *N Engl J Med*, 363(26): 2477–2481.

Pronovost, P., and Wachter, R. 2006. Proposed standards for quality improvement research and publication: One step forward and two steps back. *Quality Safety Health Care*, 15(3): 152–153.

Rouse, W. 2008. Health care as a complex adaptive system. *Bridge*, 38(1): 17–25.

Senge, P. 1990. *The Fifth Discipline.* New York: Doubleday.

Shadish, W., Cook, T., and Campbell, D. T. 2002. *Experimental and Quasi-Experimental Designs for Generalized Causal Inference.* Boston: Houghton Mifflin.

Solberg, L., Kottke, T., and Brekke, M. L. 2006. Quality improvement in primary care. In McLaughlin, C., and Kaluzny, A. (Eds.), *Continuous Quality Improvement in Health Care: Theory, Implementations, and Applications* (3rd ed.). Sudbury, MA: Jones and Bartlett Publishers.

Swensen, S. J., Meyer, G. S., Nelson, E. C., et al. 2010. Cottage industry to postindustrial care—The revolution in health care delivery. *N Engl J Med,* 362(5): e(12)1–e(12)4.

Wachter, R. M. 2004. The end of the beginning: Patient safety five years after *To Err Is Human. Health Aff (Millwood),* Suppl Web Exclusives: 534–545.

Wachter, R. M. 2010. Patient safety at ten: Unmistakable progress, troubling gaps. *Health Aff (Millwood),* 29(1): 165–173.

INDEX